PERSPECTIVES ON THEORY

for

THE PRACTICE OF OCCUPATIONAL THERAPY

Editors

Rosalie J. Miller, PhD, OTR
Associate Professor
Department of Occupational Therapy
University of Florida

and

Kay F. Walker, PhD, OTR, FAOTA
Associate Professor and Chairperson
Department of Occupational Therapy
University of Florida

AN ASPEN PUBLICATION®
Aspen Publishers, Inc.
Gaithersburg, Maryland
1993

Library of Congress Cataloging-in-Publication Data

Perspectives on theory for the practice of occupational therapy /
edited by Rosalie J. Miller and Kay F. Walker.
p.   cm.
Includes bibliographical references and index.
ISBN: 0-8342-0358-8
1. Occupational therapy—Philosophy. I. Miller, Rosalie J.
II. Walker, Kay F.
RM735.4.P47 1993
615.8'515'001—dc20
92-46385
CIP

Editorial Resources: Ruth Bloom

Library of Congress Catalog Card Number: 92-46385
ISBN: 0-8342-0358-8

Printed in the United States of America

1 2 3 4 5

We dedicate this book
to the memory of
A. Jean Ayres
July 18, 1923 — December 16, 1988
With enduring respect and admiration

Table of Contents

Contributors

Mary V. Donohue, PhD, OTR
Clinical Assistant Professor
Department of Occupational Therapy
New York University
New York, New York

Ferol Menks Ludwig, MS, OTR
Doctoral Student
Department of Occupational Therapy
University of Southern California
Downey, California

Rosalie J. Miller, PhD, OTR
Associate Professor and Graduate
  Coordinator
Department of Occupational Therapy
University of Florida
Gainesville, Florida

**Susan Denegan Shortridge, MHS,
  OTR**
President, Developmental
  HealthCare Services, Inc.
Gainesville, Florida

**Julia Van Deusen, PhD, OTR,
  FAOTA**
Professor
Department of Occupational Therapy
University of Florida
Gainesville, Florida

**Kay F. Walker, PhD, OTR,
  FAOTA**
Associate Professor and Chairperson
Department of Occupational Therapy
University of Florida
Gainesville, Florida

Preface

The first edition of this book was titled *Six Perspectives on Theory for the Practice of Occupational Therapy*. This second edition was stimulated by both the need to update information from the first and the recognition that it was now important to add Claudia Allen to the group of theorists included here. The goal of this book remains to provide a thorough review of selected theorists whose lives and works have influenced the direction and development of clinical practice in occupational therapy. Two assumptions have guided the development of the book. First, careful study of existing theoretical material is needed to provide a knowledge base for the refinement of current theories and for the development of new ones. Second, the clinical relevance of a theory can be enhanced when that theory is studied in the context of the individual theorist's attempts to solve clinical problems or address professional issues that the theorist has encountered in her or his own career.

We felt such a book was needed in the occupational therapy profession. Practicing therapists can use it to develop a frame of reference for a clinical setting, to review theory related to a new job area, to formulate justifications for practice decisions to other professionals and to third-party payers, to establish a rationale for research, or to prepare for continuing education workshops.

For the increasing numbers of therapists returning to school to obtain graduate degrees, a book was needed to provide an overview of theorists and exhaustive bibliographies for more in-depth study. Graduate students also need to identify research questions that could add to the body of knowledge and theory base for the profession.

This book is designed to help entry-level students who are in the process of formulating a professional identity. It can assist them to begin to understand the common themes and the differences among the basic theories, which so often seem elusive in this diverse profession. And because the book identifies a heritage of the outstanding ideas and exemplary careers of some of the people in the profession it can aid the development of professional self-esteem and confidence.

The book can assist educators to provide a broader conceptual base for course content and curriculum planning, as well as to impart to students an appreciation of the richness of theoretical ideas in the profession. It also can provide educators with an additional stimulus for their own scholarly research endeavors.

It is hoped that this book will also inspire all its readers by "demythologizing" the major theorists. Each theory chapter begins with a biographical sketch describing factors that influenced and motivated the theorist's growth as therapist and theorist. Theory is enlivened in the context of each theorist's personal and professional efforts to solve practical and realistic problems that confront occupational therapists.

In Chapter 1, theory is defined and its relevance to occupational therapy issues is addressed. The core of the book is organized around seven theorists, with a chapter devoted to each. These chapters follow a similar format: (1) a biographical sketch of the theorist, (2) an objective review of that person's theory, and (3) the use of that theory in occupational therapy. The impact of each theory on OT practice is revealed through the presentation of subsequent research and application of the theory by others. Comprehensive bibliographies of each theorist's works are provided to lead readers to a deeper understanding of the theorists' concepts and ideas. In the final chapter, the major themes that run through the theories are analyzed, and future theory development needs are identified.

The seven theorists included here were selected because of the impact that their work has had on the overall conceptualization and practice of occupational therapy. Certainly, there are many other people who have made and are making significant contributions to our growing theory base. It is hoped that this book will provide support and stimulus to those individuals who have already presented their ideas on OT theory, and that it will inspire others in the profession to join in this exciting search for ever greater understanding and clarity about occupational therapy.

Throughout the writing of this book the authors have kept in mind Yerxa's statement that "we deal with enormous complexity which we tend to simplify rather than clarify" (1986, p. 211). It has not been possible to address all the complex issues behind the theories presented, a reality that readers must keep in mind when reading this book. We do hope that the work we have done adds more to clarity than to simplification.

REFERENCE

Yerxa, E.J. (1986). Target tomorrow. In *Occupational therapy education: Target 2000* (pp. 209–213). Rockville, MD: American Occupational Therapy Association.

Acknowledgments

For this second edition, Gail Fidler, Anne Mosey, Lela Llorens, and Gary Kielhofner graciously provided us with updates for their biographies. Claudia Allen gave generously of her time to be interviewed and to answer follow-up questions in phone calls and letters. And Vivian Moore once again provided patient and competent assistance in preparation of the manuscript.

We are grateful to these people, to the expert crew at Aspen Publishers, and to our families of loved ones and friends who continue to lend us support and encouragement throughout this and all the other projects of our lives.

Chapter One

What Is Theory, and Why Does It Matter?

Rosalie J. Miller

WHAT IS THEORY?

In the practice of our profession a concentration on individual techniques sometimes obscures the underlying relations between the person, their function, and their world. Our view of these relationships is theory. Theory explains how some aspect of human behavior or performance is organized, and thus it enables us to make predictions about that behavior. Without a theory of human definition and capability linked to function in the world, occupational therapy as a concept could not exist.

The major structural components of a theory are *concepts*, which are ideally well defined, and *principles*, or postulates, which explain how the concepts are related to one another.

Concepts

Our unique human ability to use symbols through language enables us to develop concepts. The young child, upon seeing something unfamiliar, asks, "What is that?" and is told, "That's a cow" or "That's a pan." Through these experiences categories are formed into which one organizes things from the environment. These categories are concepts (Duldt & Giffin, 1985, p. 46).

As one grows, one develops more concept categories, relates more and more things to them, and subdivides levels of concept categories in one's mind. For instance, the large concept category of animals is subdivided into cows, dogs, cats, horses, and others. The child learns that food is subdivided into fruits, vegetables, grains, and so on, which are then further subdivided—fruits into apples, pears, grapes. . . . So one learns "to recognize things as belonging to certain categories; thus one develops a notion of concepts" (Duldt & Giffin, 1985, p. 46).

Language enables conceptualization. And because of language, we can conceptualize things that we cannot see, whether because we are out of sight of the physical thing itself, as in "cow," or "the pyramids," or because there is no physical reality to the concept, as in "self-esteem" or "motivation." Concepts such as these latter two that have no physical referent but rather are labels for intangible ideas are often called constructs.

Principles

As one learns more about concepts one also learns about ways in which concepts relate to one another. Relationships between concepts are called principles or postulates. For instance, once one learns the concepts of "2" and of "4," one learns the principle that if 2 is added to 2, the result is 4. Once one has learned the concepts of "cat," "petting," and "enjoyment," one can put together the principle that the cat enjoys being petted. One also learns reverse consequences of principles: 4 minus 2 equals 2, if one strokes the cat against the lay of the fur it objects, and so on. In all these examples one is using language symbolically to think about the relationships between concepts, and in so doing one is deriving principles (Duldt & Giffin, 1985).

Concepts and principles serve two important functions. First, they "help us understand or explain what is going on around us" (Duldt & Giffin, 1985, p. 47). For example, beginning OT students are usually somewhat confused about "what occupational therapy is." In the course of their education they learn new concepts that are used in the field, such as "neurodevelopment" and "occupation," and learn how to categorize other things and ideas (subconcepts) into these major concepts. For example, subconcepts of "ADL," "work," and "play/leisure" are categorized under the major concept of "occupation." Then the student learns principles governing the relationships among concepts: for example, "involvement in occupation is essential to normal neurodevelopment." Through this process of learning concepts and principles, students grow to better understand what occupational therapy is.

Second, according to Duldt and Giffin, established principles also help us predict future events.

> Some concepts relate to one another so consistently that predictions about future outcomes are relatively simple. For example, when we see dark clouds with lightning and we hear thunder, we know from experience that rain is approaching. We can make this prediction because we understand the relationship between the three concepts—clouds, lightning, and thunder—and because we know they usually combine in such a way that a fourth concept, rain, occurs. Using our knowledge, we can

exert some control over the situation by wearing raincoats and using umbrellas. . . . In developing theories, similar relationships are established between concepts. (1985, p. 33)

These relationships can be stated as correlational ("dark clouds are often accompanied by rain") or causal ("if you stand in the rain without a raincoat or umbrella you get wet").

From the OT principle stated earlier one can predict future events. For example, given the principle that involvement in occupation is essential to normal neurodevelopment, one can predict that a child who is in a body cast and kept in an isolated environment for a period of time will suffer setbacks in neurodevelopment. When several related principles of neurodevelopment are logically organized, the outcome can be a theory.

Theory

Theory is defined in slightly different ways by different people. Duldt and Giffin define it this way: "A theory is a related set of principles, each principle being a statement that ties two or more concepts together, usually in a correlation or causal way" (1985, p. 47).

Reed states it somewhat differently, yet she incorporates the same elements. "A theory is defined as a set of interrelated assumptions, concepts, and definitions that presents a systematic view of phenomena by specifying relationships among variables, with the purpose of explaining and predicting the phenomena" (1984, p. 677).

In this definition Reed raises a very important issue—that of assumptions. No theory is totally value free. Every person brings to the task of explaining her or his observations a particular perspective and certain basic values. Certainly most of us share the assumption that the world exists and that we can accurately perceive it through our senses. This may or may not be ultimately true, but most theories are based on these assumptions.

In occupational therapy certain assumptions are generally considered basic to the profession and influence the types and direction of theories that are introduced. In 1919 William Rush Dunton, Jr., published the "Credo for Occupational Therapists," which delineated the following basic assumptions:

That occupation is as necessary to life as food and drink.

That every human being should have both physical and mental occupation. That all should have occupations which they enjoy, or hobbies. . . . That sick minds, sick bodies, sick souls may be healed through occupation. (p. 10)

The "Philosophical Base of Occupational Therapy" adopted by the Representative Assembly (RA) of the American Occupational Therapy Association (AOTA) in 1979 states very similar assumptions in different words:

> [Humans are] active beings whose development is influenced by the use of purposeful activity. Using their capacity for intrinsic motivation, human beings are able to influence their physical and mental health and their social and physical environment through purposeful activity. . . .

> Occupational therapy is based on the belief that purposeful activity (occupation), including its interpersonal and environmental components, may be used to prevent and mediate dysfunction, and to elicit maximum adaptation. (Hopkins & Smith, 1983, p. 27)

It is important to be aware of the assumptions underlying a particular theory so that one may evaluate it thoroughly, rather than accepting it at face value. For instance, a theory may seem quite logical at first, but an examination of the assumptions on which it is based may give one cause to reject it as incompatible with one's own world view. At the same time, it is important to maintain an attitude of flexibility about one's assumptions and realize that the results of truth seeking might lead one to change an assumption from time to time.

RELATIONSHIP OF RESEARCH TO THEORY

The way one determines whether the principles relating concepts in any particular theory are valid is through the process called research. There are many legitimate ways to go about this process, a fact that even many previously "hard-line" experimental research protagonists are beginning to acknowledge. As Ottenbacher put it:

> Many investigators (myself included) have displayed a tendency to be overzealous in their use and promotion of experimental methods, much like the young child who, when first given a hammer, finds that everything he encounters needs pounding. The evolving discussion concerning the relative merits of various research strategies makes it clear that traditional designs are a valuable and viable empirical option, but that they are not the absolute ideal in every situation. The debate also helps legitimize and increase the acceptance of qualitative, idiographic, and other alternative research and evaluation strategies. It has forced investigators to focus not only on outcome but also on process, holism, ecology, and other attributes not generally afforded a high priority in the traditional experimental paradigm. (1985, p. 203)

As a practice profession OTs' research laboratories are the practice settings in which therapists interact with patients and clients. Those therapists who use theoretical principles to make practice decisions and then observe the results are engaging in a process of testing those theories and, in so doing, may also generate new ones.

Ottenbacher's statement illuminates the fact that there are many exciting ways to go about this process of both testing and generating theory. Productive debate has been growing as to the ways and means by which the theoretical propositions of occupational therapy should be generated, investigated, and tested (Carlson & Clark, 1991; Kielhofner, 1992; Mosey, 1992; Ottenbacher, 1992; Yerxa, 1991). The development of a solid theoretical and concrete knowledge base of the profession requires that occupational therapists become more knowledgeable about theory and more conscious and deliberate about the kinds of thinking and problem solving in which they are already engaged, and that they then record and share their findings.

DEVELOPMENT OF THEORY

Stages

Theory is constantly revised as new knowledge is discovered through research. Any new science, according to Lewin (1947), goes through three stages in theory development. The first stage is the speculative period, in which the field puts forth theoretical models to attempt to explain phenomena. The second stage is the descriptive period, in which the field gathers facts through research to describe what really is happening and to test the theoretical models. Lewin calls the third stage the constructive period. During this time old theories are revised and new ones developed that are grounded in facts rather than based on speculation.

Any science must and does go through these stages. Occupational therapy seems to have developed speculative theories and has begun the process of gathering facts through research. The new discipline of occupational science will stimulate this process and will speed the development of theory and research in many of the areas of concern to occupational therapy (Clark et al., 1991).

Process

Theory is generally developed in one of two ways. An individual may have many facts and then develop a theory to explain relationships among them. Darwin was a scientist who knew the facts that had been gathered up to his time about different species and their description and classification. He posited his theory of evolution as a way of explaining how these many species were related to one another and to human beings (Ostrow, 1980).

Or a person may have a flash of insight that suddenly gives him or her a whole new perspective about the relationship of certain concepts. An example of this type of theory development is Einstein's theory of relativity, which opened up new areas of research and inquiry that had not existed before because no one had ever conceptualized the possibility that energy, matter, and time could be related in the way Einstein suggested.

The way that Jean Ayres' theory of sensory integration was derived combined these two processes. Ayres saw certain developments in the cognitive, perceptual, and motor functioning of the children with whom she worked. After extensive observation and testing she presented her theory of sensory integration. Like Darwin she had accumulated a good deal of knowledge and was a scholar in her area. Also like Einstein, she went beyond the proven, the tested, and the observable to develop her theory. Ayres states:

> Exactly how SI occurs in the brain remains elusive, but that lack of knowledge should not be an excuse for avoiding an issue basic to all learning. [Lack of knowledge] must be faced and dealt with in as adequate a manner as possible with full recognition of the limitations involved and with the realization that any conceptual framework is in some aspects erroneous and will require constant revision as new knowledge unfolds. (1965, p. 43)

This willingness to take risks is an essential quality in any theorist.

Complexity and Scope

Theories range in complexity and scope along a continuum. At one end lie those that are narrow in focus and deal with specific phenomena that are fairly easily defined, and at the other end lie those that are very broad and complex and attempt to explain major areas within a discipline. The latter theories often incorporate numerous more specific theories within them (Marriner, 1986).

Parham defines this continuum as ranging from scientific theories to conceptual frameworks and says they are:

> different kinds of thinking tools for the therapist. An overarching conceptual framework allows the therapist to frame the context for intervention by sketching a general configuration of the situation, while a scientific theory leads the therapist to specify technical details of how to act on a problem once it is selected as a target for intervention. It is likely that, in the best instances of competent clinical practice, both kinds of thinking are involved. (1987, p. 558)

The model of human occupation is an example of an overarching conceptual framework that provides a perspective from which the therapist can evaluate and determine areas of function and dysfunction in a given patient or client. Ayres' theory of sensory integration is a scientific theory that guides the therapist's intervention once it has been determined that lack of sensory integration is a probable contributor to dysfunction.

The major theories in occupational therapy fall at different points along this continuum of complexity and scope, and very often in a clinical situation a therapist will use more than one theory. This is often necessary because of the complexity of the problems faced by disabled individuals. However, one must be certain when utilizing multiple theories that they are based on compatible assumptions and that their concepts fit together logically.

> Often the therapist will have to choose between competing theories that offer different points of view for understanding a single clinical situation. An appreciation of the different kinds of theories available and what each can bring to the understanding of the problem is required if a wise decision is to be made. (Parham, 1987, p. 557)

An obvious example would be a theorist working from a psychoanalytic theory base with a disturbed child, encouraging her to express her anger. It would greatly confuse that child if she were also treated from a behavioral perspective and rewarded for "good" behavior.

One of the dangers in our field today is the potential for proponents of one or another theoretical perspective to claim authority (Grady, 1987). No one theory or conceptual framework in occupational therapy has yet been subjected to enough clinical research to make such a claim. Each of the theories presented in this book offers important perspectives for the problems faced in OT practice. Familiarity with these theories and methods for applying their principles helps therapists to meet the occupational needs of their patients.

WHY DOES IT MATTER?

The therapist who is working in a clinical setting using tools learned in school to evaluate and treat patients and seeing some progress as a result may ask, "So why do we need theory anyway? I'm doing pretty well without thinking much about it, thank you, and besides I don't have the time."

There are many good reasons why it is important for occupational therapists to become conscious of, interested in, and competent with the use of theory. These reasons are described below.

To Validate and Guide Practice

The following excerpt from a 1938 editorial in the journal *Occupational Therapy and Rehabilitation* illustrates that the need for theory and research to justify our practice is not a new concern:

> The following list of questions was recently sent to us by a therapist connected with one of our large state hospitals, [the questions] having been given her by the psychologist connected with that institution. It can be recognized that they are questions which are often asked by physicians and sometimes we do not have a ready answer for them so that it is desired to hold a symposium upon them in order that all therapists may be prepared.
>
> 1. What is the occupational therapist's theory as to how occupational therapy proves of assistance in bringing about recovery?
>
> 2. What are the statistics upon which is based the statement that occupational therapy does aid recovery? (Editorial, 1938, p. 127)

These remain, today, two of the major issues in promoting and justifying the use of occupational therapy. The first question can be addressed by the therapist familiar with theories of occupational therapy, and the second can be answered by the occupational therapist who is familiar with the information derived from research in the profession.

As Clark has stated:

> The development and use of theory and theory-testing in practice can and will define the validity of occupational therapy as a professional service. The theories developed for and through practice may be evaluated in terms of their capacity to define and describe that practice, including actions and technology; and their predictive value for the outcome of practice. (1979, p. 508)

The theories that guide everyday practice may be used unconsciously. It is critical to bring those theories into the light of consciousness because they may be incomplete, contradictory, or inconsistent. Although it may at first seem threatening to risk discovering that such is the case, concern for providing the best possible care for patients and acceptance of the reality that we are all always learning should provide the necessary motivation to examine the theories one uses in making practice decisions.

As Parham put it:

> Theory is a key element in problem setting and in problem solving. It is a tool that enables the therapist to "name it and frame it." Both language

and logic are needed to identify a problem (name it) and to plan a means for altering the situation (frame it). Theory provides these by giving us words or concepts for naming what we observe, and by spelling out logical relationships between concepts. This allows us to explain what we see and to figure out how to manipulate a situation to cause change. (1987, p. 557)

And as Kielhofner states, occupational therapy practice is only becoming *more* complex.

The nature of occupational therapy practice will shift from the application of a limited number of known clinical solutions to the use of increasingly complex, autonomous decision-making and problem-solving in multifactorial situations. The therapist must, therefore, be a critical thinker, capable of evaluating and synthesizing information from a variety of sources about a wide range of phenomena. This means that the therapist must be able to draw on a well-formed body of disciplinary knowledge. (1992, p. 8)

To Justify Reimbursement

Validation of practice is directly tied to reimbursement. Those who pay for OT services are ever more demanding of substantive justification for what occupational therapists do: they want both an explanation of why something is being done and a demonstration that what is being done works. The explanation is provided through theory, the demonstration through research.

Baum has stated that in today's changing health marketplace it is important not only to develop cost-effective programs but also to "document program effectiveness using standard and reliable measures of patient/client performance" (1985, p. 24). She writes:

Is occupational therapy cost-effective? Can occupational therapy influence performance? The public expects answers to these questions, and the profession bears the responsibility for providing the answers. In the past OT has relied on the medical and basic sciences for knowledge generation and scientific inquiry. But if our contribution to health care is to be unique, it is up to us to address the important questions about health, occupation, and human performance. (1987, p. 145)

To Clarify Specialization Issues

The issue of specialization is related to theory, since occupational therapists need to be able to balance the technical aspects of practice with underlying theoretical explanations that reflect their basic assumptions and identity as occupational therapists. Otherwise, how can one explain the differences between an occupational therapist who specializes in hand therapy and a physical therapist who also specializes in hand therapy? Or, how does one explain the common connections between an occupational therapist who works with adolescent drug abusers and another one who works with elders afflicted with Alzheimer's disease?

To Enhance the Growth of the Profession and the Professionalism of Its Members

One of the major attributes of a profession is that it has a distinctive theoretical base. In 1982 the AOTA stated that one of its missions was "to encourage the development and testing of theories that contribute to the knowledge base, which will enhance the growth of the profession" (American Occupational Therapy Foundation, 1982, p. 116).

> The theoretical systems that comprise the body of knowledge of OT are generated within the profession, as well as drawn from the academic disciplines (e.g., the social and biological sciences) and other professional fields (e.g., medicine). Theories are selected, formulated, and adapted to have specific meaning to the profession's practice. So constituted, they form the body of knowledge or theoretical foundation of the profession. The body of knowledge is unique in its entirety but not in its component parts. The challenge to OT is to identify a body of knowledge that reflects its scientific base and philosophical assumptions in order to organize this knowledge in ways that serve clinical practice. (Williamson, 1977, p. 718)

The use of a theory base to guide decision making is much of what distinguishes a professional person from a technician. As Williamson goes on to state:

> Therapists vary in their level of awareness regarding the philosophical assumptions and theoretical foundations of their practice and their ability to communicate them to others. A professional is distinguished from a technician by knowledge of the propositions that guide his or her actions and the conscious selection of those propositions to influence change. In a practice based on theory, the therapist is able to ascertain the relationship between a client's need and a theoretical principle, and apply intervention procedures on the basis of accurate prediction of outcome. (1977, p. 722)

Although development of a strong theory base will not guarantee occupational therapy's acceptance and recognition by others as a profession, such acceptance and recognition will certainly not come without such a base. What seems most important in the entire controversy about professionalism is that to deliver the best service, both directly to patients and clients and indirectly through communication with other members of the health care system, occupational therapists need to feel confident about what they are doing and about their ability to communicate why they are doing it. This confidence requires a solid theoretical foundation, as well as the ability to apply that theory to facilitating the functional needs of individual patients and clients.

To Educate Competent Practitioners

Not only practitioners but also students and educators must be actively involved in the process of studying, understanding, and consciously utilizing theory. Yerxa and Sharrott state, "The person who graduates from an occupational therapy program needs to be an independent, critical thinker who is at home with principles and interrelationships among concepts; acts from a knowledge base and can articulate the theoretical support for what he or she does" (1986, p. 155). According to Shapiro and Shanahan, "One of the primary goals for educators of OT's is the preparation of independent practitioners—persons who will be able to use accepted theories, and when necessary, to generate new theories to guide their practice" (1976, p. 217).

Once they leave the classroom, students need to work with fieldwork supervisors who provide positive role models for using theory in everyday practice.

> The application of theory to practice in fieldwork education cannot occur without strong collaborative partnerships between education and practice. We must do all we can to build and reinforce an atmosphere of working together toward the same goal of a profession with strong theoretical bases and practical techniques that are adaptable in a world of changing health care systems. (McGourty, 1986, p. 128)

THEORY AS UNIFYING FOUNDATION

Our theoretical base should and can provide major connections among the various aspects of our field. One certainly should be able to explain best those theories that one uses most often. Yet possessing an understanding of the major theories that influence practice in the field is a goal to which each occupational therapist can aspire, not only in order to be well educated and better able to communicate, but also to be better able to define oneself as an occupational therapist and have confidence that what one is doing with patients, with students, and in research is well founded.

One must take care, however, in using any theory without adequate knowledge. Attempts to apply theories with only a cursory understanding of concepts and principles can lead to inaccurate assumptions and potentially harmful practice with contradictory and confusing outcomes.

SEMANTIC ISSUES

One of the major difficulties in understanding, analyzing, and comparing theories in occupational therapy is that different theorists use different words to discuss similar concepts. The same theorist may even use such terms as "theory," "model," and "paradigm" interchangeably. This can be very confusing to the reader. This problem is not unique to occupational therapy, but efforts need to be made to clarify labels, particularly at this time when the importance of understanding and utilizing theory is of such concern.

The process of clarifying and comparing these labels in a way that is consistent and true to theorists' meanings will be a lengthy one. However, it is important that the effort be made. What is presented here is merely a beginning step that, it is hoped, will assist readers to apply their own critical reasoning faculties to the effort to sort out and understand the complexities, similarities, and differences behind the labels.

Highest Levels of Conceptualization

Four of the seven theorists in this book present recommendations for conceptualizing what occupational therapy is about. The terms used to describe these overarching conceptualizations differ: consider Reilly's paradigm, Kielhofner's paradigm, Mosey's model, and Llorens' schematic. The term "paradigm" can be

> used to denote the prevailing network of science, philosophy, and theory accepted by a discipline. . . . The prevailing paradigm directs the activities of a discipline. As such, it is accepted by the majority of individuals within the discipline and suggests the areas of study of interest to the discipline and the means to study them. (Marriner, 1986, p. 22)

The concept of paradigm is much more complex than the scope of this chapter can encompass, and the reader is referred to Kuhn (1970) for greater understanding of its significance.

Reilly was the first occupational therapist to write about paradigm. Her citation as a charter member of the American Occupational Therapy Foundation (AOTF) Academy of Research lauded her "exemplary contributions to the development of a generic paradigm for practice."

Gary Kielhofner has expanded on the occupational behavior paradigm and has diverged from it in some significant ways. In the book *Health Through Occupation* (1983), Kielhofner presented contributions from many writers in the field on issues involved in paradigm development for occupational therapy. By 1992 he had derived the following definition:

> The paradigm consists of the basic assumptions and perspectives that unify the field. The paradigm defines and gives coherence or wholeness to the entire profession. It speaks to the nature and purpose of occupational therapy. Therefore, it is general and does not provide specific strategies for practice. (1992, p. 13)

Mosey uses the term "model" in the sense of

> the typical way in which a profession perceives itself, its relationship to other professions, and its association with the society to which it is responsible. The model of a profession is characterized by a description of the profession's philosophical assumptions, ethical code, theoretical foundation, domain of concern, legitimate tools, and the nature of and principles for sequencing the various aspects of practice. (1981, p. 50)

She now calls this "compilation of information" our "fundamental body of knowledge" (1992, p. 49).

Though not quite so global, Llorens' three-dimensional "schematic" for organizing the body of knowledge in the field bears resemblance to the above conceptualizations. Reilly and Kielhofner took the idea of paradigm from Kuhn, a pure sociologist; Mosey took her concept of model from the literature of the sociology of professions; and Llorens' schematic cubic representation is similar in structure to Guilford's "Structure of Intellect" model (Guilford, 1977).

Levels of Theory

Fidler, Mosey, Ayres, Llorens, and Allen all use the label "theory" to refer to a conceptual framework when trying to explain, describe, or predict phenomena of concern to occupational therapy. Kielhofner uses the term "model" to mean a conceptual framework or theory that is at the broad and complex end of the theory continuum. As Parham states, "A good conceptual framework enables the therapist to cope with the many details of a human problem by synthesizing them into a perspective of the whole" (1986, p. 121). This use of the term "model" is obviously quite different from Mosey's.

Linking Theory to Practice

> Traditionally, the function of theory is to explain, describe, and predict phenomena. Control of events is not a primary aim of scientific knowledge, although it may be a desirable outcome. . . . In the applied professional fields one is concerned with the nature of the change process and the means to influence it. Two approaches are commonly used to relate theoretical systems to intervention—practice theories and frames of reference. They are two systematic ways of organizing and applying knowledge to effect change. Both . . . are similar since they share a common goal and use components of a theory. Practice theories and frames of references serve as linking structures between theory and practice. (Williamson, 1977, p. 718)

Ayres' theory is an example of a practice theory, and Mosey has articulated frames of reference for occupational therapy.

As was stated previously, there obviously are very important differences among these concepts that one must take great care not to oversimplify or gloss over. It is hoped that this brief beginning will stimulate others to further clarify and differentiate concept labels.

The next seven chapters describe the lives and works of seven major theorists in occupational therapy. Each chapter begins with a photograph and a biographical sketch of the theorist. The intent of these is to place the person in social and professional contexts, to identify influences on her or his theory development, and to "demystify" by presenting the person behind the ideas. It is hoped that this will both enlighten the reader as to the theorist's perspective and inspire the reader to see his or her own practice and potential within a broader historical and professional context.

REFERENCES

American Occupational Therapy Foundation (1982). A long-range research plan for occupational therapy. *American Journal of Occupational Therapy, 36*, 116–118.

Ayres, A.J. (1965). Sensory integrative processes and neuropsychological learning disability. In J. Hellmuth (Ed.), *Learning disorders* (Vol. 3) (pp. 41–58). Seattle, WA: Special Child Publication.

Baum, C.M. (1985). The evolution of the U.S. health care system. In J. Blair & M. Gray (Eds.), *The occupational therapy manager* (pp. 3–26). Rockville, MD: American Occupational Therapy Association.

Baum, C.M. (1987). Nationally speaking: Research: Its relationship to public policy. *American Journal of Occupational Therapy, 41*, 143–145.

Carlson, M.E., & Clark, F. (1991). The search for useful methodologies in occupational science. *American Journal of Occupational Therapy, 45*, 235–241.

Clark, F.A., Parham, L.D., Carlson, M.E., Frank, G., Jackson, J., Pierce, D., Wolfe, R.J., & Zemke, R. (1991). Occupational science: Academic innovation in the service of occupational therapy's future. *American Journal of Occupational Therapy, 45*, 300–310.

Clark, P.N. (1979). Theoretical frameworks in contemporary occupational therapy practice, Part 1. *American Journal of Occupational Therapy, 33*, 505–514.

Duldt, B.W., & Giffin, K. (1985). *Theoretical perspectives for nursing.* Boston: Little, Brown.

Dunton, W.R. (1919). *Reconstruction therapy.* Philadelphia: W.B. Saunders.

Editorial. (1938, April). *Occupational Therapy and Rehabilitation* (Vol. 17), p. 127.

Grady, A.P. (1987). Nationally speaking: Research: Its role in enhancing the professional image. *American Journal of Occupational Therapy, 41*, 347–349.

Guilford, J.P. (1977). *Way beyond the IQ.* Buffalo, NY: Creative Education Foundation and Bearly Limited.

Hopkins, H.L., & Smith, H.D. (Eds.). (1983). *Willard and Spackman's occupational therapy* (6th ed.). Philadelphia: J.B. Lippincott.

Kielhofner, G. (Ed.). (1983). *Health through occupation: Theory and practice in occupational therapy.* Philadelphia: F.A. Davis.

Kielhofner, G. (1992). *Conceptual foundations of occupational therapy.* Philadelphia: F.A. Davis.

Kuhn, T. (1970). *The structure of scientific revolutions* (2nd ed.). Chicago: University of Chicago Press.

Lewin, K. (1947). *Principles of topological psychology.* New York: McGraw-Hill.

Marriner, A. (Ed.). (1986). *Nursing theorists and their works.* St. Louis: C.V. Mosby.

McGourty, L.K. (1986). Applying theory to practice: Fieldwork education. In *Occupational therapy education: Target 2000* (pp. 126–128). Rockville, MD: American Occupational Therapy Association.

Mosey, A.C. (1981). *Occupational therapy: Configuration of a profession.* New York: Raven Press.

Mosey, A.C. (1992). *Applied scientific inquiry in the health professions: An epistemological orientation.* Rockville, MD: American Occupational Therapy Association.

Ostrow, P.C. (1980). The foundation: The care and feeding of theories. *American Journal of Occupational Therapy, 34*, 272–273.

Ottenbacher, K.J. (1985). The foundation: Ritual, rigor, and relevance: The design of clinical research. *American Journal of Occupational Therapy, 39*, 202–203.

Ottenbacher, K.J. (1992). Confusion in occupational therapy research: Does the end justify the method? *American Journal of Occupational Therapy, 46*, 871–874.

Parham, L.D. (1986). Applying theory to practice. In *Occupational therapy education: Target 2000* (pp. 119–122). Rockville, MD: American Occupational Therapy Association.

Parham, L.D. (1987). Toward professionalism: The reflective therapist. *American Journal of Occupational Therapy, 41*, 555–561.

Reed, K.L. (1984). Understanding theory: The first step in learning about research. *American Journal of Occupational Therapy, 38*, 677–682.

Shapiro, D., & Shanahan, P.M. (1976). Methodology for teaching theory. *American Journal of Occupational Therapy, 30*, 217–224.

Williamson, G.G. (1977). A heritage of activity: Development of theory. *American Journal of Occupational Therapy, 36*, 716–722.

Yerxa, E.J. (1991). Nationally speaking: Seeking a relevant, ethical, and realistic way of knowing for occupational therapy. *American Journal of Occupational Therapy, 45*, 199–204.

Yerxa, E.J., & Sharrott, G. (1986). Liberal arts: The foundation for occupational therapy education. *American Journal of Occupational Therapy, 40*, 153–159.

Chapter Two

Gail Fidler

Ferol Menks Ludwig

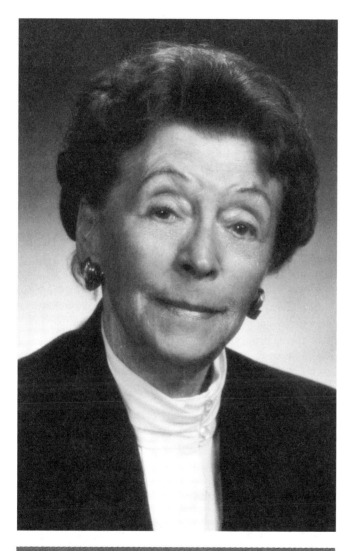

Gail Fidler

BIOGRAPHICAL SKETCH

Gail Fidler was born in Spencer, Iowa, in 1916. She is the first of four children and lived with her family in South Dakota and later in Lebanon, Pennsylvania. Her father was a high school teacher and coach who fostered her avid interest in sports. She played varsity basketball and field hockey in high school and college and later used her certification as a basketball referee to help support herself during occupational therapy school. Other activities in high school and college included being on the debating team, writing poetry for the college paper, doing art illustrations, and being a member of her local church's drama club and choral group.

Fidler earned her Bachelor of Arts degree from Lebanon Valley College in 1938 with a double major in education and psychology. After graduation she worked for six months as a high school history teacher, but she found the school system to be too constricting for her (G. Fidler, personal communication, May 13, 1982). At that time, limited financial resources prevented her from pursuing graduate work in psychology or attending medical school to become a psychiatrist. So to earn the money for tuition she worked as a hospital attendant at Wernersville State Hospital, where she discovered occupational therapy (OT). She described the director of occupational therapy as an interesting and well-educated person with whom she felt that she could connect, and she appreciated the normalizing, pleasant atmosphere of the OT clinic.

> I was impressed by the change in patients' behavior while they were in occupational therapy. They seemed almost like different persons when they were engaged in productive activity. Working as an attendant on the back wards of the state hospital was an incredible learning experience for me. It was extremely difficult, challenging and exciting, all at the same time. (G. Fidler, personal communication, July 1992)

She enrolled in the OT Certificate Program at the University of Pennsylvania in 1940 and, while attending the program, was employed as a group worker at Smith Memorial Settlement House in Philadelphia until her graduation in 1942. During a summer break she returned to work at the Wernersville State Hospital, where she met a medical student who was to become her husband in 1944.

Her first position as an occupational therapist was in 1942 at the Norristown State Hospital. She described this experience as "disturbing."

> It was quite different than my experiences with OT as a student. I had high expectations and what I was seeing in practice was certainly different. I suddenly had to confront reality in comparison to my expectations, knowing that I could not stay in OT if it was no more than I was seeing. It was quite upsetting to suspect that I had made an error in choosing

occupational therapy as a career. (G. Fidler, personal communication, May 13, 1982)

> In retrospect the department of OT at Norristown was probably the most comprehensive and best organized one that I have seen. It was highly respected and acknowledged as a valuable service to patients. What was lacking, and disturbing to me, was a rationale for practice. The why's were not being asked and the challenge of hypotheses—of theoretical explanation—was simply not being faced. (G. Fidler, personal communication, November 3, 1987)

She decided, however, that it was not wise to make a decision on the basis of sheer emotion, so she entered into a year's contract with herself to study and explore thoroughly the potential of occupational therapy in psychiatry. She clearly defined the procedures that she would follow to answer the question, "Is this all that there is to OT?" She decided that if at the end of a year she discovered that occupational therapy was no more than what was reflected in current practice, she would leave the field. During the following year she methodically attempted to find some rationale for what her 60 patients were doing and how the activities were or were not helpful. It was during this time that she conceived the idea of the activity analysis.

> Midway through my searches I was hooked and felt that at this time I could not pursue medical school or any other career. I had hold of this idea and I needed to see it through. It has been almost 40 years of seeing it through. (G. Fidler, personal communication, May 13, 1982)

During that year she also had the opportunity to learn from Dr. Alfred Noyes, a renowned psychiatrist and superintendent of Norristown State Hospital. "It was a rare privilege to see this man in action and my commitment to psychiatry and to the pursuit of a rationale for occupational therapy was reconfirmed" (G. Fidler, personal communication, May 1, 1987).

Fidler wanted to pursue graduate education in occupational therapy, but at the time no such program existed. She enrolled in the graduate clinical psychology program at New York University, but withdrew after one semester because it was not relevant to the questions that she had nor to what she wanted to do. Several years later she enrolled in social work and discontinued that for similar reasons.

> Mainly my motivation has come from a very fundamental itch that began during that first year of inquiry. This thesis is that there has to be some relationship among what people do, their interests, how they occupy their time, their state of health, and their characteristic personality patterns. (G. Fidler, personal communication, May 13, 1982)

Fidler then worked as an occupational therapist at Walter Reed Army Hospital, Washington, D.C., where the director of occupational therapy was Danish and a master weaver. She taught Fidler how to master weaving and to love it passionately. From 1944 to 1946 Fidler was chief occupational therapist at the Army Hospital in Fort Story, Virginia, and from 1946 to 1950 she was employed as a staff therapist at the Veterans' Hospital in Lyons, New Jersey.

Always stimulated by the questions raised in practice, Fidler sought more answers by attending the William Alanson White Institute of Psychiatry and Psychology in New York City from 1947 to 1951. During this time, she was significantly influenced by the work of Harry Stack Sullivan (1953), particularly his interpersonal theory and hypotheses regarding ego development, self-esteem, and competence.

From 1952 to 1955 she was an instructor with the Pennsylvania Department of Mental Health Training Programs. In that capacity she assumed a major teaching and consultant role in implementing an ongoing series of training institutes for program staff throughout the Pennsylvania mental health system.

From 1955 to 1957 she was the coordinator of the American Occupational Therapy Association (AOTA) Psychiatric Study Group, which was funded by a National Institute of Mental Health (NIMH) grant to examine, assess, and define the current concepts and practice of occupational therapy in psychiatry and to find ways to improve the preparation of future occupational therapists in this specialty area. This study culminated in the Allenbury Workshop Conference on the Function and Preparation of the Psychiatric Occupational Therapist. The proceedings of this workshop conference were published in the book *Changing Concepts and Practices in Psychiatric Occupational Therapy*, which was edited by Wilma West (1959). Fidler served as one of the editorial consultants for this book.

During this period she also taught a summer session at the Philadelphia School of Occupational Therapy and lectured on occupational therapy theory in psychiatry at New York University. She served as member-at-large for the AOTA Board of Management from 1957 to 1963.

From 1959 to 1968 Fidler served as director of professional education for the Department of Occupational Therapy at the New York State Psychiatric Institute. In that position Fidler developed and directed clinical field work study for occupational therapists and students; provided in-service education to physician residents, social workers, and nurses; supervised OT staff; initiated prevocational and work rehabilitation programs; developed patient evaluation and diagnostic measures; and collaborated with the sociology department to research and measure the nature and effect of change within institutional systems.

From there she went on to be director of the Activities Therapy Department at Hillside Hospital, where she was responsible for administration, coordination, and management of a staff consisting of occupational therapists, vocational coun-

selors, therapeutic recreators, secondary school teachers, music and dance therapists, and volunteers. She designed and implemented new service programs for the
day hospital, aftercare, and acute admission center. She served as liaison between
the city school system and the school at Hillside Hospital and planned in-service
education for teachers on working with emotionally disturbed adolescents. She
also developed undergraduate and graduate field work experiences with ten curricula and collaborated to develop a community outreach rehabilitation grant.

While working at the New York State Psychiatric Institute and Hillside Hospital, Fidler directed the master's degree programs in psychiatric occupational
therapy at New York University and at Columbia University. She also served as a
consultant to several state and hospital programs. During this time her civic activities included involvement with the League of Women Voters, United Fund Coun-
cil, Visiting Nurse Association Homemakers Program, Education Committee for
Teachers and Parents, Plainfield Public Schools, and Union County Aftercare Program. In her work with this latter group, she was instrumental in developing the
state's first psychiatric aftercare program.

In January 1971, Fidler moved into the national offices of AOTA, where she
served as associate executive director, managing the practice, education, and research divisions. She wrote grants that enabled AOTA to offer a series of training
institutes for practitioners and educators. She was instrumental in obtaining a
grant to support graduate traineeships, and she helped AOTA secure grants total-
ing over $500,000 to conduct several major studies.

Fidler served as interim executive director of the AOTA from March 1975 until
that October, when she became coordinator of AOTA's Educator Training Institutes. In that capacity she planned, organized, and implemented regional institutes
for OT academic and clinical faculty from all of the professional and technical
programs. These institutes focused on curriculum design, teaching methods, and
competency-based learning. An outgrowth of these educator institutes was the
project to revise the certified occupational therapist and the certified occupational
therapy assistant registration examinations to emphasize competency-based outcomes in preference to the accumulation of knowledge.

During the 1970s and 1980s, Fidler continued her consultative services to several psychiatric hospitals, where she planned and organized OT services and activity therapy programs and coordinated these services with vocational rehabilitation. The Department of Rehabilitation Services developed by her at Springfield
Hospital Center in Maryland was subsequently used as a model for service delivery in mental health hospitals throughout the state.

From 1980 to 1982 Fidler served as the assistant hospital administrator for programming at Greystone Park Psychiatric Hospital in New Jersey. Since 1980 she
has been a consultant in curriculum development to the New York University
Department of Occupational Therapy, and in 1982 she was appointed rehabilita-

tion consultant to the New Jersey Division of Mental Health Hospitals. During her tenure as rehabilitation consultant, she developed and had approved state standards for rehabilitation programs in mental health facilities and agencies and established staffing standards and quality assurance monitoring.

In 1984 she was appointed chief executive officer of the Hagadorn Center for Geriatrics, a New Jersey state facility. In 1987 she completed a major reorganization of the Center from a long-term nursing care facility to a geropsychiatric rehabilitation center that provides community-based day treatment and housing programs in order to sustain the elderly in the community. According to Fidler, "Hagadorn Center operates on those fundamental constructs of occupational therapy which emphasize and prioritize the meaning and value of human performance and the ability 'to do' as the quality of life and as characterizing health" (G. Fidler, personal communication, May 1, 1987).

Throughout her career, Fidler has displayed a strong dedication and enthusiasm for the education of the young professional. She introduced occupational therapists to supervision as a tutorial learning process and offered the first workshops in supervision at Columbia University in the 1950s. During the 1970s, she was a visiting professor at the University of California at San Jose, Kean College, the University of Pennsylvania, and Boston University. She continues to teach and lecture on management, the meaning and uses of activities, group process, and program design.

In the summer of 1990 she was asked by College Misericordia to assume the position of interim program director of occupational therapy. With almost 300 students in three different tracks at the school, the college found itself suddenly without a program director and with only two faculty members.

> I was indeed surprised at their request for me to help them out, since academic administration was something that I had never done. Although I had taught students, part time teaching is a far cry from academic administration and being enmeshed in the system of higher education. However, I have always looked for challenge in any position that I have ever taken; the challenge of problems, and the challenge of learning. What I discovered as Interim Program Director, very rapidly, was that there was plenty of both! (G. Fidler, personal communication, July 1992)

Because of her firm commitment to the development of occupational therapy as a profession, Fidler has been very active in volunteer professional activities from the beginning of her career. She has chaired numerous task forces within AOTA and has served on many of its committees. She has also served on the board of directors of the AOTF and on the advisory board of the *American Journal of Occupational Therapy*.

Fidler is also a member of a number of professional organizations. She has served on the advisory board of Kean College, on the board of the Coalition for the Reform of the New Jersey Mental Health System, and on the board of directors of the Union County Mental Health Association and its Professional Advisory Committee. She was also a member of the New Jersey Rehabilitation Committee and was the chair of the Monitoring Committee in the Office of the Public Advocate for the State of New Jersey.

Fidler has received the highest honors awarded by the occupational therapy profession. In 1965 she was the Eleanor Clarke Slagle Lecturer (Fidler, 1966a), and in 1980 she was presented the AOTA Award of Merit. She is also a Fellow of the AOTA.

Fidler has written over 20 articles and chapters, has authored three books, and has co-authored two books with her husband, Jay Fidler. She continues to give presentations, institutes, and workshops.

She is the mother of two children, a daughter Dagny and a son Eric. She and her husband, Jay, have recently moved to Fort Lauderdale, Florida, where they plan to spend their winters. During the warmer months of each year Gail Fidler will be a "scholar in residence" at Misericordia College in New Jersey.

Reflections on the Profession

Fidler believes that some of the obstacles to theory development in occupational therapy stem from the profession's minority position in the health care system and its subsequent difficulty in influencing the medical model of human functioning with its own concepts and constructs.

> I've always said that what we really have to deal with is double jeopardy. What we theorize and practice is not in the top priority of the medical and health care delivery system structure. It is so "mundane" and seemingly obvious that it carries very little glamour, and it is hard to convince people of the value of something that is part of their everyday life. It is hard to maintain one's professional self-respect when references are continually made to psychology, the psychiatrist, the nurse, the social worker and "others." I was an "and others" for so long it became difficult to maintain a level of ego strength and self-respect in the practice arena. (G. Fidler, personal communication, May 13, 1982)

Any success or contributions that Fidler made were often credited to her personally rather than to the profession. This angered her because she experienced it as a criticism of the profession.

According to Fidler, another barrier to the development of the OT profession is attitudes about its predominantly female composition, which tend to perpetuate its minority status and are the other half of the "double jeopardy" concept.

> We are many times our own worst enemy and there is a critical need to develop more assertive behaviors and attitudes among our members. We need to state what we do, write it, and publicize it. We need to educate and socialize students into professional behaviors, rather than reinforcing female stereotypical behaviors. (G. Fidler, personal communication, May 13, 1982)

To address this concern, Fidler sees the need to recruit young, bright, and ambitious women and men and to stimulate them by providing an assertive career role model within the profession. Fidler also has recently been offering workshops across the country teaching skills for negotiating the system and facilitating the development of leadership skills, behaviors, and attitudes based on awareness of self and on interpersonal competence. Her presentation at the 1992 AOTA conference in Houston titled "Our Search for Efficacy" dealt with these issues.

Because occupational therapy is a very complex profession, Fidler believes that a master's degree should be a prerequisite for entry-level positions in the field. To understand the constructs of the art and science of the field requires a longer term of educational socialization than is provided by baccalaureate programs. Other bona fide professions are built on graduate-level work, and their entry into practice is at the graduate level (G. Fidler, personal communication, May 13, 1982).

> Being at the beginning of the development of a profession is both exciting and scary. It means admitting that there is much that we cannot know, and acknowledging that many years of arduous development of research and of educational preparation of the professional occupational therapist may be required. I really believe that it is going to take as many years to begin to move toward realizing this potential and generating a knowledge base as it has taken medicine and law. But search and discovery are incredibly exciting. (G. Fidler, personal communication, May 1982)

Fidler is disturbed by the devaluation of activities in OT practice and their replacement with "talking groups" in mental health and with physical therapy modalities in physical dysfunction. She feels that the mimicking of other professions brings the field very close to losing what is essential and critical to occupational therapy (G. Fidler, personal communication, May 13, 1982).

On the other side of the ledger, balancing out the obstacles to her work in occupational therapy is the support she has received from others in and outside the profession.

I was indeed fortunate to have been able to work with and learn from so many very talented and famous persons in the field of psychiatry, such as Nathaniel Apter, Elvin Semiad, Alfred Noyes, and Lawrence Kolb. Another strong incentive has been the positive, challenging responses of the many young, bright occupational therapists with whom I've been privileged to work. Certainly the most positive force has been the interest and support of my husband. He has continued to be my finest advocate, teacher, and friend. (G. Fidler, personal communication, September 24, 1984)

Fidler states that many persons influenced her thinking and motivation (G. Fidler, personal communication, May 1, 1987). She credits her father with teaching her the values and attitudes of critical thinking and creative and logical problem solving. He taught her to understand that only she can be responsible for herself. Her husband, Jay Fidler, immeasurably shaped her thinking, sparked her motivation, and "clarified realities with loving care" (G. Fidler, personal communication, May 1, 1987). She credits Helen Willard with teaching her about "integrity and dignity without ever once threatening the spontaneous fun in me." She mentions Elizabeth Ridgway, whose understanding and sensitivity about the schizophrenic patient impressed her and taught her much.

Fidler describes her current viewpoint on occupational therapy.

I have not become disenchanted nor have I had any questions about the fundamental concept of OT. The longer I have looked and worked with it, the more convinced I am that there is a credibility and relevance to this perspective of human functioning that is unique and different from any other perspectives about human behavior. I have no question about that. I do have a question about how we pursue development and how we do not pursue it. (G. Fidler, personal communication, September 24, 1984)

This last statement is of great concern to her. She feels that the fundamental concept underlying occupational therapy is viable and that if the profession does not develop it and use it, other professions will.

THEORETICAL CONCEPTS

Since she entered the field of occupational therapy in 1942, Fidler has consistently believed that purposeful planned activity is the very core of the OT therapeutic process. Although her theories were derived from psychoanalytic concepts and during the first half of her career were mainly applicable to psychosocial function and dysfunction, she has continued to expand them to include new knowledge and developments in related basic and applied sciences and in occupational therapy. Likewise, she has influenced the development of other theories and theorists such as Anne Mosey.

Currently her theory concerning activity addresses the physical, neurobehavioral, cognitive, psychological, and sociocultural aspects of the individual and how purposeful activity and objects in the human and nonhuman environment might best match the needs of the individual. She believes that the meanings of activities cannot be reduced to one or two factors, but instead interact with each other at many levels. The following subsections examine these factors and their hypothesized relationships.

Nonhuman Environment and Object Relations

Searles' (1960) work on the human and nonhuman environment strongly supported Fidler's early formulations of the meaning of activity. They described how persons develop object relationships with the nonhuman environment from infancy through adulthood. These interactions serve many functions. Symbolically and realistically, they are a means of communicating feelings, needs, and ideations; they mediate between the inner and outer world; and they help one achieve a sense of self. One uses object relations to differentiate self from nonself and to learn more about both. The nonhuman environment is a source of need gratification. Ego functions are developed and strengthened by realistic encounters with objects.

Object relations and their symbolic meaning and unconscious processes (Azima, 1961; Azima & Azima, 1959; Wittkower & Azima, 1958) are key elements of Fidler's early theories. She outlined procedures for evaluating and measuring clients' responses to objects, which included responses to the therapist, the activity, and the group. Such responses provide diagnostic information regarding clients' basic needs, if and how these needs are being gratified, and clients' development of adequate ego defenses and strengths. Since this initial formulation, little has been done to develop or define these constructs and concepts further in OT evaluation and treatment. This is of great concern to Fidler (Fidler & Fidler, 1954, 1963).

Communication Process

Another purpose of activity is to express thoughts and feelings nonverbally. "Occupational therapy is in effect another language for communication with the patient" (Fidler & Fidler, 1963, p. vi). In their 1954 and 1963 texts, Gail and Jay Fidler describe this language as an expression of needs, attitudes, and emotion and explain their reasoning behind this application. "As a communication process occupational therapy is concerned with action, the meaning of action, its use in communicating feelings and thoughts, and the use of such nonverbal communication for the benefit of the patient" (Fidler & Fidler, 1963, p. 19).

Action of the patient involved in occupational therapy is more likely to reveal the unconscious. The therapist will use techniques such as uncovering, supporting, or directing to help the patient to communicate (Fidler & Fidler, 1963).

Activity Analysis

A central theme of Fidler's work throughout her career has been the analysis of the components of activities and the correlation of these components with the specific needs, interests, and abilities of the client in order to provide action-oriented learning experiences to facilitate needed skill acquisition. Her early activity analysis (Fidler, 1948; Fidler & Fidler, 1954, 1963) focused mainly on the psychodynamic properties of activities as a guide for the therapist in evaluation and treatment. Motion, procedures, materials, creativity, symbols, hostile and aggressive components, control, predictability, narcissism, sexual identification, dependence, reality testing, and group relatedness are examined because she felt that these factors provide valuable clues to what emotional needs and drives might be encouraged by particular activities. Activities should be selected that correlate with the specific needs of the client, and then the performance of those activities should be controlled and guided in order to increase their therapeutic value.

Subsequently, Fidler expanded the analysis of activities to include motor, sensory integrative, psychological, sociocultural, cognitive, and interpersonal skills (Fidler, 1958, 1981a, 1982a). Activities need to be matched to the individual's readiness to learn or to receive stimuli, to personal characteristics, to interests and abilities, and to sociocultural values and norms. The real and symbolic meanings of activities used to promote acquisition of these essential skills also need to be explored (1981a). This concept is further developed in the Fidlers' construct of "doing" (Fidler & Fidler, 1978).

Doing

The Fidlers (Fidler & Fidler, 1978) use the term "doing" to connote performing, producing, or causing purposeful action in order to (1) test a skill, (2) clarify a relationship, or (3) create an end product. The process of doing enables the development and integration of the sensory, motor, cognitive, and psychological systems; is a socializing agent; and verifies one's efficacy as a competent contributing member of one's society. Thus the occupational therapist uses doing to enable patients to learn the performance skills that they will need to care for and maintain themselves more independently, to satisfy their personal needs for intrinsic gratification, and to contribute to meeting the needs and enhancing the welfare of others within an appropriate cultural context.

At any given point in time, the level and type of performance skills and the balance among them are determined by the individual's age, developmental level, unique biology, and culture. The balance among these skill clusters is critical to a lifestyle that is health sustaining and satisfying to oneself and to significant others (Fidler & Fidler, 1978).

According to the Fidlers (Fidler & Fidler, 1978), the acquisition of skills needed to perform one's life tasks and roles is influenced both by factors in the external environment and by internal systems. Such variables as culture, economics, family constellation, social class, housing, geographical surroundings, and architectural structures affect the external environment. They can inhibit or facilitate performance skill development.

Internal systems refer to the individual's unique biology: that is, his or her sensory, motor, physical, cognitive, and psychological systems. Maturational or developmental delays or deficits caused by trauma affect these systems and thereby influence the development of performance skills learning (Fidler & Fidler, 1978).

Competence and Mastery

Fidler's hypotheses concerning the relationship of purposeful activity to competence were influenced by the works of Sullivan (1953), Arieti (1962), White (1959, 1971), and other ego psychologists who proposed an innate drive to master and explore the environment that results in survival and a sense of competence from direct successful encounters with it. The reward is intrinsic, and reinforcement from others is not necessary. Fidler (1981a; Fidler & Fidler, 1983) suggests that the more experiences of mastery one has, the stronger is one's sense of competence. Each success then reinforces more attempts to develop skills and competencies further. Thus "doing" facilitates one's sense of competence and efficacy by creating experiences with human and nonhuman objects in one's environment. One learns about one's potential and limitations through these direct, action-oriented experiences.

Fidler (1981a) believes that the profession of occupational therapy must work to relate competence, mastery, adaptation, and self-esteem to OT practice. She views competence, mastery, achievement, self-esteem, self-value, and self-worth as interrelated states that are derived from direct encounters with and successful management of elements in the environment. When each of these experiences is verified both by the resulting intrinsic gratification and by positive feedback from significant others, one's value is enhanced (1981a, 1981b). Fidler emphasizes that the feedback that one receives from the process of doing is essential to learning about the realities of the self and the world. People learn about reality and test their perception of reality from predictable learned interactions with it (Fidler, 1981a; Fidler & Fidler, 1983). Until one acts on an idea or thought there can be no distinction between reality and nonreality. It is necessary to test one's ideas and thoughts through action in order to ascertain their validity, efficacy, and relevance to one's life.

Fidler (Fidler & Fidler, 1978) considers the social feedback from doing to be important because it provides consensual validation of masteries and competencies by their value to others. Another hypothesis that she offers is germane to the meaning and use of activities and their social relevance. That is, the values and norms of a society place higher status on certain tasks and activities than on others. Some activities may have high social significance and priority, whereas others may be less important or even be seen as having negative significance or value (Fidler, 1981a). Thus when one successfully performs an activity valued by society, one's sense of esteem and value as a human being is enhanced. Likewise, when one senses a risk of failure, doing in the presence of others is threatening and may be inhibited. Activities that are not valued by society may adversely affect one's sense of worth and competence (Fidler & Fidler, 1983).

Fidler's advocacy of the use of task groups in occupational therapy is based on the hypothesis that the task selected within a group context will meet the social, developmental, and learning needs of the participants by providing feedback on the efficacy of the action within sociocultural norms. By working within the context of a task group, the patient has a chance to learn constructive and rewarding behavior patterns. Opportunities arise for the development of several different roles, and a variety of individual needs can be met simultaneously (Fidler, 1969). The client learns to use his or her existing integrative assets and capacities to develop and improve skills necessary for the assumption of successful economic and social roles in everyday life outside the hospital. Age-appropriate social skill development is a critical component of performance and is facilitated or impaired both by factors in the external environment and by internal processes.

Integrative Process

Fidler (1982a) hypothesizes that activities are an integral part of human development, represent real-life situations, and are valuable and realistic vehicles for acquiring or redeveloping skills necessary to fulfill life roles and provide a source of satisfaction. The acquisition of these functional skills is a developmental process and progresses hierarchically. Certain behaviors are prerequisite to more mature and complex performance skills.

Specific actions of an activity or task elicit distinguishable and measurable sensory integrative, motor, cognitive, psychological, and social behaviors. When these are matched with the individual's needs and capacities, opportunities are provided to learn skills and develop more functional abilities in sensorimotor integration, self-maintenance, task behaviors, and leisure skills. Thus, by engaging in purposeful activity, the development and integration of internal sensory, motor, cognitive, and psychological processes are facilitated (Fidler, 1982a).

Health and Illness

Health is viewed as the ability to perform those roles and tasks of living throughout the life cycle that are essential to care for and to maintain the self independently, satisfy one's personal needs and thus provide intrinsic gratification, and contribute to the welfare of others within a socially and age-appropriate context (Fidler, 1981a, 1981b, 1982a; Fidler & Fidler, 1978, 1983). A sense of competence and social efficacy is basic to the ability to cope and adapt. This sense of the self as competent is largely achieved through successful doing experiences that carry social value and indicate mastery and achievement.

Dysfunction results when physical, social, cognitive, or psychosocial problems or trauma impedes development or impair functions and adaptations that are fundamental to daily living skills for self-maintenance, work, and leisure (Fidler, 1984; Fidler & Fidler, 1978, 1983).

APPLICATION TO OCCUPATIONAL THERAPY PRACTICE

Fidler's theories and hypotheses were derived from and directed toward clinical practice. She developed several assessment tools to explore the meaning and use of activities and the nature and quality of the processes in occupational therapy. Her initial contribution was the "Activity Analysis," which was created to examine the psychodynamics of activity (Fidler, 1948; Fidler & Fidler, 1963). Fidler wrote that practitioners needed a thorough understanding of each component of the OT experience to become more skilled in its use. "We believe that the nature or characteristics of the action experience are of primary importance. Involvement in an activity can be either therapeutic or damaging to the patient" (Fidler & Fidler, 1963, pp. 72–73). The purpose of this activity analysis was to guide one toward an understanding of the basic and fundamental psychodynamic characteristics of a selected activity.

Assessment

Fidler's "Outline for Evaluation" (Fidler & Fidler, 1963, pp. 104–107) guides the therapist by raising questions about the psychodynamics manifested by the patient in relationship to the therapist, activity, and group. It is psychoanalytically oriented, as was most of her work until the early 1970s.

The "Diagnostic Battery" (Fidler, 1968) is made up of a drawing, a finger painting, and a clay sculpture. The client is asked to comment on each production after it is completed. The productions and responses are interpreted and used in total team treatment planning.

In 1965, Fidler further refined this tool, adapting it for use within a group context. This instrument, the "Activity Laboratory" (Fidler, 1982a, pp. 195–207), has been used since 1965 with a wide variety of clients, with numerous students, and with interdisciplinary staffs. During that time, it has undergone many refinements to enable its tasks to elicit important areas of skill components and performance more effectively. Fidler does not propose that this be the only instrument used for evaluation to determine treatment planning. Rather, it is intended to be used as an "initial tentative behavioral profile" (Fidler, 1982a, p. 196). It also explores how strengths and characteristic styles of organizing and responding can be capitalized on in treatment intervention. How the individual handles the five tasks in the "Activity Laboratory" indicates his or her predominant sensory, motor, cognitive, psychological, and social behavior needs.

In collaboration with Susan Fine in 1970, Fidler developed the "Object History" (unpublished manuscript) to help people learn about and understand the importance of objects. Fidler feels that every occupational therapist should complete an "Object History" as part of his or her education. This instrument provides a descriptive account of the ways in which certain nonhuman objects are significantly linked with phases of an individual's growth and development. The participant selects an object that has had or continues to have special meaning during a particular part of his or her life. Objects might be toys, animals, household items, nature objects, clothing, or food. The participant is then asked to describe the object, how it came to be his or hers, how it was used, its meaning and importance, how family and friends were aware of or involved with the object, and how the object relationship was ended (Activity workshop, Galveston, Texas, September 22–23, 1983).

Fidler's "Play/Activity History" (1971, unpublished manuscript) is intended to develop an individual's appreciation for cultural and sexual differences in his or her play history and to help him or her understand better the real and symbolic meanings of these activities. The person is asked to identify and briefly describe those games or activities in which he or she engaged during the childhood and adolescent years. Then the person is asked to identify who taught him or her the game, what was the most enjoyable aspect of the game, with whom it was most frequently shared, and the extent to which it was part of his or her family's culture. Next, the person describes the specific practice or learning that the game provided in such areas as sensory/perceptual, motor, self-identity, reality orientation, cognitive, dyadic, and group skills. Aspects felt to be most and least enjoyable are then explored. Then one section examines the strategies involved, the game's aesthetic elements, and the role played by chance in determining the game's outcome. Competitive elements and the game's symbolic, creative, structured, and unstructured properties are analyzed. Finally, three hobbies or activities that are an important part of the individual's present lifestyle are identified, compared with activities from earlier years, and compared to one's present job or career choice (Activity workshop, Galveston, Texas, September 22–23, 1983).

More recently, Fidler developed "The Lifestyle Performance Profile" (1982b, pp. 43–48) as part of a conceptual model that describes adaptive performance as a fundamental concern of OT practice, building on her concepts of "doing" and competence. According to Fidler, OT practice is primarily concerned with skill development and the achievement of a satisfying, health-sustaining lifestyle. To achieve those goals, one has to evaluate the individual's existing strengths and skill deficits, developmental levels, and external barriers and resources (Fidler, 1982b, pp. 43–48). "The Lifestyle Performance Profile" provides a structure to identify and organize the person's sensorimotor functions and cognitive, psychological, dyadic, and group social skills within the context of his or her sociocultural milieu and characteristic response patterns and management of life tasks. It also describes sociocultural and environmental resources that support skill development or interfere with and impede it. The therapist must assess what work, play, and self-care activities are required of this individual in his or her given environment and which of these are intact or dysfunctional. This information may be obtained from existing records, interviews, standardized tests, and observation of the patient in specifically planned tasks and activities that involve sensorimotor, cognitive, and social behaviors.

Patient evaluations and assessments are fundamental means of providing data needed to plan and set priorities among treatment goals, to measure progress, and to plan for discharge. From the evaluation and assessment information, the therapist obtains an overview of the patient's strengths and deficits in managing the everyday tasks of his or her world and of performance patterns and related functional deficits that impair coping and adaptation (Fidler, 1984, pp. 33–36).

Intervention

Fidler's early theories about intervention and application were derived mainly from a psychoanalytic frame of reference. According to that perspective, the occupational therapist is a valuable contributor to the psychotherapeutic process because of his or her use of the combination of activities, the dyadic relationship, and groups. Specific treatment guidelines, rationale, and case histories were described in several publications (Fidler, 1958; Fidler & Fidler, 1954, 1963, 1978). The Fidlers felt, and still feel, that nonverbal techniques and the use of objects and object relationships are very effective treatment methods to incorporate into the total treatment regimen for many patients.

In their second book the Fidlers (1963) developed these concepts further, describing occupational therapy as a communication process in terms of the action itself, objects used in the action process, and the end products of those actions and interpersonal relationships. The therapeutic process, goals, and case examples are described in that book as consistent with the psychodynamic theoretical constructs described earlier in this chapter.

The idea of the dyadic or therapeutic relationship (discussed as therapeutic use of self by Fidler) is based on Harry Stack Sullivan's work on interpersonal theory (1953). Therapeutic use of self involves the therapist's use of actions that will be helpful to the patient. According to the Fidlers, "The problem in therapy is to anticipate the degree and type of response that will help the patient" (Fidler & Fidler, 1963, p. 41).

Group phenomena in occupational therapy are an essential part of intervention. The group leader is responsible for the emotional atmosphere of the group. He or she sets the tone and the expectations for group behavior. Important social roles and behaviors are learned in the context of task-oriented group activity (Fidler, 1969; Fidler & Fidler, 1963).

Fidler's conceptualization of the rehabilitative process is built on her theories of meanings, both real and symbolic, of activity, and of involvement with objects. Activities are used to explore and express the unconscious, provide gratification of needs, teach adaptive ego defenses and functional skills, provide a base for reality testing, and explore interpersonal relationships (Fidler, 1948, 1957, 1966b; Fidler & Fidler, 1963; Ridgway & Fidler, 1955). Activities may also be used to sustain and protect intact functions and abilities and to prevent further disability. The therapist selects those that provide experiences that enable the individual to use existing interests and skills for personal growth, to experience intrinsic gratification, and to meet needs for acceptance, achievement, creativity, autonomy, and social relationships. Activities and tasks are also chosen that will promote and enhance work skills and habits and teach and encourage independent functioning in activities of daily living. The therapist also introduces new activities that will provide compensatory learning and practice for the skills the patient needs to assume for his or her roles in community life. The individual is able to develop new interests and explore potentials because of his or her new experiences with activities. The client comes to see himself or herself as the doer, and the end product is tangible evidence of his or her ability to achieve (Fidler, 1981a).

As Fidler developed her theory further to include new developments in the art and science of occupational therapy, more implications for practice emerged. Purposeful activity is an organizing construct for practice and the distinguishing characteristic of occupational therapy (Fidler, 1981b). Purposeful activity, as expanded into concepts of "doing" and competence, became an essential link in the treatment process. The Fidlers relinquished the term "treatment" because it connoted changing and altering pathology and adopted instead the terms of "habilitation" or "remediation" (Activity workshop, Galveston, Texas, September 22–23, 1983).

When pathology is identified, doing must be used in the service of personality integration via performance skill development and reinforcement with treatment modalities that are adaptive and relevant to the performance skill demands and expectations of the home setting. An understanding of the nature and complexity of these performance skills and their interrelationship with internal and external processes is required. These skills are needed to enable one to feel that one is a productive, contributing, and needed member of society (Activity workshop, Galveston, Texas, September 22–23, 1983).

Action is directed toward (1) testing a skill, (2) clarifying a relationship, or (3) creating an end product. As discussed earlier, activities and doing experiences must be analyzed and matched to the individual's developmental needs and skill readiness in motor, sensorimotor integration, cognitive, psychological, and interpersonal components in ways that are relevant and significant to the needs and values of the person's sociocultural group and satisfying to the self (Fidler & Fidler, 1983, pp. 267–280). The fit between the individual and an activity is crucial if (1) integration of these systems and an adaptive response are to occur and (2) if choices of leisure, work, and self-maintenance activities are to result in intrinsic gratification, pleasure, and social efficacy of the individual (Fidler & Fidler, 1978).

Fidler's future goals for her theory development are to reach a sophisticated understanding of the nonhuman environment and nonhuman objects, the complex process of engagement with and manipulation of the environment, and the "doing" process as a facilitative process. Fidler encourages occupational therapists to go out into the community and create environments that are less stressful and more supportive of the individual. She is convinced that our future is dependent on fuller development of these constructs through doctoral and postdoctoral studies and research.

Fidler wrote *Design of Rehabilitation Services in Psychiatric Hospital Settings* (1984) as a result of her work as a consultant with the Mental Hygiene Administration of the Maryland State Department of Health and Mental Hygiene at Springfield Hospital Center and at Greystone Park Psychiatric Hospital in New Jersey. The book is a comprehensive guide to program design of rehabilitation services primarily for public psychiatric hospitals, but it is also relevant to private hospitals and community mental health centers. It shows how rehabilitation services can be integrated into the program of a psychiatric hospital by describing policies and procedures for rehabilitation services, clarifying the rationale and focus of the program design, and giving guidelines for practice and administration of a rehabilitation program. The goal of rehabilitation services is to develop and support functional skills that patients need to perform basic everyday living tasks and social roles as independently as possible so that they can cope with their environmental demands in ways that are satisfying to themselves and to significant others. Fidler describes in detail how to organize a number of specialized services to achieve this goal, focusing on program principles, staffing and supervisory patterns, referral guidelines, evaluations and assessments, program evaluation, budget, planning, and task and activity group programs and protocols.

In her most recent book, *Recapturing Competence: A System's Change for Geropsychiatric Care* (1992), Fidler presents her efforts to apply these and other ideas to an entire system. The book is a case presentation of her three years as CEO at Hagadorn, a 188-bed long-term nursing care facility for chronically mentally ill elders. After three years the Hagadorn Center had evolved into a comprehensive treatment and rehabilitation hospital. As Fidler states:

> This endeavor involved the generation of fundamental changes in the institution's organization and administrative functions, its clinical policies and practices, its definition of patient needs, intervention strategies, and priorities. These alterations finally brought about significant change in both patient and staff expectations regarding autonomy, achievement, and productivity. (Fidler, 1992, p. 1)

APPLICATION TO THE OCCUPATIONAL THERAPY PROFESSION

Fidler has posed many hypotheses and raised numerous questions about OT.

> I have always believed that defining the question and pursuing the question is far more important than coming up with an answer. The writing that I have done has pushed for clarifying the question because I think that once the question is clarified, this will inevitably lead to answers. (G. Fidler, personal communication, May 13, 1982)

She has spent most of her professional life pursuing these questions through her writings, grants, workshops, seminars, and clinical and educational activities. She has taught and challenged others to clarify and search out the questions and answers. She has affected the practice and education of occupational therapists in their everyday activities, as well as the work of other theorists, by her relentless search for the meaning of activities and their application in occupational therapy. With her husband she wrote the first major texts for occupational therapists in psychiatric settings. For almost 20 years these works remained as the only texts. She educated therapists about object relationships and developed several assessment tools and guides for treatment planning. Her conceptualization of doing further supported the importance of activities as therapeutic agents and their relationship to competence, mastery, self-worth, and achievement.

RESEARCH

Though informal surveys done during "Mental Health Focus" workshops in the 1980s indicated that at that time many therapists based their practice on her work, the questions raised by Fidler about the OT process and the nature of purposeful activity have been the subject of very little subsequent research. What she wrote thirty years ago is still true:

> To date, there has been very little effort to study activities with a standardizing process to list the most common types of response. It is possible to give people a variety of activities and have them express their subjective experience while they are involved in the activity. (Fidler & Fidler, 1963, p. 36)

Fidler urged that research be done with many people in a variety of settings as she has been doing with her "Activity Laboratory" since 1965. Each of her many hypotheses regarding doing are awaiting validation through further research and empirical testing. Each construct and theory of "doing" needs to be translated into researchable questions and hypotheses and systematically developed and pursued. "There is a need to pursue investigation into the neurologic, perceptual, and social components of action in relation to mental health" (Fidler & Fidler, 1983, p. 273).

One hallmark of a good theory is that it is flexible and internally consistent enough to allow new information to be incorporated into it. Fidler has steadily incorporated new information into her theories and consistently expanded them to include a more comprehensive view of occupational therapy.

Another feature of a good theory is that it enables one to organize phenomena and make predictions. Fidler's work has provided a structure for conceptualizing the OT process that has many direct applications to practice. What is needed is empirical testing of these hypotheses and constructs. Such research will be long term and will require many investigators to do empirical work and replication. Each study will need to focus on only a small part of Fidler's theories. Yet the gratification from such a task is long term and builds upon itself and the work of others. It is essential to test hypotheses generated by her work and the predictions of her theory to measure its significance.

REFERENCES

Arieti, S. (1962). Psychotherapy of schizophrenia. *Archives of General Psychiatry, 6*, 232–239.

Azima, H. (1961). Dynamic occupational therapy. *Diseases of the Nervous System Monograph Supplement, Section 2, 22*(4), 138–142.

Azima, H., & Azima, F. (1959). Outline of a dynamic theory of occupational therapy. *American Journal of Occupational Therapy, 13*, 215–221.

Fidler, G.S. (1948). Psychological evaluation of occupational therapy activities. *American Journal of Occupational Therapy, 2*, 284–287.

Fidler, G.S. (1957). The role of occupational therapy in a multidisciplinary approach to chronic illness. *American Journal of Occupational Therapy, 11*, 8–12.

Fidler, G.S. (1958). Some unique contributions of occupational therapy in the treatment of the schizophrenic. *American Journal of Occupational Therapy, 12*, 9–12.

Fidler, G.S. (1966a). Learning as a growth process: A conceptual framework for professional education. The 1965 Eleanor Clarke Slagle lecture. *American Journal of Occupational Therapy, 20*, 1–8.

Fidler, G.S. (1966b). A second look at work as a primary force in rehabilitation. *American Journal of Occupational Therapy, 20*, 72–74.

Fidler, G.S. (1968). Diagnostic battery-scoring and summary. In *Final report* (Rehabilitation Services Administration Grant No. 123-T-68 for Field Consultant in Psychiatric Rehabilitation). Washington, DC: U.S. Government Printing Office.

Fidler, G.S. (1969). The task-oriented group as a context for treatment. *American Journal of Occupational Therapy, 23*, 43–48.

Fidler, G.S. (1971). *Play/activity history*. Unpublished manuscript.

Fidler, G.S. (1981a). From crafts to competence. *American Journal of Occupational Therapy, 35*, 567–573.

Fidler, G.S. (1981b). *Overview of occupational therapy in mental health*. Prepared by the American Occupational Therapy Task Group of the American Psychiatric Association on Psychiatric Therapies.

Fidler, G.S. (1982a). The activity laboratory: A structure for observing and assessing perceptual, integrative, and behavioral strategies. In B. Hemphill (Ed.), *The evaluation process in psychiatric occupational therapy* (pp. 195–207). Thorofare, NJ: Charles B. Slack.

Fidler, G.S. (1982b). The lifestyle performance profile: An organizing frame. In B. Hemphill (Ed.), *The evaluation process in psychiatric occupational therapy* (pp. 43–47). Thorofare, NJ: Charles B. Slack.

Fidler, G.S. (1984). *The design of rehabilitation services in psychiatric hospital settings*. Laurel, MD: Ramsco.

Fidler, G.S., with Bristow, B.J. (1992). *Recapturing competence: A system's change for geropsychiatric care*. New York: Springer.

Fidler, G.S., & Fidler, J.W. (1954). *Introduction to psychiatric occupational therapy*. New York: Macmillan.

Fidler, G.S., & Fidler, J.W. (1963). *Occupational therapy: A communication process in psychiatry*. New York: Macmillan.

Fidler, G.S., & Fidler, J.W. (1978). Doing and becoming: Purposeful action and self-actualization. *American Journal of Occupational Therapy, 32*, 305–310.

Fidler, G.S., & Fidler, J.W. (1983). Doing and becoming: The occupational therapy experience. In G. Kielhofner (Ed.), *Health through occupation: Theory and practice in occupational therapy* (pp. 267–280). Philadelphia: F.A. Davis.

Fidler, G.S., & Fine, S.B. (1962). The occupational therapist and psychotherapy. In R. Morehouse (Ed.), *Transitional programs in psychiatric occupational therapy* (pp. 14–20). Dubuque, IA: William Brown.

Fidler, G.S., & Fine, S.B. (1970). *Object history.* Unpublished manuscript.

Ridgway, E.P., & Fidler, G.S. (1955). Occupational therapy: Laboratory for living. *Mental Health Views, 3*(3).

Searles, H. (1960). *The nonhuman environment.* New York: International University Press.

Sullivan, H.S. (1953). *The interpersonal theory of psychiatry.* New York: W.W. Norton.

West, W.L. (Ed.). (1959). *Changing concepts and practices in psychiatric occupational therapy.* New York: American Occupational Therapy Association.

White, R.W. (1959). Motivation reconsidered: The concept of competence. *Psychiatric Review, 66,* 297.

White, R.W. (1971). The urge toward competence. *American Journal of Occupational Therapy, 25,* 271–274.

Wittkower, E.D., & Azima, H. (1958). Dynamic aspects of occupational therapy. *Archives of Neurology and Psychiatry, 79,* 706–711.

BIBLIOGRAPHY

1948

Fidler, G.S. (1948). Psychological evaluation of occupational therapy activities. *American Journal of Occupational Therapy, 2,* 284–287.

1953

Fidler, G.S. (1953). Comments on a study of a task directed and a free choice group. *American Journal of Occupational Therapy, 7,* 124, 130.

1954

Fidler, G.S., & Fidler, J.W. (1954). *Introduction to psychiatric occupational therapy.* New York: Macmillan.

1955

Ridgway, E.P., & Fidler, G.S. (1955). Occupational therapy: Laboratory for living. *Mental Health Views, 3*(3).

1957

Fidler, G.S. (1957). The role of occupational therapy in a multidisciplinary approach to chronic illness. *American Journal of Occupational Therapy, 11,* 8–12.

1958

Fidler, G.S. (1958). Some unique contributions of occupational therapy in the treatment of the schizophrenic. *American Journal of Occupational Therapy, 12,* 9–12.

1962

Fidler, G.S., & Fine, S.B. (1962). The occupational therapist and psychotherapy. In R. Morehouse (Ed.), *Transitional programs in psychiatric occupational therapy* (pp. 14–20). Dubuque, IA: William Brown.

1963

Fidler, G.S. (1963). Educational experiences for the occupational therapist. *Journal of the South African Occupational Therapy Association.*

Fidler, G.S., & Fidler, J.W. (1963). *Occupational therapy: A communication process in psychiatry.* New York: Macmillan.

1964

Fidler, G.S. (1964). A guide to planning and measuring growth experience in the clinical affiliation. *American Journal of Occupational Therapy, 18,* 240–243.

1966

Fidler, G.S. (1966). Learning as a growth process: A conceptual framework for professional education: The Eleanor Clarke Slagle lecture. *American Journal of Occupational Therapy, 20,* 1–8.

Fidler, G.S. (1966). A second look at work as a primary force in rehabilitation. *American Journal of Occupational Therapy, 20,* 72–74.

1968

Fidler, G.S. (1968). Diagnostic battery-scoring and summary. In *Final report* (Rehabilitation Services Administration Grant No. 123-T-68 for Field Consultant in Psychiatric Rehabilitation). Washington, DC: U.S. Government Printing Office.

Fidler, G.S. (1968). The task-oriented group as a context for treatment. In *Final report* (Rehabilitation Services Administration Grant No. 123-T-68 for Field Consultant in Psychiatric Rehabilitation). Washington, DC: U.S. Government Printing Office.

1969

Fidler, G.S. (1969). The task-oriented group as a context for treatment. *American Journal of Occupational Therapy, 23,* 43–48.

1970

Fidler, G.S., & Fine, S.B. (1970). *Object history.* Unpublished manuscript.

1971

Fidler, G.S. (1971). *Play/activity history.* Unpublished manuscript.

1977

Fidler, G.S. (1977). From plea to mandate. *American Journal of Occupational Therapy,* 31, 653.

1978

Fidler, G.S., & Fidler, J.W. (1978). Doing and becoming: Purposeful action and self-actualization. *American Journal of Occupational Therapy, 32,* 305–310.

Fidler, G.S. (1978). Professional or non-professional. In *Occupational therapy: 2001 AD* (pp. 31–36). Rockville, MD: American Occupational Therapy Association.

1979

Fidler, G.S. (1979). Specialization. *American Journal of Occupational Therapy, 33*, 34.

1981

Fidler, G.S. (1981). From crafts to competence. *American Journal of Occupational Therapy, 35*, 567–573.

Fidler, G.S. (1981). *Overview of occupational therapy in mental health.* Prepared by the American Occupational Therapy Task Group of the American Psychiatric Association on Psychiatric Therapies.

1982

Fidler, G.S. (1982). The activity laboratory: A structure for observing and assessing perceptual, integrative, and behavioral strategies. In B. Hemphill (Ed.), *The evaluation process in psychiatric occupational therapy* (pp. 195–207). Thorofare, NJ: Charles B. Slack.

Fidler, G.S. (1982). The lifestyle performance profile: An organizing frame. In B. Hemphill (Ed.), *The evaluative process in psychiatric occupational therapy* (pp. 43–47). Thorofare, NJ: Charles B. Slack.

1983

Fidler, G.S., & Fidler, J.W. (1983). Doing and becoming: The occupational therapy experience. In G. Kielhofner (Ed.), *Health through occupation: Theory and practice in occupational therapy* (pp. 267–280). Philadelphia: F.A. Davis.

1984

Fidler, G.S. (1984). *The design of rehabilitation services in psychiatric hospital settings.* Laurel, MD: Ramsco.

1990

Fidler, G.S. (1990). Reflections on choice. *Occupational Therapy in Mental Health, 10*, 77–84.

1991

Fidler, G.S. (1991). The challenge of change to occupational therapy practice. *Occupational Therapy in Mental Health, 11*, 1–10.

1992

Fidler, G.S., with Bristow, B.J. (1992). *Recapturing competence: A system's change for geropsychiatric care.* New York: Springer.

Chapter Three

Anne Cronin Mosey

Ferol Menks Ludwig

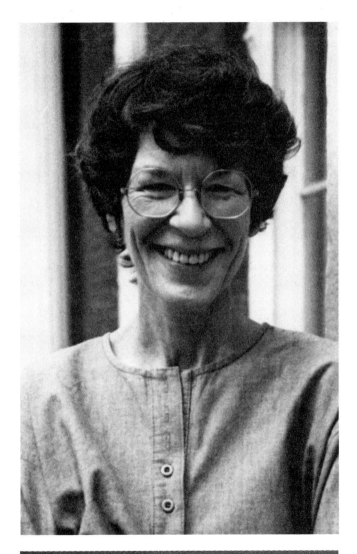

Anne Cronin Mosey

BIOGRAPHICAL SKETCH

Anne Cronin Mosey was born in 1938 and was raised in Minneapolis, Minnesota. She is the third in a family of seven children. As a child, she read extensively, helped with cooking for nine people, and had long talks with her father about the state of the world. She asserts that "life picked up" when she discovered boys and she began to date (A.C. Mosey, personal communication, August 4, 1985).

After graduation from high school, she attended the University of Minnesota, where she pursued a double major in sociology and psychology. Her Irish family background did not permit young ladies to work, so during the summer of her junior year she did volunteer work at the Veteran's Hospital in Minneapolis. At the suggestion of the coordinator of volunteer services, she worked in the occupational therapy department on the psychiatric unit.

Although she had not really understood what occupational therapy was about, she had enjoyed the work, so she changed her major to occupational therapy when she returned to college. In 1961, she earned her BS degree in occupational therapy from the University of Minnesota School of Medicine. Mosey credits Marvin Lepley, her advisor at the University of Minnesota, with playing an important role in her professional development through his confidence in her and his encouragement (A.C. Mosey, personal communication, October 4, 1984; Richert, 1989).

After graduation, Mosey worked for several months at Glenwood Hills Hospital in Minneapolis. She then moved to New York City to work with and learn from Gail Fidler. She joined the OT department at New York State Psychiatric Institute, where she remained for five years until August 1966. As her supervisor, Fidler encouraged Mosey to think, read, and broaden her horizons about clinical practice and to focus on patient needs.

Mosey decided after a few years that she wanted to be an educator. She began graduate studies in occupational therapy at New York University and earned her MA degree in 1965. She then enrolled in Human Relations and Community Studies, also at New York University, and was awarded her PhD in 1968. Professor Lloyd Barenblatt, one of her instructors and chair of her dissertation committee, helped her "to refine skills in critical thinking" (A.C. Mosey, personal communication, October 4, 1984).

From 1966 to 1968, she was on the faculty of Columbia University as an instructor in occupational therapy. During this period she (1) realized that "teaching is something one must learn how to do and is a difficult task" (A.C. Mosey, personal communication, May 3, 1987), (2) developed the idea and structure of the frame of reference, (3) wrote *Three Frames of Reference for Mental Health* (1970), and (4) completed her dissertation. She then joined the faculty at New York University and moved upward through the academic ranks to her current status as Professor of Occupational Therapy with tenure. From 1972 to 1980 she served as department chairperson and in 1977 was the acting head of the Division of Health.

Mosey has served AOTA in several leadership capacities on the state and national levels. Since 1979 she has been a continuous reviewer of proposed presentations for AOTA Annual Conferences. She was a member of the Panel of Experts of the AOTA Continuing Education Program in Mental Health from 1984 to 1988. More recently, she was a member of the Scholars Group for the Directions for the Future Project of AOTA/AOTF (1988–1991). She is a member of the Panel for Review of Research Proposals of AOTF and is an AOTF research consultant. She also serves on the Editorial Board of the journal *Occupational Therapy in Mental Health*. Mosey participated in the development of the newest AOTA Self Study Series on Cognitive Rehabilitation (1992) (A.C. Mosey, personal communication, September 20, 1992).

Dr. Mosey has also shared her experience and knowledge by serving as a consultant to several hospitals and state mental health systems. From 1966 to 1969 she was a consultant for the Massachusetts Department of Mental Health. She was a faculty member for the AOTA Regional Institutes from 1966 to 1967. As an invited participant, she was involved with the Theory Building Seminar for AOTA in 1967. She also served as consultant to: the Division of Rehabilitation Education at New York University, Hillside Hospital Professional Examination Services, the Family Centered Research Project, the Institute of Pennsylvania Hospital, the Greater Trenton Mental Health Center, and Christopher House.

Mosey has published 15 papers and 6 books and has given numerous presentations and workshops. One of her articles is a collection of four poems about the thoughts of an occupational therapist arriving home late on a dark winter night after a long and exhausting day (Mosey, 1976). As the therapist looks out the window at the blinking city lights below, she tries to put into words the thoughts and feelings of four patients. These sensitive and insightful poems demonstrate empathy, understanding, and caring.

Numerous students and therapists have learned from Mosey and sought her guidance. She has supervised master's and doctoral research projects since 1968. Recently she has been teaching more international students, a task that she finds to be "a tough, fun, insightful, and interesting learning experience" (A.C. Mosey, personal communication, August 4, 1985).

Her profession honored her in 1973 by naming her a Fellow of the AOTA. In 1975 she received the Distinguished Service Award from the National Association of Activity Therapy, and in 1985 she was awarded the AOTA's Eleanor Clarke Slagle Lectureship. The title of her lecture was "A Monistic or a Pluralistic Approach to Professional Identity?"

Mosey lives in Greenwich Village. She is divorced and has a grown son whom she considers to be her best critic (A.C. Mosey, personal communication, May 3, 1987). She is interested in history and anthropology and enjoys the theater, concerts, being with friends, and being alone to think, read, and "contemplate the nature of the world" (A.C. Mosey, personal communication, August 4, 1985). Her current professional interest is examining and attempting to identify what areas need to be addressed in the philosophical study of health professions, and constructing a philosophy of applied science (A.C. Mosey, personal communication, September 20, 1992).

THEORETICAL CONCEPTS

Throughout her career, Mosey has been concerned with laying the groundwork for the OT evaluation and intervention process. She has searched for answers to the questions of where we are now and how we got here. She has investigated the building blocks of the profession in a scholarly manner and has organized them into a taxonomy of the profession. Three main themes can be seen in her work: (1) the articulation of frames of references for occupational therapy in mental health, (2) the process of structuring and translating theories of psychosocial dysfunction into frames of reference to apply to practice, and (3) the development of a taxonomy that identifies the various elements of the profession and their relationship to each other.

Frames of Reference for Mental Health

Recapitulation of Ontogenesis

One of the three main strands of Mosey's work, that of articulating frames of reference for occupational therapy in mental health, began with her proposal, in "Recapitulation of Ontogenesis: A Theory for the Practice of Occupational Therapy" (1968b), of a developmental frame of reference for evaluation and treatment. Its theoretical base is derived from a variety of personality and developmental theories proposed by Sullivan (1953), Piaget (Flavell, 1963), Bruner (1966), Sigmund Freud (1949), Anna Freud (1965), Llorens (Llorens & Beck, 1966), Schilder (1950), Searles (1960), Sechehaye (1951a, 1951b), Ayres (1958, 1961, 1963, 1964) and Hartman (1958). Her clinical work with Fidler also was influential in this frame of reference's development. The biological term "ontogenesis," referring to the biological development of an individual organism, is used by psychologists to denote the individual's progression through developmental stages. Mosey's frame of reference is specifically concerned with the development of basic adaptive skills that build on each other and must be learned in proper sequence, beginning with the most elementary components and moving on to the more complex (Mosey, 1968b, 1986).

Mosey (1968b) proposes that the individual is a being who seeks equilibrium. Disequilibrium results from changing psychological and physical needs and new environmental demands. It motivates one to learn adaptive skills needed to reestablish a state of equilibrium. Mosey describes seven adaptive skills—each of which has component subskills—in the sequential order in which they are learned: (1) perceptual-motor skills, (2) cognitive skills, (3) drive object skills, (4) dyadic interaction skills, (5) primary group interaction skills, (6) self-identity skills, and (7) sexual identity interaction skills. When all of the component subskills of a given skill have been integrated, the person has achieved full maturity in that skill.

A state of function is characterized by integrated learning of those adaptive skill components needed for successful participation in the social roles expected of the individual in his or her usual setting. Minimal and maximal limits are usually set by one's cultural group. Adaptive skill performance enables one to obtain gratification and meet environmental demands.

Dysfunction results when necessary skill components are not learned because of (1) abnormalities or lack of maturation of physical structures, (2) severe environmental stress, or (3) lack of environmental elements necessary for the development of these skill components. Failure to learn skill components needed for the fulfillment of social roles may result in unproductive interactions with the social system or learned maladaptive patterns such as depression or hyperactivity (Mosey, 1968b). There is a continuum of function/dysfunction.

To evaluate the patient, one must observe him or her in roles and activities that will elicit adaptive skills and then identify whether particular skill components are present or absent. The therapist needs to collaborate with the patient and other staff to learn more about what skills are needed in the person's expected environment.

Patients can move from a state of dysfunction to a state of function through activities that are similar to those object interactions responsible for normal skill development. It is the role of the therapist to select these activities. He or she helps the patient grow from where normal development ceased by providing experiences that take the person through the developmental stages of skill acquisition and facilitate learning of the needed skills. Thus therapy recapitulates ontogenesis, the normal sequence of individual development, and enables the patient to complete that sequence. Activities are interactive, and the objects with which the patient interacts will vary according to the component that needs to be learned. Symbolic activities may be used, but reality and the here and now are stressed. In particular, the more mature skill components must employ reality-oriented activities (Mosey, 1968b).

The long-term goal of this developmental approach is to help the person partici-pate fully in his or her expected social roles and environment. The short-term goal is to learn the skill component.

Mosey's next publication (1969) provides a developmental frame of reference, consistent with her recapitulation of ontogenesis frame of reference (1968b), for the evaluation and treatment of pathological distortion of body image. Normal development of body image is crucial to the control and development of normal motor behavior, purposeful movement, and body mastery. It also determines whether one is accepted or rejected by one's peers. Mosey argues that defective experiences during the developmental process may lead to pathological distortion of body image. Drawing on the work of Schneider (1960), Ayres (1958, 1961, 1963, 1964), Schilder (1950), Sigmund Freud (1949), Anna Freud (1965), Pearce and Newton (1963), Sechehaye (1951a, 1951b), and the Fidlers (1963), she pro-poses that the transition from an undifferentiated body image to an adult body image is a complex process that can be disrupted by factors both internal and external to the self. One such factor is physical trauma that causes loss of function of a body part or parts. Another is children's incorporation of their parents' idio-syncratic and cultural norms, values, and attitudes about the body or any of its parts. Children may learn either to value the body or to view it, or any of its parts, negatively—for example, to see it as "dirty." They may deny a particular body part or focus on it excessively.

Acceptance of sexuality and sexual parts of the body is especially important to the attainment of a mature body image. When people reject their sexuality, they divert large amounts of libidinal energy to the control of internal conflicts. This may cause de-egotization of the body or any of its parts and even depersonaliza-tion. Self-mutilation, perception of the self as a tree, or egotization of less threat-ening objects may result.

Evaluation of the client is based on observation and interpretation of behavior to identify whether body image distortion is present and, if so, the type and extent. Such distortion is expressed by the client's wearing clothes that are too large, too tight fitting and revealing, childish, or sexually undifferentiated; covering the face with hair and excessive makeup; emphasizing, denying, or rejecting a body part; or making rigid, uncoordinated, or stylized movements (Mosey, 1969).

Treatment is based on the theory that distortion of body image may be corrected by providing similar experiences to those believed responsible for the normal de-velopment of body image. In keeping with her recapitulation of ontogenesis frame of reference, Mosey proposes the use of developmental groups for persons who lack primary group interaction skills (1970a). The position of a client on the func-tion/dysfunction continuum is determined by his or her achievement of primary group interaction skills and skill components. Developmental groups are defined as groups that are structured to simulate the various types of nonfamilial groups usually experienced in the normal developmental process. Mosey describes a progression through five levels of developmental groups: (1) parallel group, (2) project group, (3) egocentric group, (4) cooperative group, and (5) mature group. Learning occurs as the individual experiences the consequences of his or her behavior in the structured group setting. The type of behavior to be learned is clearly spelled out: adaptive behavior is reinforced and maladaptive behavior is not.

Developmental groups can be used to treat deficiencies in other adaptive skill components that can be either partially or completely learned through nonfamilial groups. The group must be structurally similar to the type of group in which these components are normally acquired. Developmental groups can also be used to satisfy mental health needs (Mosey, 1970a).

Three Frames of Reference

Mosey's book *Three Frames of Reference for Mental Health* was written "to plead a case for the conscious use of theoretical frames of reference as a basis for the treatment of psychosocial dysfunction" (1970b, p. v), and it has served for many years as a basic text on the subject. The three frames of reference that it considers are: (1) analytical, (2) developmental, and (3) acquisitional (1970b).

The analytical perspective is concerned with concepts of need fulfillment, expression of primitive impulses, and control of inherent drives. It is based on the theories of Sigmund Freud (1949), Anna Freud (1965), Maslow (1962), Erikson (1950), and Jung (1933, 1964).

The developmental frame of reference is the one set forth in "Recapitulation of Ontogenesis: A Theory for the Practice of Occupational Therapy" (1968b). Freud's stages of psychosexual development and Erikson's eight stages are classified here. Skills in the developmental frame of reference are interdependent, qualitative, and stage-specific. They are usually acquired in the normal developmental process in growth-facilitating environments.

The acquisitional frame of reference, as opposed to the developmental frame of reference, concerns skills and abilities that are independent of each other, quantitative, and nonstage-specific. It is based on learning theories, such as those of Bandura (1969), Wolpe and Lazarus (1966), Dollard and Miller (1950), and ego theories, such as that of Sullivan (1953). It is also based on the work of such occupational therapists as Sieg (1974), Diasio (1968), and Smith and Tempone (1968).

Mosey still regards these three frames of reference as the major current frames of reference in occupational therapy in psychosocial dysfunction. In her book *Psychosocial Components of Occupational Therapy* (1986), she refines them and develops their application further. She also analyzes the work of other researchers in occupational therapy, such as Fidler, King, Llorens, Reilly, and Kielhofner, and has integrated their thinking into the frames of reference that she has outlined. Thus she considers Reilly (1962, 1974), Banus (1979), Llorens (1976), Kielhofner

(1977, 1983), Rood, Brunnstrom, and Bobath to be contributors to the developmental frame of reference, and she has included the biomechanical and rehabilitative approaches of Trombly and Scott (1977) in her acquisitional frame of reference category.

Activities Therapy

In Mosey's *Activities Therapy* (1973a), the sequence, principles, and case examples of the evaluation and treatment process discussed are consistent with her *Three Frames of Reference for Mental Health* (1970b). Mosey also describes the kinds of psychiatric treatment centers in which this type of treatment might be applicable.

Activities Therapy (Mosey, 1973a) was written to show how therapy that uses immediate, action-oriented interactions can help persons designated as mentally ill learn to be a part of their community and to cope with the stresses of daily life. This book is based on the assumption that psychosocial dysfunction is due to a lack of one or more of the following abilities: to plan and carry out a task, to interact comfortably in a group, to identify and satisfy needs, to express emotions in an acceptable manner, to attain a fairly accurate perception of the self and the human and nonhuman environment, to establish a value system that allows the person to meet his or her needs without infringing on the rights of others, to perform activities of daily living skills, to work at a relatively satisfying job, to enjoy avocational and recreational activities, and to interact comfortably in relationships with family and friends. Any deficits in these abilities limit one's effective performance in the community. Deficit learning or learning of inappropriate behaviors can be treated by teaching more effective behaviors.

As in her earlier works, Mosey stresses the importance of learning through doing in the here and now. Activities are used to provide realistic situations that help participants learn new skills, identify faulty patterns of behavior, and recognize the feelings and values that support these maladaptive patterns. The therapist is concerned with the (1) greater understanding of self and (2) development of skills.

Human beings have three facets: basic skills, the private self, and the public self. Basic skills are those that a person must have to function satisfactorily in the community with others. They include task and group interaction skills. The private self is composed of those aspects that cannot be directly seen or experienced by others, such as cognitive processes, needs, emotions, and values. The public self involves aspects of the individual that can be observed by others and can be a point of contact. Activities of daily living, work, recreation, and intimacy are essential components of the public self (1973a). The teaching-learning process and group dynamics that use action-oriented experiences help the client learn necessary skills.

Theory and Frame of Reference

Mosey's second major concern has been to explore the process of structuring and translating theory into frames of reference for use in practice. In *Three Frames of Reference for Mental Health*, she defines theory as a set of statements that describes the relationship among events and makes predictions about these events. A theoretical frame of reference is derived from theory and makes use of concepts, definitions, and postulates from a theory or theories. It is composed of principles to guide action that are derived from scientific postulates regarding change. Whereas a theory is merely descriptive, a theoretical frame of reference provides principles for action and is prescriptive. It applies to daily situations and can guide the decisions of the practitioner.

Frames of reference should be comprehensive, internally consistent, and stated in an organized and logical manner (Mosey, 1970b, p. 9). Mosey uses a four-part structure for a frame of reference that she derived from Ford and Urban (1963). The first part is a theoretical base that is drawn from theory or theories from such fields as psychology, sociology, and neuroscience. It specifies the nature of human beings, the environment, and their relationship to each other and identifies the parameters of the frame of reference. It is the basis from which all other parts are deduced.

The second part is made up of function and dysfunction continua and operational definitions of verbal and nonverbal behaviors that are indicative of function or dysfunction. These are derived from the theoretical base's assumptions concerning health and dysfunction, and will vary according to the frame of reference selected. The behaviors are what the therapist will assess in the evaluation process.

Evaluation, the third part of the frame of reference, is the process of identifying whether an individual is in a state of function or a state of dysfunction. It is used as a basis for treatment. Evaluation tools and techniques serve as stimuli to elicit observable and measurable behaviors that differentiate between function and dysfunction. Procedures and rules to interpret the data are determined by the frame of reference selected.

Prescriptive statements derived from the postulates of the theoretical base make up the fourth part of the frame of reference. They state the principles by which an individual is aided in moving from a state of dysfunction to one of function. They guide the therapist in arranging his or her interaction with the client and the nonhuman environment. Ideally, these postulates have been empirically tested. Similar activities may be used with different frames of reference or postulates, but they will differ in the ways they are structured and utilized. For example, both analytical and developmental task groups might use fingerpainting. However, the analytical group might be using fingerpainting to express primitive impulses, whereas the developmental group might be working on primary social skill interaction.

Treatment is aimed at effecting predetermined change in the patient's limitations so that he or she may be a more productive member of a social system. It is a planned collaborative interaction between the patient, therapist, and nonhuman environment (Mosey, 1970b).

The criteria for a frame of reference are stringent and are a statement of the ideal rather than the actual. Mosey has painstakingly synthesized theories and developed them into three frames of reference according to this four-part structure. She does not consider them to be complete, but has proposed them to stimulate thinking about frames of reference and what they should and should not include, to identify a goal for continued work in the area, and to give an orientation for classification of frames of reference that are currently available.

Taxonomy of the Profession

Mosey's position as program director of the OT curriculum at New York University led her to widen her focus to the profession of occupational therapy as a whole. She began to search for its common elements in order to describe and analyze the profession's form and structure and the ways in which its parts relate to one another (A.C. Mosey, personal communication, October 4, 1984). This has been the third main focus of her work.

Biopsychosocial Model

In 1974 Mosey developed a biopsychosocial model as an alternative to the medical or health models for occupational therapy. She argued that the medical model is not relevant to the OT process because occupational therapists are not concerned with diagnosis of disease or elimination of pathology. The health model is too vague. Because it focuses primarily on assets rather than limitations or dysfunction, it is useful for prevention and community practice, but is too limiting for remediation. Neither model permits the complete organization of the theoretical base of occupational therapy.

The biopsychosocial model, in contrast, focuses on the body, mind, and environment of the individual. It views the individual as a physical being who suffers the effects of illness and injury; a person with thoughts, emotions, needs, and values; and a player of many and varied social roles. This model is concerned with the skills, knowledge, abilities, and values that the individual must learn in order to function productively with others in his or her expected environment. The therapist effects change in the individual primarily by identifying learning needs and guiding the teaching-learning process. The teaching-learning process, as described in Mosey's earlier works (1968b, 1970b, 1973b), and in her 1981 book *Occupational Therapy: Configuration of a Profession*, may be based on any of a variety of theories about learning, such as operant conditioning and social learning theory. The therapist, as the teacher, begins where the learner is and moves at a rate that is comfortable for the learner. He or she provides opportunities for trial and error, imitation, repetition, and practice in different situations so that the learner can observe and experience the consequences of an action. The learner needs to understand both what is to be learned and the rationale for learning.

Mosey (1974) initially felt that this model would be useful for practice because it (1) provides a method to systematize OT knowledge, (2) provides a holistic statement of the profession's goals and theories of change, (3) is oriented to the development of skills needed by the client or patient for fuller participation in the community setting, (4) helps clarify the role of occupational therapy in relationship to medicine and the other health-related professions, and (5) is well suited to community-based programs and the meeting of health needs. However, six years after presenting the biopsychosocial model, she wrote that "it became evident that the biopsychosocial model did not provide sufficient structure and content to give a holistic view of occupational therapy" (1980, p. 11). She continued with her quest for a model for the profession, refining the biopsychosocial model in an attempt to provide a holistic or generic approach to the philosophical and scientific foundation for the practice of occupational therapy. "My goal was and remains the identification of those factors which give unity to the profession and a firm base for the further development of areas of specialization" (Mosey, 1980, p. 11).

Characteristics of a Professional Model

Mosey further researched the occupational therapy literature and primary sources most frequently cited by occupational therapists, and discussed this issue with faculty, students, and clinicians. Based on this further study, and on philosophical and sociological literature of what constitutes a profession, she defined and described the structure, function, and characteristics of a model for professions in general and one specific to occupational therapy (1980, 1981, 1986). A model for a profession describes the way in which a profession perceives itself, its relationship to other professions, and its relationship to society, as well as the profession's responsibility to society, methods, and rationale. A model applies to the entire profession rather than to any particular area of specialization. A model defines and delineates the nature of the profession and is accepted by its members and by society. It is dynamic, and its content is continually changing. Some of the changes result from changes in the body of knowledge and expertise of the profession, the domain of concern of other professions, and the needs, mandate, or acceptance of society. Each part of the model is interrelated, and a change in one part affects change in others. Mosey cautions that a profession takes great risks in expanding its model beyond the limits of its present theoretical foundation and domain of concern. More may be claimed than can be delivered, and this may result in a loss of respect for the profession (Mosey, 1981, pp. 52–57).

The structure and characteristics of a model seem to be similar for all health professions. Some content, such as theories of human growth and development, may be shared by several professions. However, each profession's model has its own specific content. A profession's model is composed of the following six elements: (1) philosophical assumptions basic to practice, (2) ethical code, (3) theoretical foundation (later referred to as a body of knowledge), (4) domain of concern, (5) nature of and principles for sequencing the various aspects of practice, and (6) legitimate tools. Mosey (1980, 1981, 1986) describes each of these components in detail in terms of its composition, structure, and relation to and influence on other components.

In Mosey's model for occupational therapy, the first element—philosophical assumptions—contains seven basic beliefs about the individual, his or her relationship with the human and nonhuman environment, and the profession's goals or purpose. They are as follows:

1. Each individual has the right to a meaningful existence; to an existence that allows one to be productive; to experience pleasure and joy; to love and be loved; and to live in surroundings that are safe, supportive, and comfortable.

2. Each individual is influenced by stage-specific maturation of the species, the social nature of the species, and the cognitive structure of the species.

3. Each individual has inherent needs for work, play, and rest that must be satisfied in a relatively equal balance.

4. Each individual has the right to seek his or her potential through personal choice within the context of some social constraints.

5. Each individual is only able to reach his or her potential through purposeful interaction with the human and nonhuman environment.

6. Each individual is only able to be understood within the context of his or her environment of family, community, and cultural group.

7. Occupational therapy is concerned with promoting functional independence through intervention directed toward facilitating participation in major social roles (occupational performances) and the development of the physical, cognitive, psychological, and social skills (performance components) that are fundamental to these roles. The extent to which intervention is focused on occupational perform-

ances or performance components is dependent on the needs of a particular client at any given point in time. (Mosey, 1986, p. 6)

The profession's ethical code comprises principles of human conduct regarding what is moral behavior toward clients, students, and colleagues. Mosey refers the reader to AOTA's Code of Ethics (1981, pp. 64–70).

The profession's body of knowledge, which is also referred to as its theoretical foundation, contains the scientific basis for the profession. It is derived from an ordered set of selected theoretical systems from a variety of different disciplines, as well as from the profession itself. Although professions may share some knowledge with other fields, each profession selects from outside its boundaries knowledge of particular relevance to it and develops its own unique combinations and adaptations of this knowledge. Occupational therapy's body of knowledge comes from the biological sciences, behavioral sciences, the arts, medicine, and occupational therapy (Mosey, 1980, 1981, 1986).

The domain of concern, the fourth element, is the profession's areas of expertise. Though the concept of domain of concern and the subconcepts of performance components and areas of occupational performance had been identified and labeled by an AOTA task force, Mosey conducted her own survey of the literature, including the writings of Reilly (1962, 1974), Llorens (Llorens, 1976, Llorens & Beck, 1966), Kielhofner (1977, 1983), and many others, to identify those areas of human function that occupational therapists believed they could successfully influence. She lists the components of performance as motor function, sensory integration, visual perception, cognitive function, psychological function, and social interaction. Occupational performances include family interaction, activities of daily living, school/work, play/leisure/recreation, and temporal adaptation. The clients' chronological and developmental age and cultural, social, and physical environment all interact with performance components and occupational performances. (See Figure 3-1.)

Fifth, the nature of and principles for sequencing the various aspects of practice (1980, 1981, 1986) describe the problem-identification and problem-solving processes used to evaluate and treat clients. Mosey wrote about these in her earlier works (1970b, 1973a) mainly as applicable to frames of reference. In *Occupational Therapy: Configuration of a Profession* (1981) and in *Psychosocial Components of Occupational Therapy* (1986) she builds on and integrates these principles into the larger concept of a model.

Legitimate tools, the sixth part of the model, are the modalities that the profession uses to achieve its goals. From her review of the OT literature Mosey identifies the following six tools: (1) nonhuman environment, (2) conscious use of self, (3) the teaching-learning process, (4) purposeful activity, (5) activity groups, and (6) activity analysis and synthesis (Mosey, 1981, 1986).

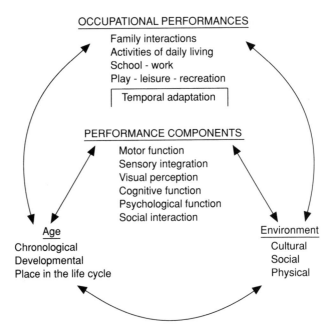

OCCUPATIONAL PERFORMANCES
Family interactions
Activities of daily living
School - work
Play - leisure - recreation

Temporal adaptation

PERFORMANCE COMPONENTS
Motor function
Sensory integration
Visual perception
Cognitive function
Psychological function
Social interaction

Age
Chronological
Developmental
Place in the life cycle

Environment
Cultural
Social
Physical

Figure 3-1 Domain of concern for occupational therapy. *Source:* From *Occupational Therapy: Configuration of a Profession* (p. 75) by A.C. Mosey, 1981, New York: Raven Press Ltd. Copyright 1981 by Raven Press Ltd. Adapted by permission.

Models and Frames of Reference

Since frames of reference are derived from a theoretical base, they may be said to derive from the model of the profession that includes that base. In 1986, Mosey provided an expanded definition of "frame of reference": it is a set of interrelated, internally consistent concepts, definitions, and postulates derived from or compatible with empirical data that provide a systematic description of, or prescription for, a practitioner's interaction within a particular aspect of a profession's domain of concern for the purpose of facilitating evaluation and effecting change (p. 376). The professional model provides the linkages among the various frames of reference to the profession as a whole.

Frames of reference are more limited than models. They link theory and practice in only a small area of the profession's body of knowledge and domain of concern, whereas a model defines the whole profession. A model is almost universally accepted by the profession and the society to which it is responsible. In contrast, a frame of reference has more limited acceptance by practitioners, and more than one frame of reference may be applied to the same portion of the domain of concern in the profession. The conflict and disagreement that may ensue can lead to clarification of concepts and further research. Whereas a frame of reference guides the practitioner in his or her daily interaction with clients, a model gives overall direction to the profession.

Professional Configuration

According to Mosey (1981, 1986), both a profession's model and its frames of reference are basic elements of a larger *professional configuration*. This configuration is a loop with six parts: (1) philosophical foundation, (2) model, (3) frames of reference, (4) practice, (5) data, and (6) research (see Figure 3-2).

Philosophical assumptions, ethics, art, and science are basic elements of all professions. It is from each profession's particular philosophical foundation that a unique professional model develops. Various frames of reference are deduced from this model and serve as a guide for practice. Practice then produces data that enable one to evaluate their effectiveness and to refine the profession's body of knowledge. Thus the arrows flow in two directions among data, research, and model. In Mosey's configuration, there is no direct relationship between research

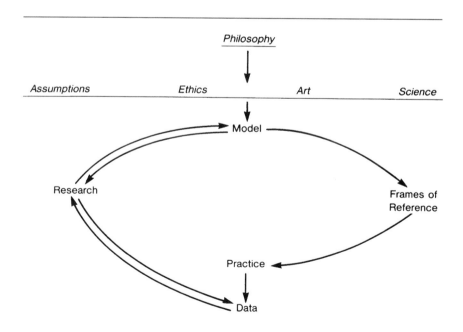

Figure 3-2 Occupational Therapy Loop. *Source:* From *Occupational Therapy: Configuration of a Profession* (p. 42) by A.C. Mosey, 1981, New York: Raven Press Ltd. Copyright 1981 by Raven Press Ltd. Reprinted by permission.

and practice or between research and frames of reference. Research only directly influences the body of knowledge component of the model by modifying or supporting its theoretical base. When a theory is altered by research findings, changes are effected in frames of reference that utilize that base. These in turn lead to changes in practice. Thus research can influence practice only after it is integrated into the professional model and relevant frames of reference. The professional model also influences research because a theoretical foundation should be continually evaluated (Mosey, 1981, 1986).

Mosey has also discussed the five areas of specialization recognized by AOTA—(1) mental health, (2) physical disabilities, (3) developmental disabilities, (4) gerontology, and (5) sensory integration—in terms of the special problems that occupational therapy can address.

APPLICATION TO OCCUPATIONAL THERAPY

Use of Theory

Mosey (1973b) regards clinical practice as the process of using science and applying theories. The therapist must consciously select theories and use them as a guide for action. The therapist's actions may be guided by one or more theories. Such an eclectic approach is acceptable, but the postulates need to be logically compatible. Mosey objects to therapists' doing what they feel is right intuitively without reference to any particular theoretical system.

Until more refined techniques of measurement are developed and researched, no one frame of reference can claim authority. Therefore, Mosey encourages therapists to develop their own individual frame of reference and techniques for patient care to suit their style of practice. The frame of reference needs to be a part of the self in order to be a useful guide for action, but it cannot be part of the self if it is incompatible with the self. The frame of reference selected also needs to be appropriate to the client's cultural norms and background. She suggests that the beginning therapist study and use a variety of frames of reference with a nonjudgmental attitude. Initial efforts to apply frames of reference should be done under competent supervision.

In a (1971) review of the growth of the rehabilitation movement from 1942 to 1960, Mosey concludes that during that period occupational therapists functioned primarily as technicians rather than as professionals. Emphasis was placed on technique, not on theory. She sees little change as of 1970: practice continues without the conscious use of a theoretical base. To remedy this state of affairs, researchers must systematically organize the considerable amount of available knowledge basic to practice. This will enable practitioners to eliminate the irrelevant and help them identify what knowledge is lacking and what is available, thereby facilitating the organization of theory and research.

Mosey herself has begun this work in her book *Psychosocial Components of Occupational Therapy* (1986). It reviews, synthesizes, and systematizes the literature basic to psychosocial occupational therapy from within the field and from related disciplines and professions. Mosey writes that "its purpose is to provide an overview of the psychosocial components—both the body of knowledge and approaches to evaluation and intervention" (Mosey, 1986, p. vii).

Mosey feels that psychosocial components are applicable to all areas of specialization because they are "fundamental to the understanding of our clients, ourselves as therapists, and the tools that we use in practice" (Mosey, 1986, p. vii). She examines the knowledge, skills, and attitudes basic to adaptation regardless of the person's current physical condition. Consistent with her thinking is the pluralistic approach and use of a variety of frames of reference. Mosey encourages occupational therapists to select frames of reference best suited to their own theoretical and philosophical positions and consistent with their clients' needs. Through her excellent synthesis of the theoretical base of the profession as a whole and her taxonomy of its specific parts, the therapist is provided with the structure needed to make the transition from theory to practice.

Health Needs

Mosey, using a concept similar to Maslow's, defines health needs as "inherent human requirements that must be met for an individual to experience a sense of physical, psychological, and social well-being" (1973b, p. 14). All persons, regardless of their state of health, have these needs. Mosey encourages therapists to re-emphasize the importance of meeting health needs in occupational therapy, the institution, and the community. This becomes increasingly important as therapists move into community-based practice. The occupational therapist's knowledge of human growth and development and recognition of the individual's need for satisfying interaction with the human and nonhuman environment provide excellent support for this focus. The occupational therapist needs to ask whether the patient's environment (the occupational therapy clinic, the institution, the community) offers the opportunity for those types of need satisfaction that the patient requires. Further study of the process of meeting health needs is necessary (Mosey, 1973b, 1986).

APPLICATION TO THE OCCUPATIONAL THERAPY PROFESSION

Much of Mosey's work has focused on developing and articulating occupational therapy's professional identity and exploring how this identity influences practice. Mosey argues that this kind of professional self-questioning is a natural and necessary process that "occurs in cycles and provides a healthy means for reexamination, revitalization, and change" (1981, p. 120). In her book *Psychosocial Components of Occupational Therapy* (1986), a chapter entitled "Historical Perspective" traces a history of changes in types of intervention, frames of reference, and techniques employed by occupational therapy, and discusses the profession's "search for identity" from its initial reliance on medicine to its development of frames of reference.

In her Eleanor Clarke Slagle lecture in 1985, Mosey explored monism and pluralism as two approaches that professions can take to form their identity. Monism is an attempt to define a profession by one of its elements or a facet of an element that is considered primary and that governs all other elements. A pluralistic approach is much broader and takes into consideration all of the elements of a profession. The whole is defined by the totality of its parts, and each of these parts is distinct and different.

A monistic approach usually takes the form of a comprehensive theory (Mosey, 1985). The profession has one theoretical base and one method for applying it to its domain of concern. Some of the approaches that have been considered for a comprehensive theory for occupational therapy have been developmental theory as proposed by Llorens (1976), occupational behavior as described by Reilly (1962, 1974), purposeful activity as discussed by Fidler and Fidler (1978), King's theory of adaptive response (1978), and the model of human occupation as proposed by Kielhofner (1983). Mosey (1985) states that a monistic approach may exclude important facts, ignore important social needs, and discourage creative, divergent thinking. A comprehensive theory may oversimplify the profession's body of knowledge, domain of concern, and practice, or it may be too complex and intricate to be easily understood. It may also inhibit research if the concepts cannot be operationalized and made into variables for empirical testing to assess the theory's validity or the effectiveness of interventions derived from that theory.

Therefore, Mosey has consistently advocated a pluralistic approach in her development of frames of reference. The pluralistic approach regards all the elements of a profession as being of equal importance. The legitimate tools of the profession are as important as the theories that underlie their application and vice versa. Mosey feels that the pluralistic model is more flexible and can more readily allow for change as new ideas, knowledge, and beliefs emerge to meet the changing needs of society. Diversity in orientations is healthy and potentially more adaptive (Mosey, 1985, 1986).

Mosey suggests a taxonomy for the articulation of a pluralistic identity (1985). Each of the elements of the profession—philosophical assumptions, ethical code, theoretical foundation, domain of concern, principles for sequencing various aspects of practice, and legitimate tools—needs to be clearly defined and the various contents outlined. By making clear the content of each element, this taxonomy would allow researchers to readily identify incongruence among elements. It would also enable occupational therapists to recognize what their many specialties have in common. Content could be added or deleted as appropriate. Professional identity would be derived from all of the elements. This pluralistic approach would provide a structure that would make it easier for occupational therapists to analyze their philosophical assumptions critically, select or develop new theories, make changes in their domain of concern, consider alternative legitimate tools, and formulate more definitive and additional frames of reference. Mosey argues that an important part of this effort must be the exploration of current theories generated by other disciplines such as neurophysiology and their integration into occupational therapy.

Epistemology

Mosey's latest work has been in the wider realm of philosophies about knowledge, or epistemology. In her newest book, *Applied Scientific Inquiry in the Health Professions: An Epistemological Orientation* (1992), she articulates existing points of view about knowledge generation and presents the neopositivistic orientation as the one most relevant for the health professions. She argues that applied scientists, such as occupational therapists, need to understand theory both to determine which theories are suitable for their use and to apply them; therefore, she devotes a chapter to explaining how theory is developed and tested.

Mosey explains that whereas basic scientific inquiry has as its sole purpose the generation of theory and the discovery of new knowledge, applied scientific inquiry is concerned with immediate practical ends. She also distinguishes two types of applied scientific inquiry: Type I, the goal of which is to develop guidelines for practice, and Type II, the goal of which is to find the best answer to a particular practical problem. Examples from occupational therapy illustrate how guidelines for practice, or frames of reference, are formulated (1992).

SUBSEQUENT RESEARCH AND APPLICATION BY OTHERS

Mosey's work has contributed immeasurably to an understanding of the profession's parts and wholeness. However, because her major work has been to develop a taxonomy, and now an epistemology, it is difficult to evaluate subsequent research and application of her work. The structure of a frame of reference is hard to live within, and many therapists are generally more comfortable operating intuitively. Mosey's pluralistic model has received support, but whether researchers and practitioners will actually adopt it remains to be seen. It is more difficult to work with and combine various frames of reference than just to use one. Mosey's view of her own influence is modest:

> It takes a long time for professions to change and I present my ideas and people can accept or not accept them. I have no driving need for people to accept my ideas. I am not a public person. The thrill and reward come from playing with ideas and putting ideas together and knowing that eventually it will help our patients. (A.C. Mosey, personal communication, August 4, 1985)

Mosey has repeatedly emphasized that occupational therapists need to test the theories and theoretical foundations that they have and use them as a basis for practice, translate them into frames of reference, and evaluate their effectiveness (1968a, 1968b, 1970b, 1980, 1981, 1986). She has painstakingly given the profession the framework with which to do this. Through the research process, data generated from practice can systematically lead to tentative hypotheses that will refute, develop, refine, or verify the theoretical bases. This can help researchers evaluate frames of reference and their theoretical base. According to Mosey (1986, 1992), when the theoretical base is altered by research findings, changes in frames of reference result, and these in turn lead to changes in practice. Researchers who wish to engage in this process will find Mosey's works an invaluable tool.

REFERENCES

Ayres, J. (1958). The visual-motor function. *American Journal of Occupational Therapy, 12*, 130–139.

Ayres, J. (1961). Development of body scheme in children. *American Journal of Occupational Therapy, 15*, 99–102.

Ayres, J. (1963). The development of perceptual motor disabilities. *American Journal of Occupational Therapy, 17*, 221–225.

Ayres, J. (1964). Tactile function. *American Journal of Occupational Therapy, 18*, 6–11.

Bandura, A. (1969). *Principles of behavior modification.* New York: Holt, Rinehart, & Winston.

Banus, B. (Ed.). (1979). *The developmental therapist.* Thorofare, NJ: Charles B. Slack.

Bruner, J. (1966). *Studies in cognitive growth.* New York: John Wiley & Sons.

Diasio, K. (1968). Psychiatric occupational therapy: A search for a conceptual framework in light of psychoanalytic, ego psychology, and learning theory. *American Journal of Occupational Therapy, 22*, 400–407.

Dollard, J., & Miller, N. (1950). *Personality and psychotherapy.* New York: McGraw-Hill.

Erikson, E. (1950). *Childhood and society.* New York: Norton.

Fidler, G., & Fidler, J. (1963). *Occupational therapy: A communication process in psychiatry.* New York: Macmillan.

Fidler, G., & Fidler, J. (1978). Doing and becoming: Purposeful action and self-actualization. *American Journal of Occupational Therapy, 32*, 305–310.

Flavell, J. (1963). *The developmental psychology of Jean Piaget.* New York: D. Van Nostrand.

Ford, D., & Urban, H. (1963). *Systems of psychotherapy.* New York: John Wiley & Sons.

Freud, A. (1965). *Normality and pathology in childhood.* New York: International University Press.

Freud, S. (1949). *An outline of psychoanalysis.* New York: Norton.

Hartman, H. (1958). *Ego psychology and the problems of adaptation.* New York: International University Press.

Jung, C. (1933). *Modern man in search of a soul.* New York: Harcourt, Brace and World.

Jung, C. (1964). *Man and his symbols.* New York: Doubleday.

Kielhofner, G. (1977). Temporal adaptation: A conceptual framework for occupational therapy. *American Journal of Occupational Therapy, 31,* 235–242.

Kielhofner, G. (Ed.). (1983). *Health through occupation: Theory and practice in occupational therapy.* Philadelphia: F.A. Davis.

King, L.J. (1978). Towards a science of adaptive responses. *American Journal of Occupational Therapy, 32,* 429–437.

Llorens, L. (1976). *Application of a developmental theory for health and rehabilitation.* Rockville, MD: American Occupational Therapy Association.

Llorens, L., & Beck, G. (1966, March). *Training methods for cognitive-perceptual-motor dysfunction.* Paper presented at the Therapy Seminar on Normal Growth and Development with Deviations, St. Louis.

Maslow, A. (1962). *Toward a psychology of being.* Princeton, NJ: D. Van Nostrand.

Mosey, A. (1968a). *Occupational therapy: Theory and practice.* Medford, MA: Pothier Brothers Press.

Mosey, A. (1968b). Recapitulation of ontogenesis: A theory for the practice of occupational therapy. *American Journal of Occupational Therapy, 22,* 426–432.

Mosey, A. (1969). Treatment of pathological distortion of body image. *American Journal of Occupational Therapy, 23,* 413–416.

Mosey, A. (1970a). The concept and use of developmental groups. *American Journal of Occupational Therapy, 24,* 272–275.

Mosey, A. (1970b). *Three frames of reference for mental health.* Thorofare, NJ: Charles B. Slack.

Mosey, A. (1971). Involvement in the rehabilitation movement 1942–1960. *American Journal of Occupational Therapy, 25,* 234–236.

Mosey, A. (1973a). *Activities therapy.* New York: Raven Press.

Mosey, A. (1973b). Meeting health needs. *American Journal of Occupational Therapy, 27,* 14–17.

Mosey, A. (1974). An alternative: The biopsychosocial model. *American Journal of Occupational Therapy, 28,* 137–140.

Mosey, A. (1976). The night of January twenty-seven. *American Journal of Occupational Therapy, 30,* 648–649.

Mosey, A. (1980). A model for occupational therapy. *Occupational Therapy in Mental Health, 1,* 11–32.

Mosey, A. (1981). *Occupational therapy: Configuration of a profession.* New York: Raven Press.

Mosey, A. (1985). A monistic or a pluralistic approach to professional identity. Eleanor Clarke Slagle lecture. *American Journal of Occupational Therapy, 39,* 504–509.

Mosey, A. (1986). *Psychosocial components of occupational therapy.* New York: Raven Press.

Mosey, A.C. (1992). *Applied scientific inquiry in the health professions: An epistemological orientation.* Rockville, MD: American Occupational Therapy Association.

Pearce, J., & Newton, S. (1963). *The conditions of human growth.* New York: Citadel Press.

Reilly, M. (1962). Occupational therapy can be one of the great ideas of 20th century medicine. *American Journal of Occupational Therapy, 16,* 1–9.

Reilly, M. (Ed.). (1974). *Play as exploratory learning.* Beverly Hills: Sage Publications.

Richert, G.Z. (1989). An interview with Anne Cronin Mosey. *Occupational Therapy in Mental Health, 9,* 1–15.

Schilder, P. (1950). *The image and appearance of the human body.* New York: John Wiley & Sons.

Schneider, A. (1960). *Personality development and adjustment in adolescence.* Milwaukee: Bruce Publishing Company.

Searles, H. (1960). *The nonhuman environment.* New York: International University Press.

Sechehaye, M. (1951a). *Symbolic realization.* New York: International University Press.

Sechehaye, M. (1951b). *A new psychotherapy in schizophrenia.* New York: Grune & Stratton.

Sieg, K. (1974). Applying the behavioral model to occupational therapy. *American Journal of Occupational Therapy, 7,* 421–428.

Smith, A., & Tempone, V. (1968). Psychiatric occupational therapy within a learning theory context. *American Journal of Occupational Therapy, 22,* 415–425.

Sullivan, H.S. (1953). *The interpersonal theory of psychiatry.* New York: Norton.

Trombly, C., & Scott, A.D. (1977). *Occupational therapy for physical dysfunction.* Baltimore: Williams & Wilkins.

Wolpe, J., & Lazarus, A. (1966). *Behavior therapy techniques.* New York: Pergamon Press.

BIBLIOGRAPHY

1968

Mosey, A.C. (1968). *Occupational therapy: Theory and practice.* Medford, MA: Pothier Brothers Press.

Mosey, A.C. (1968). Recapitulation of ontogenesis: A theory for the practice of occupational therapy. *American Journal of Occupational Therapy, 22,* 426–432.

1969

Mosey, A.C. (1969). Treatment of pathological distortion of body image. *American Journal of Occupational Therapy, 23,* 413–416.

1970

Mosey, A.C. (1970). The concept and use of developmental groups. *American Journal of Occupational Therapy, 24,* 272–275.

Mosey, A.C. (1970). *Three frames of reference for mental health.* Thorofare, NJ: Charles B. Slack.

1971

Mosey, A.C. (1971). Involvement in the rehabilitation movement 1942–1960. *American Journal of Occupational Therapy, 25,* 234–236.

1973

Mosey, A.C. (1973). *Activities therapy.* New York: Raven Press.

Mosey, A.C. (1973). Meeting health needs. *American Journal of Occupational Therapy, 27,* 14–17.

1974

Mosey, A.C. (1974). An alternative: The biopsychosocial model. *American Journal of Occupational Therapy, 28,* 137–140.

Corry, S., Sebastian, V., & Mosey, A.C. (1974). Acute short-term treatment in psychiatry. *American Journal of Occupational Therapy, 28,* 401–406.

1976

Mosey, A.C. (1976). The night of January twenty-seven. *American Journal of Occupational Therapy, 30,* 648–649.

1980

Mosey, A.C. (1980). A model of occupational therapy. *Occupational Therapy in Mental Health, 1,* 11–32.

Katz, G.M., & Mosey, A.C. (1980). Fieldwork performance, academic grades and pre-selection criteria of occupational therapy students. *American Journal of Occupational Therapy, 34,* 794–800.

1981

Mosey, A.C. (1981). The art of practice. In B.C. Abreu (Ed.), *Physical disabilities manual* (pp. 1–3). New York: Raven Press.

Mosey, A.C. (1981). *Occupational therapy: Configuration of a profession.* New York: Raven Press.

1985

Mosey, A.C. (1985). A monistic or a pluralistic approach to professional identity? Eleanor Clarke Slagle lecture. *American Journal of Occupational Therapy, 39,* 504–509.

Mosey, A.C. (1985). *Psychosocial components of occupational therapy.* New York: Raven Press.

1989

Mosey, A.C. (1989). The proper focus of scientific inquiry in occupational therapy: Frames of reference. *Occupational Therapy Journal of Research, 9,* 195–201.

1991

Mosey, A.C. (1991). Letter to the editor. Common vocabulary. *Occupational Therapy Journal of Research, 11,* 67–68.

1992

Mosey, A.C. (1992). *Applied scientific inquiry in the health professions: An epistemological orientation.* Rockville, MD: American Occupational Therapy Association.

Mosey, A.C. (1992). The issue is: Partition of occupational science and occupational therapy. *American Journal of Occupational Therapy, 46,* 851–853.

Chapter Four

Lela A. Llorens

Susan Denegan Shortridge and Kay F. Walker

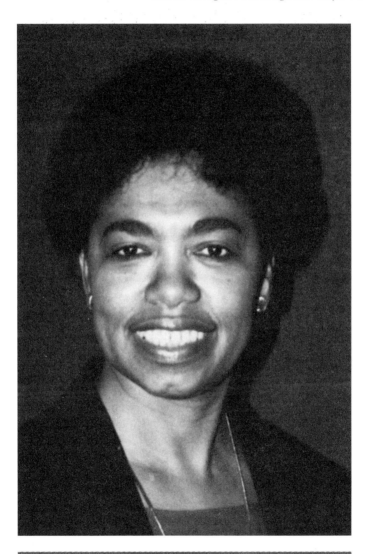

Lela A. Llorens

BIOGRAPHICAL SKETCH

Lela A. Llorens (née Williams) was born in Shreveport, Louisiana, in 1933 during an era when women were not expected to have careers. In addition to the gender stereotypes of the times, she experienced the cultural limitations imposed on black women in the Southern community of her childhood. Segregation of the races in schools was the norm in the South at that time, and educational opportunities available to black children were severely limited. Recognizing the impact of these barriers on the family, her father moved them to Detroit, Michigan, in search of a better life and more accessible education for the children.

A review of the career achievements and written works of Lela Llorens and the authors' experiences of having worked closely with her as an academic colleague brings to mind many possible reasons for her successes. Perhaps the lessons of her early struggles as a black female child contributed to her lifelong determination and motivation for excellence. She cites her father's goal orientation, his insistence on thinking ahead and planning what you are going to do and then doing it, as a definite influence in her approach to life. When she and her sister entered school in Detroit, they were placed in a lower grade because they had come from a school in the South. Her father urged the school to give his daughters the opportunity to demonstrate their ability. Llorens noted, "We successfully passed the grade to which we advanced, and I was then advanced two grades" (L.A. Llorens, personal communication, September 14, 1992).

Her achievements may also be due to her brilliant intellect and ability to analyze, synthesize, and communicate information. Jean Ayres once remarked at an informal gathering that many of us (herself included) have either a well-developed right or a well-developed left cerebral hemisphere. "Lela," she pointed out, "has both hemispheres fully developed, integrated, and operating."

Perhaps Lela Llorens has achieved so much because of her ability to balance professional and personal sides of her life. She achieves a balance of work and play through recreational and creative outlets such as travel with her husband, visits with her daughter, cooking, and sewing her own clothes.

The key to her success is that she makes people a high priority in her life. Never too busy to attend to people issues, she is a caring and unpretentious person. Students at Texas Women's University named themselves the "Lela A. Llorens Class of 1976," stating, "Her warm, open manner and genuine interest in everyone she meets immediately sets people at ease so that a sharing of interests, knowledge, and ideas can take place."

Her positive attitude and sense of humor have also been sustaining traits in her achievements. She tells about how she was marked down by one of her internship supervisors because she smiled too much and seemed too happy. However, she remains able to bring a lightheartedness to otherwise discouraging situations.

These reasons for her exemplary career are speculative. What is known is that Lela A. Llorens has achieved greatness in her professional and personal life.

Education

Llorens identified occupational therapy as her career choice when she read the University of Puget Sound college catalog description of occupational therapy and realized that this matched her natural abilities in arts and crafts and her interest in medicine. She began her studies at Puget Sound in 1949 and received her Bachelor of Science degree in Occupational Therapy from Western Michigan University in 1953. In order to support her practice goals with educational advancement, she pursued graduate work at Wayne State University, where she received a Master of Arts degree in Vocational Rehabilitation. She chose this degree program because its flexibility enabled her to elect course work that complemented her effectiveness as a therapist and as a supervisor.

Desiring to develop stronger research skills, Llorens entered a doctoral program at the University of the Pacific in Stockton, California, in 1970. However, she found that the program's emphasis in educational psychology did not satisfy her need to learn more about research while maintaining her commitment to occupational therapy. At Walden University, Minneapolis, Minnesota, with its campus in Naples, Florida, Llorens was able to design and complete a doctoral program that met her educational goals. She received the Doctor of Philosophy degree in Education/Occupational Therapy in 1976.

Employment

Llorens' first position as an occupational therapist was as a staff therapist at the site of one of her internships, Wayne County General Hospital. Here she developed programs for adult psychiatric patients within a general hospital setting. She began to identify and articulate what occupational therapy was providing through these programs. Llorens remained in this position for four years (1953–1957).

Despite a decrease in salary and an increase in travel time, Llorens accepted a staff position at Northville State Hospital in Michigan because it enabled her to increase her patient contact with children. Although she was there for only one year (1957–1958), this experience confirmed her interest in pediatrics. As she stated:

> I really was fascinated with emotionally disturbed children and what occupational therapy could do for them. There was not very much in the literature regarding pediatrics . . . it was a matter of figuring out what the profession had to offer based on what was already known about adults. (L.A. Llorens, personal communication, September 2, 1983)

Llorens' next professional move was to the Lafayette Clinic (1958–1968) as supervisor of OT services in child psychiatry. She eventually became head of the OT department and supervised therapists practicing with adult psychosocial and neurological patients in addition to her practice in child psychiatry. Here she delineated the role of occupational therapy in a psychotherapeutic setting.

From 1968 to 1971, Llorens served as consultant to the Comprehensive Child Care Project at Mount Zion Hospital in San Francisco. This project enabled her to explore the consultant role and the expansion of OT services into community and nontraditional settings. While working on this project, she began to address cultural variables in health care delivery. She also explored the limits of occupational therapy's effectiveness in a pediatric population. This work experience confirmed for her that occupational therapy has a knowledge base that can be expanded and is viable in diverse settings such as public schools, community agencies, and outpatient clinics.

After about 18 years in OT, Llorens began to reflect on her original choice of profession and to explore other vocational possibilities. She went so far as to take vocational tests and found that her test profiles were almost identical to ones from her college years that had confirmed her decision to become a health care professional. From this time of reflection came her decision that she should change her focus from clinical practice to academia.

Llorens had already acquired teaching experience throughout her employment history. For example, one of her responsibilities during the Mount Zion Project was to teach growth and development to medical pediatric interns and residents. Although the Department of Pediatrics wanted her to continue to do this teaching, she was faced with a career decision.

> I really felt that if I was going to teach full-time, I should be teaching occupational therapists. I had about 18 years experience and there were not many people around with that kind of clinical experience. . . . I felt that it should be passed on. (L.A. Llorens, personal communication, September 2, 1983)

While seeking a teaching position, Llorens investigated many OT programs. Her decision to accept an appointment as an associate professor at the University of Florida was based on several critical factors. These included the opportunity to be involved in the development of a graduate program, the developmental hierarchy inherent in the design of the existing curriculum, and a deep respect for the chair, Dr. Alice Jantzen, who was to become an important mentor.

This new phase of involvement in academic occupational therapy appeared to be a significant reawakening of ambition and direction for Llorens. From 1971 to 1974 she was occupied with responsibilities as an associate professor and graduate coordinator.

In 1975, when Jantzen retired, Llorens assumed a new academic role, the position of acting department chair. In the next two years, she was promoted to the rank of professor and was officially appointed as the chair for the Department of Occupational Therapy at the University of Florida. She maintained this position for six years, during which time she contributed greatly to the department's development by facilitating the articulation of the department's frame of reference for occupational therapy education and practice and refining the OT graduate program. In addition to promoting graduate students' interest in research, Llorens had a profound influence on the professional development of less experienced faculty.

In 1982, after 11 years at the University of Florida, Llorens became professor and coordinator of Graduate Studies at the Department of Occupational Therapy, San Jose State University. The following year, she was elected by the faculty to serve as chair of that department and has been re-elected for the ensuing terms. In 1990, she was appointed co-director of the Division of Health Professions in addition to her role as chair. She also serves as core faculty of the Geriatric Education Center at Stanford University School of Medicine.

Written Work

The questions "What is OT?" and "What does OT do?" have occupied most of Llorens' written work, and the challenge of these questions dates to her early experiences in the field as a student and young therapist. As a student she was dissatisfied with not being able to explain or define occupational therapy. As a new therapist, she saw that many therapists could "demonstrate" the value of occupational therapy but could not articulate frames of reference or theory related to it.

Graduate school became the arena where Llorens could explore the questions that were uncovered during her working day. She states:

> Term papers that I was doing for classes were essentially significant learning experiences. They were not just papers that were handed in to fulfill an assignment or requirements for a degree. (L.A. Llorens, personal communication, September 2, 1983)

Llorens' first article, "Psychological Tests in Planning Treatment Goals," was published in 1960. It revealed the impact of schooling on her professional work as well as the influence of a mentor (Eli Rubin) and an interdisciplinary team in a work environment that promoted scholarly inquiry. As she said:

> My first publication resulted from a term paper that I did for my masters degree. Although I was the single author on this paper, Eli contributed a great deal to the structure and the content. He helped me to organize— which was probably the beginning of a framework or orientation to organize behaviors that we were seeing in occupational therapy. I initially

used more of a psychological framework because that seemed to offer some way of beginning to look at the behaviors that we were seeing clinically. (L.A. Llorens, personal communication, September 2, 1983)

In this paper Llorens attempts to integrate evaluation data gathered from psychological testing with behavior observations made in occupational therapy. She states:

> For occupational therapy to contribute to the therapeutic community it must be capable of contributing a specific commodity . . . [it must] participate cooperatively . . . and must be capable of a collaborative relationship. For many years, occupational therapy has maintained a dependent role to medical staff and a rivalrous, conflicting role to nursing . . . . Occupational therapy has a specific contributive function which can be realized through effective evaluation and comprehensive programming. (1960, p. 89)

Since her first publication, Llorens has authored/edited 7 books and authored 8 book chapters, 48 refereed journal articles, 8 newsletter articles and 12 proceedings publications. What began as a term paper has become a written legacy of her efforts to present her answers to the "what is" of occupational therapy.

Mentors

Llorens credits several key persons who have served as mentors in her career. Mentors played an important role in her career moves, and in each new position she sought significant people within the work setting from whom to learn. As she stated, "The positions I've held have contributed to my continued growth, interest and direction in the field. This has been partly deliberate and partly opportunity" (L.A. Llorens, personal communication, September 2, 1983).

While attending Western Michigan University (1950–1953), she was a student of Marion R. Spear, chair and founder of that department, and was impressed by the high leadership expectations for graduates of that department. She also cites her supervisor in her first job, Mae McGiverin at Wayne County General Hospital, as a significant person in encouraging her interest in mental health occupational therapy.

However, when asked to identify persons who provided long-term guidance, she named four: Eli Rubin, Wilma West, Alice Jantzen, and Richard Whitlock (Robertson, 1992). While at the Lafayette Clinic, Llorens worked with a research team, an experience that added a new dimension to her writing and treatment capabilities. She developed a strong collaborative relationship with Eli Rubin, clinical psychologist and then coordinator of children's services at the Lafayette Clinic. Rubin encouraged her to write, conduct research, and present at conferences. He endorsed her as a part-time faculty member in her first academic teaching appointment.

Throughout her career, Llorens has been inspired by Wilma West, who has served as an important mentor. West was long active in the AOTA and worked in administration, education, research, and consultation. According to Llorens, "Wilma West's vision, her ability to articulate the promise of occupational therapy, and her belief in my ability to make a significant contribution to the profession were inspirational to me" (L.A. Llorens, personal communication, September 2, 1983). On West's recommendation, Llorens became consultant to the Mount Zion Project. West continued to serve as "long-distance advisor" to Llorens in the consultant role at Mount Zion and in subsequent appointments throughout her career.

Llorens' relationship with Dr. Jantzen proved to be a significant factor in guiding her academic career toward success. As she describes:

> I would also have to name Dr. Jantzen as one of my mentors. I learned a great deal from her as a strong leader within the profession, as well as in the college and department at the University of Florida. It was important to me that she was planning to remain for a number of years after I arrived. My goals, while they included a future academic administrative position, also included some other things that I thought I needed to learn. I learned about academia from Dr. Jantzen. I learned how to "mentor" young faculty and how to run an academic program as contrasted to a rehabilitative program. I learned about higher education as viewed by the academy, which has a different value system than that held by "helping" professions. I learned how to be an academician, as well as a therapist, teacher, and writer. (L.A. Llorens, personal communication, September 2, 1983)

Finally, Llorens names Dr. Richard Whitlock at San Jose State University. He assisted her in learning the system at San Jose State. She notes that:

> He extended the education that I began at the University of Florida with Alice Jantzen. The environment of a comprehensive university with a liberal arts and sciences focus and no medical school was considerably different from that which I had previously known. Dick Whitlock was instrumental in helping me avoid the land mines while moving positively ahead toward my career goals. (Robertson, 1992, p. 27)

Honors

For her leadership in theory, education, and research, Llorens has been awarded many honors, including the highest accolades that are bestowed in the profession of occupational therapy. Recognition of her outstanding performance began as early as her undergraduate work at Western Michigan University when she received the Marion R. Spear Scholastic Award in 1953.

Llorens was awarded the AOTA Eleanor Clarke Slagle Lectureship in 1969. Her preparation for this lectureship initiated the evolution of her own developmental theory. The lecture created a time pressure, and as Llorens explicitly stated at the time of its presentation:

> Preparing for this moment has been an arduous task. Many of my colleagues and friends have checked on my progress during the year and the answer most given was "We're living with it." We, including my family, have literally lived with the "Lecture" this year and the breakthrough that I was struggling for did not come until late summer during our trip to West Africa. When it did, it came in the form of ten premises which express a developmental theory of occupational therapy. (1970, p. 93)

Llorens' influence in the area of OT education was recognized at university and state levels. One of Llorens' more noteworthy responsibilities was as chair for the Research Advisory Committee of the American Occupational Therapy Foundation. Her abilities as a researcher and leader in the field were apparent in her repeated election to this position (1978 to 1989). Awards granted by the American Occupational Therapy Association, in addition to the Eleanor Clarke Slagle Lectureship, include the Roster of Fellows in 1973, the Award of Merit in 1986, and a Service Award in 1989. Awards granted by the American Occupational Therapy Foundation include the Certificate of Appreciation in 1981, the A. Jean Ayres Award for research in 1988, and a Meritorious Service Award in 1989.

Llorens is also an invited keynote speaker and presenter at conferences and meetings. She has also been honored as a visiting scholar at Wayne State University, 1991; Texas Women's University, 1991; University of Wisconsin-Madison, 1991; Medical University of South Carolina, 1990; and Western Michigan University, 1987. The Michigan State Senate awarded her the Certificate of Merit in 1991. In 1991, she was invited to submit her written works for preservation in the Women's Collection at Texas Women's University.

THEORETICAL CONCEPTS

Developmental Theory for the Practice of Occupational Therapy

Llorens' first conceptualization of a developmental theory was based on 15 years of experience in occupational therapy practice and research in the OT and human development literature. As a new therapist and then in her subsequent positions, Llorens was challenged by the need for a clear description of occupational therapy that would lend credibility to the profession and to the role of occupational therapy. The task of writing the lecture for the Eleanor Clarke Slagle Lectureship presented her with the opportunity to provide that description. As she states:

> The theory . . . has been an outgrowth of my experiences and research in the field of psychiatry, both pediatric and adult . . . in pediatric general medicine and community health. . . . These experiences have stimulated my desire to think through the function and purpose of occupational therapy as I have experienced it. (1970, p. 93)

Ten Premises

Llorens' theory was developed from the following thesis:

> That occupational therapy is a facilitation process which assists the individual in achieving mastery of life tasks and the ability to cope as efficiently as possible with the life expectations made of him through the mechanisms of selected input stimuli, and availability of practice in a suitable environment. (1970, p. 93)

This thesis is based on the following ten premises:

1. That the human organism develops horizontally (simultaneously) in the area of neurophysiological, physical, psychosocial, and psychodynamic growth and in the development of social language, daily living, and sociocultural skills at specific periods of time.

2. That the human organism develops longitudinally (chronologically) in each of these areas in a continuous process as one ages.

3. That mastery of particular skills, abilities, and relationships in each of the areas of neurophysiological, physical, psychosocial, and psychodynamic development, social language, daily living, and sociocultural skills, both horizontally and longitudinally, is necessary to the successful achievement of satisfactory coping behavior and adaptive relationships.

4. That such mastery is usually achieved naturally in the course of development.

5. That the fundamental endowment of the individual and the stimulation of experiences received within the environment of the family come together to interact in such a way as to promote positive early growth and development in both the horizontal (simultaneous) and longitudinal (chronological) planes.

6. That later influences of extended family, community, social, and civic groups assist in the growth process.

7. That physical or psychological trauma related to disease, injury, environmental insufficiencies, or intrapersonal vulnerability can interrupt the growth and development process.

8. That such growth interruption will cause a gap in the developmental cycle, resulting in a disparity between expected coping behavior and adaptive facility and the necessary skills and abilities to achieve the same.

9. That occupational therapy, through the skilled application of activities and relationships, can provide growth and development links to assist in closing the gap between expectation and ability by increasing skills, abilities, and relationships in the neurophysiological, physical, psychosocial, psychodynamic, social language, daily living, and sociocultural spheres of development as indicated both horizontally and longitudinally.

10. That occupational therapy, through the skilled application of activities and relationships, can provide growth experiences to prevent the development of potential maladaptation related to insufficient nurturing in neurophysiological, physical, psychosocial, psychodynamic, social language, daily living, and sociocultural spheres of development both horizontally (simultaneously) and longitudinally (chronologically).*

Schematic Representation of Facilitating Growth and Development

Llorens' Schematic Representation of Facilitating Growth and Development expands on the ten premises by portraying both developmental and behavioral expectations and the activities and relationships that facilitate these expectations (Llorens, 1970, 1976). The schematic is organized into three sections (see Table 4-1).

Section I depicts developmental expectations, behaviors, and needs and their simultaneous (horizontal) and chronological (longitudinal) progression. Stage-specific development categories of human growth include those of Ayres (neurophysiological development), Gesell (physical, social language, sociocultural, and daily living development), Erikson (psychosocial development), and Freud

*Source: From "Facilitating Growth and Development: The Promise of Occupational Therapy" by L.A. Llorens, 1970, The American Journal of Occupational Therapy, 24, pp. 93–94. Copyright March 1970 by American Occupational Therapy Association, Inc. Reprinted by permission.

Table 4-1 Schematic Representation of Facilitating Growth and Development

SECTION I
Developmental Expectations, Behaviors, and Needs
(Selected for Illustrative Purposes)

Neurophysiological- Sensorimotor Ayres	Physical-Motor Gesell	Psychosocial Erikson

0–2 Sensorimotor
Tactile functions
Vestibular functions
Visual, auditory, olfactory,
    gustatory functions
	0–2
	Head sages
	Fisting
	Gross motion
	Walking
	Climbing
		Basic Trust vs. Mistrust/Oral
		    Sensory
		Ease of feeding
		Depth of sleep
		Relaxation of bowels

6 mo.–4 Integration of Body Sides
Gross motor planning
Form and space perception
Equilibrium response
Postural and bilateral integration
Body scheme development
	2–3
	Runs
	Balances
	Hand preference
	    established
	Coordination
		Autonomy vs. Shame and Doubt/
		    Muscular-Anal
		Conflict between holding on and
		    letting go

3–7 Discrimination
Refined tactile
Kinesthetic, visual, auditory,
    olfactory, gustatory functions
	3–6
	Coordination more
	    graceful
	Muscles develop
	Skills develop
		Initiative vs. Guilt/Locomotor-
		    Genital
		Aggressiveness
		Manipulation
		Coercion

3– Abstract Thinking
Conceptualization
Complex relationships
Read, write, numbers
	6–11
	Energy development
	Skill practice to attain
	    proficiency
		Industry vs. Inferiority/Latency
		Wins recognition through
		    productivity
		Learns skills and tools

Continue development
    Conceptualization
    Complex relationships
    Read, write, numbers
	11–13
	Rapid growth
	Poor posture
	Awkwardness
		Identity vs. Role Confusion/
		    Puberty and Adolescence
		Identification
		Social roles

Development presumably
    maintained
	Growth established and
	    maintained
		Intimacy vs. Isolation/Young
		    Adulthood
		Commitments
		Body and ego mastery

Alterations begin to occur in
    sensory functions,
    conceptualization, and memory
	Alterations begin to occur
	    in motor behavior,
	    strength, and endurance
		Generativity vs. Stagnation/
		    Adulthood
		Guiding next generation
		Creative, productive

Alterations in sensory functions,
    conceptualization, and memory
	Alterations in motor
	    behavior, strength, and
	    endurance
		Ego Integrity vs. Despair/Maturity
		Acceptance of own life cycle

continues

Table 4-1 continued

SECTION I
Developmental Expectations, Behaviors, and Needs
(Selected for Illustrative Purposes)

Psychodynamic Hall Grant, Freud	Socio-Cultural Gesell	Social-Language Gesell	Activity of Daily Living Gesell
0–4 Oral Dependency Initially aggressive Oral erotic activity	Individual mothering person most important Immediate family group important	Small sounds Coos Vocalizes Listens Speaks	Recognizes bottle Holds spoon Holds glass Controls bowel
0–4 Anal Independence Resistiveness Self-assertiveness Narcissism Ambivalence	Parallel play Often alone Recognizes extended family	Identifies objects verbally Asks "why?" Short sentences	Feeds self Helps undress Recognizes simple tunes No longer wets at night
3–6 Genital Oedipal Genital interest Possessiveness of opposite sex parent Antagonistic to same sex parent Castration fears	Seeks companion-ship Makes decisions Plays with other children Takes turns	Combines talking and eating Complete sentences Imaginative Dramatic	Laces shoes Cuts with scissors Toilets indepen-dently Helps set table
6–11 Latency Primitive struggles quiescent Initiative in mastery of skills Strong defenses	Group play and team activities Independence of adults Gang interests	Language major form of communication	Enjoys dressing up Learns value of money Responsible for grooming
11– Adolescence Emancipation from parents Occupational decisions Role experiment Re-examine values	Team games Organization important Interest in opposite sex	Verbal language predominates	Interest in earning money
Outgrow need for parent validation Identify with others	Group affiliation Family, social, civic interest	Non-verbal behavior also used to communicate	Concern for personal grooming, mate, family
Emotional responsibilities may lessen Physical and economic indepen-dence accepted Shift from survival to enjoyment			Accepting and adjusting to changes of middle age
Continued growth after middle age Inner trend toward survival			Adjusting to changes after middle age

Table 4-1 continued

SECTION II
Facilitating Activities and
Relationships (Selected)

	Sensorimotor Activities	Developmental Activities	Symbolic Activities	Daily Life Tasks	Interpersonal Relationships
E	Tactile stimulation Visual, auditory, olfactory, gustatory	Dolls Animals Sand Water	Biting Chewing Eating Blowing	Recognize food Hold feeding equipment Use feeding	Individual interaction
V	stimulation	Excursions	Cuddling	equipment	
A	Physical exercise Balancing Motor planning	Pull toys Playground Clay Crayons Chalk	Throwing Dropping Messing Collecting Destroying	Feeding Dressing Toileting	Individual interaction Parallel play
L	Listening Learning Skilled tasks and games	Being read to Coloring Drawing Painting	Destroying Exhibiting	Feeding Dressing Toileting Simple chores	Individual interaction Play small groups
U					
A	Reading Writing Numbers	Scooters Wagons Collections Puppets Building	Controlling Mastery	Feeding Dressing Grooming Spending	Individual interaction Groups Teams Clubs
T	All of the above available to be recycled	Weaving Machinery tasks Carving Modeling	All of the above to be recycled	Feeding Dressing Grooming Prevocational skills	Individual interaction Groups Teams
I		Arts Crafts Sports Club and interest groups Education Work		Feeding Dressing Grooming Life role, skills	Individual interaction Groups
O					
N					

continues

Table 4-1 continued

SECTION III
Behavior Expectations
and Adaptive Skills

Developmental Tasks Havighurst	Ego-Adaptive Skills Mosey, Pearce, and Newton	Intellectual Development Piaget

Learning to:
  Walk
  Talk
  Take solids
Elimination
	Ability to respond to
	  mothering
	Mastering of gross motor
	  responses
		Motor skills
		Integrated

Sex difference
To form concepts of social and
  physical reality
To relate emotionally to others
Right
Wrong
	Ability to respond to routines
	  of daily living
	Mastery of 3 dimensional
	  space
	Sense of body image
		Investigative
		Imitative
		Egocentric

To develop a conscience	Ability to
	  Follow directions
	  Tolerate frustrations
	  Sit still
	  Delay gratification
		Egocentricism reduced, social
		  participation increases
		Language replaces motor
		  behavior

Learn physical skills Getting along Reading, writing Values Social attitudes	Ability to perceive, sort, organize, and utilize stimuli Work in groups Mastery of inanimate objects	Orders experiences Relates parts to wholes Deductive reasoning

More mature relationships
Social roles
Selecting occupation
Achieving emotional independence
	Ability to accept and
	  discharge responsibility
	Capacity for love
		Systematic approach to
		  problems
		Sense of equality supersedes
		  submission to adults

Selecting a mate
Starting family
Marriage, home
Congenial social group
	Ability to function indepen-
	  dently
	Control drives
	Plan and execute
	Purposeful motion
		Development established and
		  maintained

Civic and social responsibility
Economic standard of living
Develop adult leisure activities
Adjust to aging parents
	Obtain, organize, and use
	  knowledge
	Participate in primary group
	Participate in variety of
	  relationships
		Alterations in other areas may
		  affect

Adjust to decreasing physical health,
  retirement, death
Age group affiliation
Meeting social obligations
	Experience self as acceptable
	Participate in mutually
	  satisfactory heterosexual
	  relations	

Source: From *Application of a Developmental Theory for Health and Rehabilitation* (pp. 32–33) by L.A. Llorens, 1976, Rockville, Md.: American Occupational Therapy Association, Inc. Copyright 1976 by American Occupational Therapy Association, Inc. Reprinted by permission.

(psychodynamic development). Although each theorist is recognized for a particular area of expertise, Llorens stresses that these areas of growth "overlap and interweave" and should not be viewed in a "segmental" fashion. For example, although Piaget was recognized primarily for his work in cognitive development, he linked such development closely to the acquisition of sensorimotor and sociocultural skills.

In Section III, behavior expectations and adaptive skills include those coping skills that help the individual deal effectively with life and life roles. The behavior expectations and adaptive skills presented are derived from the works of Havighurst (development tasks); Pearce, Newton, and Mosey (ego-adaptive skills); and Piaget (intellectual development). Although behavior expectations in Section III are separated from developmental expectations in Section I of the chart, Llorens feels that they occur simultaneously. Growth in developmental tasks is facilitated by the family, environment, extended family, community, and social and civic groups.

Using the chart, one can view development as a tapestry, with each area of development overlapping and interwoven horizontally and vertically, creating a stable base for the human organism to mature. If any one area is interrupted, a thread becomes weakened, and the growth and development process is no longer stable. Physical or psychological trauma in any one of the horizontal or longitudinal parameters can disrupt the development cycle. This creates disparity between developmental expectations (Section I) and behavioral expectations and adaptive skills (Section III).

Section II depicts the role of occupational therapy in providing facilitating activities and relationships to bridge this developmental gap. The first step in the intervention process is evaluation, which includes testing, interviews, record review, and systematic clinical observation. From these evaluation procedures the therapist determines "at what level the individual is functioning in the various aspects along the developmental continuum and . . . program[s] for facilitating growth and development . . . in accordance with the needs of the individual and the demands of his age" (Llorens, 1970, p. 100).

The therapist then chooses tasks from sensorimotor activities, developmental play activities, symbolic activities, daily life tasks, and interpersonal relationships to facilitate the growth process and narrow any developmental discrepancy (Llorens, 1970). Llorens emphasizes that although special attention may be placed on facilitating the process of growth in any one particular parameter, all parameters of development must be acknowledged for an integrating growth experience to occur.

An appropriate facilitation program should meet the client's needs and the demands of the client's age and life roles. The intervention process for prevention of health problems is different from that for conditions of acute illness or temporary or permanent disability. Llorens (1970) believes that "intervention at a stage that can be identified before trauma becomes overwhelming will allow the individual to continue his growth process with a minimum of interruption and continue toward the achievement of ego-adaptive skills" (p. 100). In treatment geared toward identifiable acute illness or temporary or permanent disability, facilitation of development tasks and ego-adaptive skills must be viewed in relationship to the client's needs and limitations and geared to a realistic level of attainment.

DEVELOPMENTAL THEORY AND OCCUPATIONAL THERAPY RESEARCH

Llorens' developmental theory was both derived from and applied to her research in such fields as child psychiatry, community health, and gerontology.

Child Psychiatry

Although Llorens has published in a variety of areas, including vocational rehabilitation (Llorens, 1961, 1966a, 1981e; Llorens, Levy, & Rubin, 1964), sensory integration (Llorens, 1968b, 1983; Llorens & Burris, 1981; Llorens & Sieg, 1975), community health practice, and practice with the elderly, she is most well known for her work in child psychiatry. Her early works focused on emotional disturbance in children (Llorens, 1967a, 1968b; Llorens & Rubin, 1962, 1967) and occupational therapy treatment for psychosocial dysfunction (Llorens, 1960, 1968a; Llorens & Johnson, 1966; Llorens & Rubin, 1961, 1962). With her colleagues in the interdisciplinary treatment and research team at the Lafayette Clinic, Llorens also described cognitive-perceptual-motor (CPM) dysfunction in children and made recommendations about its treatment (Beck et al., 1965; Braun et al., 1965; Braun, Rubin, Llorens, & Beck, 1967; Llorens, 1966b, 1967a; Llorens & Beck, 1966; Llorens, Rubin, Braun, Beck, & Beall, 1969; Llorens, Rubin, Braun, Mottley, & Beall, 1964; Rubin, Braun, Beck, & Llorens, 1972).

To demonstrate that occupational therapy for children with emotional disturbances was therapeutic, Llorens had to establish a baseline delineating the effects of emotional disturbance on children's development (Llorens & Rubin, 1961). Thus even very early in her career Llorens began to address what would become a central theme in her developmental theory (premises 7 and 8): the influence of physical or psychological trauma on the developmental process. In her work on CPM dysfunction she would similarly explore the adverse effect of this condition on growth and development (Beck et al., 1965) and hypothesize that CPM deficits could create an inability to cope with the demands of the environment (Llorens, Levy, & Rubin, 1964).

In her early writings on emotional disturbance, Llorens recognized that the absence of emotional problems resulted in the acquisition of skills through practice and mastery. She hypothesized that these skills later became problem-solving methods that directly affected the child's self-confidence, self-concept, and self-esteem (Llorens & Rubin, 1961). As a stronger relationship between emotional disturbance and CPM deficits emerged in the Lafayette team's research, it became apparent that mastery must be an integral part of the treatment protocol for CPM dysfunction:

> Many of the activities are those which children usually master through maturation and environmental stimulation. However, since some children do not, for a variety of reasons, such as inadequate experiences, master them successfully, the retraining process provides a sequence through which the child can progress artificially, thus enabling him to correct his deficit in primary adaptive functions. (Beck et al., 1965, pp. 236–237)

The importance of mastery would later be elaborated on in premises 3 and 4 of Llorens' developmental theory.

Llorens' involvement with CPM research also led her to address the relationship of environmental factors to the child's CPM dysfunction. Such factors included parental attitude, early schooling, and environmental feedback (Braun et al., 1967). A definitive move from the medical model can be seen in Llorens' involvement with the Lafayette research team's effort to clarify environmental causes of deficits and put aside classification according to diagnostic category. This recognition of the effects of the environment on developmental process would be incorporated into premises 5 and 6 of the developmental theory.

Community Health

Llorens' appointment as consultant to the Comprehensive Child Care Project at Mount Zion Hospital led her to explore in even more depth the role of environmental factors in child development. She argued, for example, that child rearing and health care practices in the black community, which were themselves influenced by larger social factors, had a profound impact on the psychological development of black children:

> All children must master specific developmental tasks and ego adaptive skills between infancy and adolescence. . . . Some of these skills will be learned in school. In this society, the combination of financial means, the lifestyle of the family, and its aspirations, along with knowledge of and availability of resources, play a large part in influencing the extent

to which black children are able to develop in these areas. (1971a, p. 148)

Llorens' research concerns produced a book on community-based health care, *Consultation in the Community: Occupational Therapy in Child Health* (1973b); articles on community child health (Llorens, 1971b, 1974, 1975); the effect of sociological and cultural variables in health care delivery for children (Llorens, 1971a, 1971b, 1973b) and elders (Llorens, 1988; Llorens, Hikoyeda, & Yeo, 1992; McCormack, Llorens, & Glogoski, 1991; Ross, Washington, & Llorens, 1990); and ecology of environment and individual (Llorens, 1984).

Gerontology

Although Llorens is usually identified with pediatric practice, her developmental theory is a lifespan theory and, as such, includes aging. She described the expected decline in certain functions, especially physical, with age and the ways in which OT intervention can foster continued growth and adaptation (Llorens, 1970, 1977, 1991). In 1990 and 1991, she served as presenter and facilitator at conferences and meetings that addressed elder and ethnic issues. Topics have included ethnogeriatrics, cultural diversity and the aging work force, and intergenerational issues and minority aging. Llorens' publications in the area of aging include articles on the culturally diverse elderly (McCormack, Llorens, & Glogoski, 1991), activities of daily living and self-esteem (Bolding & Llorens, 1991; Shiotsuka, Burton, Pedretti, & Llorens, in press), self-feeding (Hames-Hahn & Llorens, 1989), and health care for ethnic elders (Llorens, 1988). Llorens currently is part of a certificate in gerontology program at San Jose University.

DEVELOPMENTAL THEORY AND OCCUPATIONAL THERAPY PRACTICE

Occupational Therapy Process

Llorens (1981b) described the occupational therapy process shown in Exhibit 4-1 (Killingsworth, Llorens, Southam, Down, & Schwartz, 1992) as beginning with the client who has a condition: illness, wellness, disability, or dysfunction. Through the evaluation process, the occupational therapist determines how the client is functioning and whether intervention is indicated. Evaluations include observation, interview, history, and testing. Intervention will include one or more types of intervention: prevention, health education, modification of maladaptive behavior, adaptive change, health maintenance, or rehabilitation. Intervention includes purposeful activity *and* interpersonal relationships on an individual, group,

Exhibit 4-1 A Schematic Outline of the Occupational Therapy Process

Patient/Client with a Condition
Wellness (preventive needs)
Illness (due to disease, stress, etc.)
Disability (secondary to a chronic condition, trauma, etc.)
Dysfunction (occupational role performance)

Patient/Client Occupational Roles
Worker, student, volunteer, homemaker, parent, son, daughter, mate, sibling, peer, and best friend/chum.

Evaluation
From the evaluation results of the areas listed below and a consideration of the age and gender of the patient/client, the need or lack of need for occupational therapy services is determined based on occupational dysfunction indicated by problems in the occupational performance skill areas or in occupational performance subskills.

A. <u>Occupational performance skill areas</u>	<u>Determined by:</u>
Self-care/self-maintenance	Observation of performance
Work/education	Interview/questionnaire
Play/leisure	History taking/review
Rest/relaxation	Testing (standardized and
	nonstandardized) of self-care, time
	utilization, job/work, other
B. <u>Occupational performance subskills</u>	<u>Determined by:</u>
Neurosensory function	Observation of performance
Physical/motor performance	Interview/questionnaire
Psychological state/skills	History taking/review
Social/interpersonal skills/adaptation	Testing specific to performance, subskills,
	functions for specific age groups
C. <u>Environmental factors</u>	<u>Determined by:</u>
Physical setting (home, job)	Results from above assessments and
Support system (family, friends, agencies, etc.)	community/home survey
Culture	
Religion/spiritual system	
Socioeconomic status	
General community aspects (mores, values, etc.)	

Goal Setting
If treatment is needed, whether for prevention, modification of behavior, maintenance, habilitation, or rehabilitation, then *intervention should begin at the level(s) at which the patient/client can succeed and/or benefit.* The patient/client should be actively involved in the selection and establishment of goals. These goals should then be *monitored, graded, continuously re-evaluated,* and changed, as necessary.

continues

Exhibit 4-1 Continued

Intervention/Treatment
Treatment/intervention includes enabling purposeful and functional activity and enhancement of sensory, motor, psychological, social/interpersonal, and cognitive abilities. It also includes a variety of activities to facilitate self-care, pre-work and work, education, and play/recreation/ leisure performance. Intervention occurs on a one-to-one basis, in small and large groups, and through indirect learning experiences to facilitate change in the desired direction(s). Multiple options are given for selection and choice to involve the person actively in the treatment/intervention process. Rehabilitation may include the use of adaptive equipment, splinting, and other compensatory techniques to assist the patient/client to achieve his/her highest level of function in all possible areas.

Outcome(s)
Learning of new functions/activities (habilitation)
Maintenance of present function (maintenance)
Restoration of function (rehabilitation)
Improvement of function (rehabilitation)
Loss of function (with adaptation as loss occurs)

Research
Research is needed in all phases of this process for validation.

Source: Adapted from A. Killingsworth, L.A. Llorens, M. Southam, J. Down, and K. Schwartz (1992). Course reader, OCTH 113: *Human adaptation.* Department of Occupational Therapy, San Jose State University, San Jose, CA. Reproduced with permission of Lela A. Llorens.

or indirect service basis. Intervention is a dynamic process and is developmentally based. It is begun at the level at which the client can succeed or benefit and is monitored, graded, continuously evaluated, and changed accordingly. Outcomes of intervention are observed as improvement of function, restoration of function, maintenance of function, and/or retrogression of function.

Activity and Activity Analysis

Llorens (1970) described the OT process as the "skilled application of activities and relationships" (p. 94). She explained why occupational therapists use activities, tasks, and occupations and how these activities make a difference in a client's functioning (Llorens, 1981b, 1981c). She described activity programs for emotionally disturbed children (Llorens & Bernstein, 1963; Llorens & Rubin, 1962, 1965; Llorens & Young, 1960) and adolescent girls (Hardison & Llorens, 1988) and the use of activities in evaluation in child psychiatry (Llorens 1967b, 1967d).

In the application of activity, Llorens emphasized the need for gradation, the presentation of activity at the client's level, and the use of specific activities for specific goals (Llorens, 1967a; Llorens & Beck, 1966; Llorens & Johnson, 1966; Llorens & Rubin, 1962). She recommended that treatment procedures be activities that "begin at a level commensurate with the child's ability, allow for successful accomplishment and mastery, and present opportunities to raise the child's level of skill" (Llorens & Rubin, 1962, p. 287).

Activity analysis is used to guide the decision making in activity selection. By analyzing what is required to perform a task, activity, or occupation, the therapist can decide how a given task will meet certain therapeutic goals. Activity analysis provides the therapist with a rationale for what the activity does in the therapeutic process (Llorens, 1981b).

Llorens provides a framework (Figure 4-1) for analyzing activities (Llorens, 1973a, 1981b, 1986; Llorens & Burris, 1981) and for explaining the influence of activity on life task performance (Llorens, 1991). Activities, tasks, occupations, and personal interaction provide stimuli to the central nervous system (CNS). These activities or interactions have input to the CNS via the sensory systems: tactile, visual, auditory, vestibular, gustatory, and olfactory. These sensory systems can stimulate, facilitate, inhibit, or motivate thoughts, emotions, perceptions, or cognition in the CNS. This internal action of the CNS is observable through motor responses (or lack of responses) that are generated through muscular, joint,

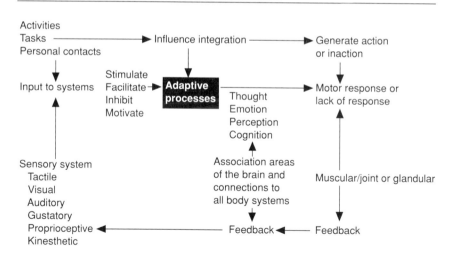

Figure 4-1 Influence of Activity on Human Performance. *Source:* From "Performance Tasks and Roles throughout the Life Span" by L.A. Llorens in *Occupational Therapy: Overcoming Human Performance Deficits*, C. Christiansen and C. Baum (Eds.), p. 50, 1991, Thorofare, NJ: Charles B. Slack, Inc. Copyright 1991 by Charles B. Slack, Inc. Reprinted by permission.

or glandular activity in the organism. This motor response generates feedback to the organism, which is conveyed to the CNS as new input. Llorens' activity analysis emphasizes the need for therapists to be aware of impact upon the organism when they introduce activities and interactions, and to be able to explain the rationale for using activity.

Occupational Performance and Occupational Performance Components

Llorens described *occupational performance areas and occupational performance components* as the focus of occupational therapy evaluation and intervention (Llorens, 1976, 1982a). These terms had first been defined in a terminology developed by the AOTA Task Force on Target Populations and published in the *Project to Delineate the Roles and Functions of Occupational Therapy Personnel* (AOTA, 1972). Their work had been an attempt to define the parameters of occupational therapy and to establish a uniform terminology for the profession. Llorens completed a comprehensive literature review on occupational performance and occupational performance components and has since developed these concepts (Llorens, 1982c, 1991).

In her descriptions of normal development, Llorens often refers to the concept of mastery as the means to achieve and to measure human development. It is mastery of developmental tasks that results in achievement of behavior expectations and adaptive skills. Although different phases of development gain primacy at specific periods of time during the developmental life span, Llorens (1970) believes that in order to "achieve in the adaptive areas of functioning, it is necessary . . . to experience satisfaction and mastery" in all areas of development (p. 95). Health and wellness are viewed in terms of the individual's ability to master developmental tasks successfully and thus achieve appropriate adaptive skills. This achievement is viewed as a healthy state, with recognition of normal deviations that may occur. Moreover, the "achievement of competence, mastery and adaptation is central to occupational performance" (Llorens, 1991, p. 46).

Llorens defines occupational performance as the "accomplishment of tasks related to self-care/self-maintenance; work/education; play/leisure; and rest/relaxation" (1991, p. 46). Occupational performance components or subskills, such as sensory perception, sensory integration, motor coordination, psychosocial and psychodynamic responses, sociocultural development, and social language responses, enable one to achieve competence, mastery, and adaptation in the tasks of occupational performance. These, in turn, enable one to function in one's occupational roles, such as worker, parent, sibling, or mate. (See Exhibit 4-2.) Llorens uses the concepts of occupational roles, occupational performance, and occupational performance enablers in her Developmental Analysis Evaluation and Intervention Schedule (1976) and her OT Sequential Client Care Record (1982c).

Exhibit 4-2 Levels of Mastery for Successful Adaptation

Level 3	**Occupational Roles** Worker • Student • Volunteer • Homemaker • Parent • Son • Daughter • Mate • Sibling • Peer • Best Friend/Chum
Level 2	**Activities and Tasks of** **Occupational Performance** Skill Areas: Self-Care/Self-Maintenance • Play/Leisure • Work/Education • Rest/Relaxation
Level 1	**Occupational Performance Enablers** Subskills: Sensory Perception • Sensory Integration • Motor Coordination • Psychosocial and Psychodynamic Responses • Sociocultural Development • Social Language Responses

Source: From "Performance Tasks and Roles throughout the Life Span" by L.A. Llorens in *Occupational Therapy: Overcoming Human Performance Deficits*, C. Christiansen and C. Baum (Eds.), p. 47, 1991, Thorofare, NJ: Charles B. Slack, Inc. Copyright 1991 by Charles B. Slack, Inc. Reprinted by permission.

Developmental Analysis Evaluation and Intervention Schedule (DAEIS)

In her book *Application of a Developmental Theory for Health and Rehabilitation*, Llorens (1976) restated her developmental theory and described its application to clients ranging from children to the elderly. She presented the Developmental Analysis Evaluation and Intervention Schedule (DAEIS) for use in developmental case analysis.

The DAEIS provides therapists with a framework for applying the developmental theory. It guides the therapist through the OT process and brings to conscious awareness the thinking processes that the therapist uses in evaluation and treatment planning. Using the DAEIS, the therapist considers the "client as a biological, psychological and social being" (Llorens, 1982c, p. 3); the OT goals; the areas of human development that are affected by the client's condition; and the OT evaluation and intervention approaches.

Llorens (1976) applied the DAEIS to 15 clients whose growth and development had been adversely affected. Her case analyses described clients of all ages and with varied areas of disruption. Occupational therapy tools used in the treatment or facilitation process were described, and standardized and nonstandardized assessment procedures were differentiated. Activity analysis provided the theoretical rationale for the use of sensorimotor activities, developmental activities, and interpersonal relationships.

OT Sequential Client Care Record (SCCR)

To improve the usefulness of the DAEIS as a data collection tool for occupational therapy, Llorens incorporated the Problem-Oriented Medical Record (POMR) (Weed, 1971) into the DAEIS to produce a client care record with a stronger scientific base. This became the Sequential Client Care Record (SCCR) (Llorens, 1982c). Subsequent research on the record's usefulness found that the variables of completeness, organizational sequence, and understandability for research and education were statistically significant (Llorens & Schuster, 1977).

The SCCR documents the OT process systematically while providing a viable communication tool to be used with colleagues, clients, and clients' families. It can be used to monitor quality care and accountability of OT services. The SCCR has served as an educational tool for occupational therapy students. Use of the SCCR as a record-keeping system for clients served in OT could potentially provide a large national data base for research (Llorens, 1982c).

APPLICATIONS TO THE OCCUPATIONAL THERAPY PROFESSION

OT Research

Llorens has promoted occupational therapy research in her academic career, her work with the American Occupational Therapy Foundation, and her publications. She recently co-authored a research guide for the health science professional (Oyster, Hanten, & Llorens, 1987). She has identified areas of research that need to be initiated by occupational therapists (Llorens, 1981d, 1984; Llorens & Gillette, 1985; Llorens & Snyder, 1987) and has encouraged professional responsibility in the area of research (Llorens, 1979, 1990; Llorens & Donaldson, 1983). Her OT Sequential Client Care Record provides a framework for collecting data for OT research.

Llorens has been a long-term advocate for the development of occupational therapy as an academic discipline, the science of "occupationology" (Llorens & Gillette, 1985). She has emphasized the need to define the existing body of OT knowledge and to validate and expand this knowledge through research. As she has stated:

> Within the practice of our profession, there are predictable aspects relative to cause and effect in the use of activities and the application of relationships which must be identified, applied repeatedly in a system-

atic manner, analyzed and documented in order to establish their validity. (1970, p. 101)

Three-Dimensional Model for Organizing OT Knowledge and the Study of OT

Llorens (1981b) proposed a three-dimensional model for organizing the knowledge and study of occupational therapy by client age or developmental stage, by practice phase, and by therapy techniques and outcomes (Figure 4-2). Occupational therapy client groups are organized into seven categories: infants, children, adolescents, young adults, middle adults, mature adults, and aged adults. Practice phases include prevention, treatment/therapy, and rehabilitation/health maintenance. Occupational therapy techniques can be organized into screening/evaluation, intervention, and outcomes. Llorens contends that ". . . occupational therapy has a rich body of knowledge that needs to be organized for study. Through categorization and classification, the body of knowledge becomes accessible for collective appraisal" (1981b, p. 10).

An example of how this three-dimensional model can be used for selecting and designing a study of an area of occupational therapy is included in Figure 4-3. First, the infant client group and the prevention phase of OT practice are selected as the areas for study from the first two dimensions of the model. Then a study is designed to investigate a question regarding screening and evaluation, intervention modalities, or therapy outcomes from the third dimension of the model. Thus a given study would address one unit of the model: for example, therapy outcomes of OT prevention with infants.

OT Education

Llorens has served as a leader in OT education throughout her academic career. Her publications in this area cover such topics as student learning and growth (Llorens, 1967c, 1982b; Llorens & Adams, 1976) and educator competency (Canfield, Williams, Llorens, & Wroe, 1973; Llorens, 1981a, 1982a).

OT Consulting

Drawing on her background as a consultant in community health practice, Llorens wrote several articles to guide other OTs in the same field. She described the OT's consulting role (1973b, 1992a) and outlined a problem-solving process that consultants could use to determine how OT could best serve a new environment. In these publications, Llorens emphasized that the key to success in commu-

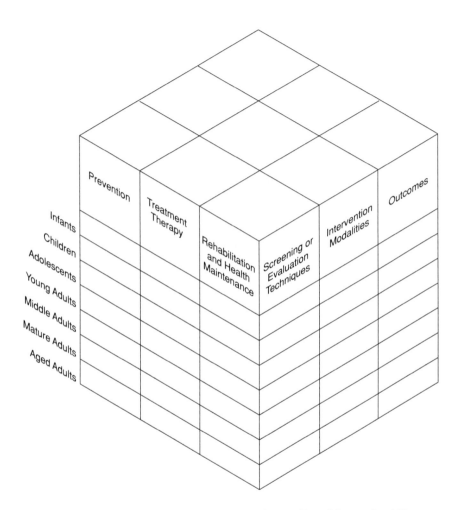

Figure 4-2 Categorization of Practice Technology. *Source:* From "Occupational Therapy: State of the Art, Potential for Development" by L.A. Llorens in *Proceedings of the New Zealand Association of Occupational Therapists Annual Conference*, p. 13, 1981, Auckland, New Zealand: New Zealand Association of Occupational Therapists. Reprinted by permission.

nity health practice was the therapist's appreciation of the cultural milieu of the clients. Knowledge of clients' ethnic characteristics, socioeconomic status, and value system was needed in order to communicate effectively with clients and negotiate within their community.

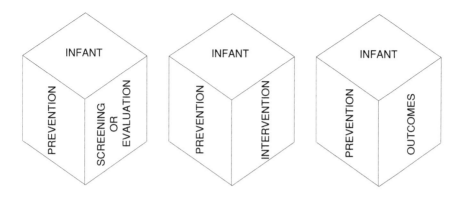

	Prevention	Screening/ Evaluation	Intervention	Outcomes
SCREENING/ EVALUATION	Identify risks for dysfunction in occupational performance and occupational performance components	Universal techniques plus infant tests		
INTERVENTION	Prevent dysfunction in occupational performance and occupational performance components specific to infancy		Activity prescription and administration, rehabilitation aids, adaptive equipment, counseling specific to infancy	
OUTCOMES	Prevent dysfunction in occupational performance and occupational performance components			Functioning at highest potential

Figure 4-3 Example of Llorens' "3-Dimensional Schemata for Knowledge Organization" in Which Knowledge in the Area of Prevention and the Age Group of Infancy Can Be Addressed in Terms of Screening/Evaluation, Intervention, or Outcomes

CRITIQUE

A critical analysis of Llorens' developmental theory reveals several identifiable strengths. The theory has made an enduring and significant contribution to the field of occupational therapy. It provides a frame of reference that is applicable to all clients along the developmental continuum and a framework that the occupational therapist can use to conceptualize his or her practice. A review of Llorens' publications reveals her consistency, her common sense, and a distinct progression and refinement of her theoretical constructs. Llorens organizes material in a logical, clear, and orderly fashion and presents schematic representations that lend visual clarity to her concepts.

Llorens' commitment to writing, research, and education has enhanced her theory's credibility by making it accessible to the profession. She circulates her information to new audiences by selecting a variety of communication methods, such as workshops, journals, newsletters, and lectureships, to convey her concepts. Through these modes, Llorens has contributed to making theory development an integral aspect of OT knowledge generation and practice.

A deliberate process of educational advances and career moves reveals Llorens' career development to be that of an organized and goal-directed professional. Preparation, planning, and timetables have been integral parts of her decision making. These organizational skills have helped her complete numerous publications and participate in many professional activities. Her roles have been varied and have included such titles as distinguished lecturer, consultant, chair, board member, grants reviewer, division editor, visiting scholar, principal investigator, and wife and mother.

Although her theory purports to be applicable to clients of all ages, it can be more easily applied to the younger client. This weakness stems from the lack of human growth and development research that was available on the adult when the theory was first developed. Llorens (1970) alluded to this weakness in the theory's initial presentation as an Eleanor Clarke Slagle lecture.

Many of the concepts in Llorens' theory have long been accepted by the OT profession, but these concepts have not yet been clearly substantiated or refuted through systematic study. An inherent weakness in theory development exists when the hierarchy on which it is built is not scientifically consistent.

Therapists seeking techniques for evaluation and treatment may find Llorens' theory lacking because she has not created new modalities. Instead, she has provided a way to describe and conceptualize the OT process, a way "to think through the function and purpose of occupational therapy as [she has] experienced it" (Llorens, 1970, p. 93). As she states:

> The theory has served me well as a way to conceptualize occupational
> therapy and to approach patients, both as practitioner and in attempting

to teach the practice discipline to undergraduate and graduate students. (L.A. Llorens, personal communication, September 2, 1983)

Future of Occupational Therapy

In speculating on the future direction of occupational therapy, Llorens hypothesizes that occupational therapy will "identify a common core from the numerous formulations that have been advanced . . . synthesized and analyzed . . . [and] will emerge with a universal theory of occupational therapy" (L.A. Llorens, personal communication, September 2, 1983). More than one frame of reference will be applied to different populations. Through this organizational process, the profession will be able to identify and organize evaluation and intervention techniques that are "congruent with the theoretical base and frames that are established" (L.A. Llorens, personal communication, September 2, 1983).

Dr. Lela A. Llorens has contributed greatly to the OT profession. She has advanced the philosophical idea of a universal theory for the profession, and she has contributed to this theory herself by organizing the principles and concepts of a developmental theory. When asked, "What advice would you give to therapists struggling to identify their professional frame of reference?" she replied:

> Try to be in touch with what you have been doing right as a practicing therapist . . . recognize the history of occupational therapy and theory development, there is more of that available to look at now, than there was. . . . It is important to struggle with the analysis and synthesis of one's own practice, values, and belief systems and to try to know what those are in relationship to the prevailing theoretical frames of reference, and theory of occupational therapy. What you will find is that the ideas that you have and the values you have shared are common with many who have written or with whom you are working. You will begin to be able to identify with the community of occupational therapy, rather than seeing yourself as an isolated therapist in a practice setting. (L.A. Llorens, personal communication, September 2, 1983)

REFERENCES

American Occupational Therapy Association (1972). *Project to delineate the roles and functions of occupational therapy personnel.* Rockville, MD: Author

Beck, G.R., Rubin, E.Z., Braun, J.S., Llorens, L.A., Beall, D., & Mottley, N. (1965). Educational aspects of cognitive-perceptual motor functions in children—A suggested change in approach. *Psychology in Schools, 2*(3), 233–238.

Bolding, D.J., & Llorens, L.A. (1991). The effects of habilitative hospital admission on self-care, self-esteem and frequency of physical care. *American Journal of Occupational Therapy, 45,* 796–800.

Braun, J.S., Rubin, E.Z., Llorens, L.A., & Beck, G.R. (1967). Cognitive motor deficits—Definition and intervention. *Proceedings of the International Convention on Learning Disabilities.* Pittsburgh: Crippled Children's Home.

Braun, J.S., Rubin, E.Z., Llorens, L.A., Beck, G.R., Beall, D., & Mottley, N. (1965). Cognitive perceptual motor function in school children: A suggested change in approach. *Journal of School Psychology, 3,* 1–5.

Canfield, A.A., Williams, M.R., Llorens L.A., & Wroe, M.C. (1973). Competencies for allied health educators. *Journal of Allied Health, 2* (4), 180–186.

Hames-Hahn, C.S., & Llorens, L.A. (1989). Impact of a multisensory occupational therapy program on components of self-feeding behavior in the elderly. *Physical and Occupational Therapy in Geriatrics, 6* (3/4), 63–86.

Hardison, J., & Llorens, L.A. (1988). Structured craft group activities for adolescent girls. *Occupational Therapy in Mental Health, 8* (3), 101–118.

Killingsworth, A., Llorens, L.A., Southam, M., Down, J., & Schwartz, K. (1992). *Course reader, OCTH 113: Human adaptation.* Department of Occupational Therapy, San Jose State University, San Jose, CA.

Llorens, L.A. (1960). Psychological tests in planning treatment goals. *American Journal of Occupational Therapy, 14,* 243–246.

Llorens, L.A. (1961). Bridging the gap: Vocational rehabilitation counseling in a psychiatric setting. *Michigan Rehabilitation Association Digest, 2,* 24–26.

Llorens, L.A. (1966a). Aspects of pre-vocational evaluation with psychiatric patients. *Canadian Journal of Occupational Therapy, 33,* 5–12.

Llorens, L.A. (1966b). Cognitive-perceptual-motor dysfunction. Evaluation and training. In J.M. Kiernat (Ed.), *Perceptual motor dysfunction evaluation and training* (pp. 271–292). Madison, WI: University of Wisconsin.

Llorens, L.A. (1967a). Cognitive-perceptual-motor dysfunction and training. *Selected papers from professional program segments of the United Cerebral Palsy's Annual Conference.* New Orleans: United Cerebral Palsy Association.

Llorens, L.A. (1967b). An evaluation procedure for children 6 to 10 years of age. *American Journal of Occupational Therapy, 21,* 64–69.

Llorens, L.A. (1967c). Gauging emotional, intellectual and professional growth in students. *Educational Newsletter, 2* (2), 2.

Llorens, L.A. (1967d). Projective technique in occupational therapy. *American Journal of Occupational Therapy, 21,* 226–229.

Llorens, L.A. (1968a). Changing methods in treatment of psychosocial dysfunction. *American Journal of Occupational Therapy, 22,* 26–29.

Llorens, L.A. (1968b). Identification of the Ayres' syndrome in children with behavior maladjustment. *American Journal of Occupational Therapy, 22,* 286–288.

Llorens, L.A. (1970). Facilitating growth and development: The promise of occupational therapy. Eleanor Clarke Slagle lecture. *American Journal of Occupational Therapy, 24,* 93–101

Llorens, L.A. (1971a). Black culture and child development. *American Journal of Occupational Therapy, 25,* 144–148.

Llorens, L.A. (1971b). Occupational therapy in community child health. *American Journal of Occupational Therapy, 25,* 335–339.

Llorens, L.A. (1972). Problem-solving the role of occupational therapy in a new environment. *American Journal of Occupational Therapy, 26,* 234–238.

Llorens, L.A. (1973a). Activity analysis for cognitive-perceptual-motor dysfunction. *American Journal of Occupational Therapy, 27*, 453–456.

Llorens, L.A. (Ed.). (1973b). *Consultation in the community: Occupational therapy in child health.* Dubuque, IA: Kendall-Hunt Publishing.

Llorens, L.A. (1974). Learning disability, occupational therapy and community programming. *Proceedings of the Sixth International Congress World Federation of Occupational Therapists*, World Federation of Occupational Therapy.

Llorens, L.A. (1975). Consultation in occupational therapy programs for children. *Canadian Journal of Occupational Therapy, 41*, 114–116.

Llorens, L.A. (1976). *Application of a developmental theory for health and rehabilitation.* Rockville, MD: American Occupational Therapy Association.

Llorens, L.A. (1977). A developmental theory revisited. *American Journal of Occupational Therapy, 31*, 656–657.

Llorens, L.A. (1979). Thinking research in occupational therapy. *Development Disabilities SIS Newsletter, 2*, 1.

Llorens, L.A. (1981a). Maintaining credibility: The academic occupational therapist. *OT Education Bulletin*, 10–11.

Llorens, L.A. (1981b). Occupational therapy: State-of-the-art, potential for development. *Proceedings of the New Zealand Occupational Therapy Association* (pp. 9–17). Auckland, New Zealand: Aukland Metro.

Llorens, L.A. (1981c). On the meaning of activity in occupational therapy. *Journal of the New Zealand Association of Occupational Therapists, 32*, 3–6.

Llorens, L.A. (1981d). Research in occupational therapy: The need, the response. *Occupational Therapy Journal of Research, 1*, 3–6.

Llorens L.A. (1981e). The role of occupational therapy in vocational rehabilitation. *Mental Health Special Interest Section Newsletter, 4* (3).

Llorens, L.A. (1982a). Continuing clinical competency for the occupational therapy educator. *Journal of the New Zealand Association of Occupational Therapists*, Summer.

Llorens, L.A. (1982b). Facilitating achievement of higher level behaviors. In J.H. Henry (Ed.), *Readings in clinical education: A resource manual for clinical instructors.* Augusta, GA: Medical College of Georgia.

Llorens, L.A. (1982c). *Occupational therapy sequential client care record.* Laurel, MD: Ramsco Publishing.

Llorens, L.A. (1983). The DSM III, sensory integration and child psychiatry: Implications for treatment and research. *Sensory Integration Special Interest Section Newsletter, 6* (1), 2.

Llorens, L.A. (1984). Changing balance: Environment and individual. *American Journal of Occupational Therapy, 38*, 29–34.

Llorens, L.A. (1986). Activity analysis: Agreement among factors in a sensory processing model. *American Journal of Occupational Therapy, 40*, 103–110.

Llorens, L.A. (Ed.). (1988). *Health care for ethnic elders: The cultural context.* Proceedings of Stanford Geriatric Education Center Conference. (Available from Stanford Geriatric Education Center, 703 Welch Road, Palo Alto, CA 94305.)

Llorens, L.A. (1990). Research utilization: A personal/professional responsibility. *Occupational Therapy Journal of Research, 10* (1), 3–6.

Llorens, L.A. (1991). Performance tasks and roles throughout the life span. In C. Christiansen & C. Baum (Eds.), *Occupational therapy: Overcoming human performance deficits* (pp. 45–66). Thorofare, NJ: Charles B. Slack.

Llorens, L.A. (1992a). Program consultation for children and adults. In E. Jaffe & C.F. Epstein (Eds.), *Occupational therapy consultation: Theory, principles and practice* (pp. 356–363). St. Louis, MO: C.V. Mosby.

Llorens, L.A. (1992b). Roles for occupational therapist consultation in higher education. In E. Jaffe & C.F. Epstein (Eds.), *Occupational therapy consultation: Theory, principles and practice* (pp. 496–500). St Louis, MO: C.V. Mosby.

Llorens, L.A., & Adams, S.P. (1976). Entering behavior: Student learning styles. In C.W. Ford & M.K. Morgan (Eds.), *Teaching in the allied health professions* (pp. 86–93). St. Louis: C.V. Mosby.

Llorens, L.A., & Beck, G.R. (1966). Treatment methods for cognitive-perceptual motor dysfunction. In M.J. Fehr (Ed.), *Normal growth and development with deviations in the perceptual motor and emotional areas* (pp. 155–177). St. Louis, MO: Washington University.

Llorens, L.A., & Bernstein, S.P. (1963). Fingerpainting for the compulsive child. *American Journal of Occupational Therapy, 17,* 120–121.

Llorens, L.A., & Burris, B. (1981). Development of sensory integration in learning disabled children. In J. Gottlieb & S. Strichart (Eds.), *Development theories and research in learning disabilities* (pp. 57–79). Baltimore: University Park Press.

Llorens, L.A., & Donaldson, K. (1983). Documentation of occupational therapy: A process model. *Canadian Journal of Occupational Therapy, 50,* 171–175.

Llorens, L.A., & Gillette, N.P. (1985). Nationally speaking: The challenge for research in a practice profession. *American Journal of Occupational Therapy, 39,* 143–146.

Llorens, L.A., Hikoyeda, N., & Yeo, G. (Eds.). (1992). Diabetes among elders: Ethnic considerations. *Proceedings of Stanford Geriatric Education Center Conference.* (Stanford Geriatric Education Center, 703 Welch Road, Palo Alto, CA 94305, available on request.)

Llorens, L.A., & Johnson, P.A. (1966). Occupational therapy in ego-oriented milieu. *American Journal of Occupational Therapy, 20,* 178–181.

Llorens, L.A., Levy, R., & Rubin, E.Z. (1964). The work adjustment program: A prevocational experience. *American Journal of Occupational Therapy, 18,* 15–19.

Llorens, L.A., & Rubin, E.Z. (1961). Occupational therapy is therapeutic: A research study with emotionally disturbed children. *Proceedings of 1961 AOTA National Conference.* Detroit, MI: American Occupational Therapy Association.

Llorens, L.A., & Rubin, E.Z. (1962). A directed activity program for disturbed children. *American Journal of Occupational Therapy, 16,* 287–290.

Llorens, L.A., & Rubin, E.Z. (1965). A directed activity program for emotionally disturbed children. In J.C. Gowan & G.D. Demos (Eds.), *The guidance of exceptional children* (pp. 168–174). New York: David McKay.

Llorens, L.A., & Rubin, E.Z. (1967). *Developing ego functions in disturbed children: Occupational therapy milieu.* Detroit, MI: Wayne State University Press.

Llorens, L.A., Rubin, E.Z., Braun, J.S., Beck, G.R., & Beall, C.D. (1969). The effects of cognitive-perceptual-motor training approach on children with behavior maladjustment. *American Journal of Occupational Therapy, 23,* 502–512.

Llorens, L.A., Rubin, E.Z., Braun, J.S., Mottley, N., & Beall, D. (1964). Training in cognitive-perceptual-motor functions: A preliminary report. *American Journal of Occupational Therapy, 18,* 202–209.

Llorens, L.A., & Schuster, J.J. (1977). Occupational therapy client care recording system: A comparative study. *American Journal of Occupational Therapy, 31*, 367–371.

Llorens, L.A., & Sieg, K.W. (1975). A profile for managing sensory integrative test data. *American Journal of Occupational Therapy, 29*, 205–208.

Llorens, L.A., & Snyder, N.V. (1987). Nationally speaking: Research initiatives for occupational therapy. *American Journal of Occupational Therapy, 41*, 491–493.

Llorens, L.A., & Young, G.G. (1960). Fingerpainting for the hostile child. *American Journal of Occupational Therapy, 14*, 306–307.

McCormack, G., Llorens, L., & Glogoski, C. (1991). The culturally diverse elderly. In J. Kiernat (Ed.), *Occupational therapy for the older adult: A clinical manual* (pp. 11–24). Gaithersburg, MD: Aspen Publishers.

Oyster, C.K., Hanten, W.P., & Llorens, L.A. (1987). *Introduction to research: A guide for the health science professional.* Philadelphia: J.B. Lippincott.

Robertson, S.C. (1992). *Find a mentor or be one.* Rockville, MD: American Occupational Therapy Association.

Ross, H.S., Washington, W.N., & Llorens, L.A. (1990). Health promotion in a multicultural community. *Health Education*, March/April.

Rubin, E.Z., Braun, J.S., Beck, G.R., & Llorens, L.A. (1972). *Cognitive-perceptual motor dysfunction: From research to practice.* Detroit, MI: Wayne State University Press.

Shiotsuka, W., Burton, G., Pedretti, L., & Llorens, L.A. (In press). An examination of performance scores on activities of daily living between elders with right and left cerebrovascular accident. *Physical and Occupational Therapy in Geriatrics.*

Weed, L.L. (1971). *Medical records, medical education and patient care.* Chicago: Year Book Medical Publishers.

BIBLIOGRAPHY

1960

Llorens, L.A. (1960). Psychological tests in planning treatment goals. *American Journal of Occupational Therapy, 14*, 243–246.

Llorens, L.A., & Young, G.G. (1960). Fingerpainting for the hostile child. *American Journal of Occupational Therapy, 14*, 306–307.

1961

Llorens, L.A. (1961). Bridging the gap: Vocational rehabilitation counseling in a psychiatric setting. *Michigan Rehabilitation Association Digest, 2*, 24–26.

Llorens, L.A., & Rubin, E.Z. (1961). Occupational therapy is therapeutic: A research study with emotionally disturbed children. *Proceedings of 1961 AOTA National Conference.* Detroit, MI: American Occupational Therapy Association.

1962

Llorens, L.A., & Rubin, E.Z. (1962). A directed activity program for disturbed children. *American Journal of Occupational Therapy, 16*, 287–290.

1963

Llorens, L.A., & Bernstein, S.P. (1963). Fingerpainting for the compulsive child. *American Journal of Occupational Therapy, 17*, 120–121.

1964

Llorens, L.A., Levy, R., & Rubin, E.Z. (1964). The work adjustment program: A prevocational experience. *American Journal of Occupational Therapy, 18*, 15–19.

Llorens, L.A., Rubin, E.Z., Braun, J.S., Mottley, N., & Beall, D. (1964). Training in cognitive-perceptual-motor functions: A preliminary report. *American Journal of Occupational Therapy, 18*, 202–209.

1965

Beck, G.R., Rubin, E.Z., Braun, J.S., Llorens, L.A., Beall, D., & Mottley, N. (1965). Educational aspects of cognitive-perceptual motor functions in children—A suggested change in approach. *Psychology in Schools, 2* (3), 233–238.

Braun, J.S., Rubin, E.Z., Llorens, L.A., Beck, G.R., Beall, D., & Mottley, N. (1965). Cognitive perceptual motor function in school children: A suggested change in approach. *Journal of School Psychology, 3*, 1–5.

Llorens, L.A., & Rubin, E.Z. (1965). A directed activity program for emotionally disturbed children. In J.C. Gowan & G.D. Demos (Eds.), *The guidance of exceptional children* (pp. 168–174). New York: David McKay.

1966

Llorens, L.A. (1966). Aspects of pre-vocational evaluation with psychiatric patients. *Canadian Journal of Occupational Therapy, 33*, 5–12.

Llorens, L.A. (1966). Cognitive-perceptual-motor dysfunction. Evaluation and training. In J.M. Kiernat (Ed.), *Perceptual motor dysfunction evaluation and training* (pp. 271–292). Madison, WI: University of Wisconsin .

Llorens, L.A., & Beck, G.R. (1966). Treatment methods for cognitive-perceptual motor dysfunction. In M.J. Fehr (Ed.), *Normal growth and development with deviations in the perceptual motor and emotional areas* (pp. 155–177). St. Louis, MO: Washington University.

Llorens, L.A., & Johnson, P.A. (1966). Occupational therapy in ego-oriented milieu. *American Journal of Occupational Therapy, 20*, 178–181.

1967

Braun, J.S., Rubin, E.Z., Llorens, L.A., & Beck, G.R. (1967). Cognitive motor deficits—Definition and intervention. *Proceedings of the International Convocation on Learning Disabilities.* Pittsburgh: Crippled Children's Home.

Llorens, L.A. (1967). Cognitive-perceptual-motor dysfunction and training. *Selected papers from professional program segments of the United Cerebral Palsy's Annual Conference.* New Orleans: United Cerebral Palsy Association.

Llorens, L.A. (1967). An evaluation procedure for children 6 to 10 years of age. *American Journal of Occupational Therapy, 21*, 64–69.

Llorens, L.A. (1967). Gauging emotional, intellectual and professional growth in students. *Educational Newsletter, 2*(2), 2.

Llorens, L.A. (1967). Projective technique in occupational therapy. *American Journal of Occupational Therapy, 21*, 226–229.

Llorens, L.A., & Rubin, E.Z. (1967). *Developing ego functions in disturbed children: Occupational therapy on milieu.* Detroit, MI: Wayne State University Press.

1968

Llorens, L.A. (1968). Changing methods in treatment of psychosocial dysfunction. *American Journal of Occupational Therapy, 22*, 26–29.

Llorens, L.A. (1968). Identification of the Ayres' syndrome in children with behavior maladjustment. *American Journal of Occupational Therapy, 22*, 286–288.

1969

Llorens, L.A. (1969). The role of the occupational therapist in a children and youth project. *Proceedings of the National Conference of Children and Youth Projects*, Southern California Occupational Therapy Association.

Llorens, L.A. (1969). The occupational therapist in a community health program. *Proceedings of SCOTA Annual Conference.*

Llorens, L.A., Rubin, E.Z., Braun, J.S., Beck, G.R., & Beall, C.D. (1969). The effects of cognitive-perceptual-motor training approach on children with behavior maladjustment. *American Journal of Occupational Therapy, 23*, 502–512.

1970

Llorens, L.A. (1970). Facilitating growth and development: The promise of occupational therapy. Eleanor Clarke Slagle lecture. *American Journal of Occupational Therapy, 24*, 93–101.

1971

Llorens, L.A. (1971). Black culture and child development. *American Journal of Occupational Therapy, 25*, 144–148.

Llorens, L.A. (1971). Occupational therapy in community child health. *American Journal of Occupational Therapy, 25*, 335–339.

1972

Llorens, L.A. (1972). Facilitating growth and development: The promise of occupational therapy. In *Eleanor Clarke Slagle Lectures 1966–1972* (pp. 191–208). Dubuque, IA: Kendall Hunt Publishing.

Llorens, L.A. (1972). Problem-solving the role of occupational therapy in a new environment. *American Journal of Occupational Therapy, 26*, 234–238.

Rubin, E.Z., Braun, J.S., Beck, G.R., & Llorens, L.A. (1972). *Cognitive-perceptual motor dysfunction: From research to practice.* Detroit, MI: Wayne State University Press.

1973

Canfield, A.A., Williams, M.R., Llorens, L.A., & Wroe, M.C. (1973). Competencies for allied health educators. *Journal of Allied Health, 2* (4), 180–186.

Llorens, L.A. (1973). Activity analysis for cognitive-perceptual-motor dysfunction. *American Journal of Occupational Therapy, 27*, 453–456.

Llorens, L.A. (1973). A case presentation: Billy. In E.K. Oremland & J.D. Oremland (Eds.), *Effects of hospitalization on children.* Springfield, IL: Charles C Thomas.

Llorens, L.A. (Ed.). (1973). *Consultation in the community: Occupational therapy in child health.* Dubuque, IA: Kendall-Hunt Publishing.

Llorens, L.A. (1973). What journal editors want. In M.K. Morgan, D.M. Filson, & A.A. Canfield (Eds.), *Publishing in the health professions.* Gainesville, FL: University of Florida.

1974

Henderson, A., Llorens, L., Gilfoyle, E., Myers, C., & Prevel, S. (Eds.). (1974). *The development of sensory integrative theory and practice.* Dubuque, IA: Kendall-Hunt Publishing.

Llorens, L.A. (1974). The effects of stress on growth and development. *American Journal of Occupational Therapy, 28*, 82–86.

Llorens, L.A. (1974). Learning disability, occupational therapy and community programming. *Proceedings of the Sixth International Congress World Federation of Occupational Therapists.*

1975

Llorens, L.A. (1975). Consultation in occupational therapy programs for children. *Canadian Journal of Occupational Therapy, 41,* 114–116.

Llorens, L.A. (1975). Occupational therapy consultation in community programs for children. *Proceedings from Consultation in the Community: A Conference for Occupational Therapists.*

Llorens, L.A., & Sieg, K.W. (1975). A profile for managing sensory integrative test data. *American Journal of Occupational Therapy, 29,* 205–208.

1976

Llorens, L.A. (1976). *Application of a developmental theory for health and rehabilitation.* Rockville, MD: American Occupational Therapy Association.

Llorens, L.A., & Adams, S.P. (1976). Entering behavior: Student learning styles. In C.W. Ford & M.K. Morgan (Eds.), *Teaching in the allied health profession* (pp. 86–93). St. Louis: C.V. Mosby.

1977

Llorens, L.A. (1977). A developmental theory revisited. *American Journal of Occupational Therapy, 31,* 656–657.

Llorens, L.A., & Schuster, J.J. (1977). Occupational therapy client care recording system: A comparative study. *American Journal of Occupational Therapy, 31,* 367–371.

1978

Llorens, L.A., & Adams, S.P. (1978). Learning style preferences of occupational therapy students. *American Journal of Occupational Therapy, 32,* 161–164.

1979

Llorens, L.A. (1979). Thinking research in occupational therapy. *Development Disabilities SIS Newsletter, 2,* 1.

1981

Llorens, L.A. (1981). Maintaining credibility: The academic occupational therapist. *OT Education Bulletin,* 10–11.

Llorens, L.A. (1981). Occupational therapy: State-of-the-art, potential for development. *Proceedings of the New Zealand Occupational Therapy Association* (pp. 9–17). Auckland, New Zealand: Aukland Metro.

Llorens, L.A. (1981). On the meaning of activity in occupational therapy. *Journal of the New Zealand Association of Occupational Therapists, 32,* 3–6.

Llorens L.A. (1981). Research in occupational therapy: The need, the response. *Occupational Therapy Journal of Research, 1,* 3–6.

Llorens, L.A. (1981). The role of occupational therapy in vocational rehabilitation. *Mental Health Special Interest Section Newsletter, 4* (3).

Llorens, L.A., & Burris, B. (1981). Development of sensory integration in learning disabled children. In J. Gottlieb & S. Strichart (Eds.), *Development theories and research in learning disabilities* (pp. 57–79). Baltimore: University Park Press.

1982

Llorens, L.A. (1982). Continuing clinical competency for the occupational therapy educator. *Journal of the New Zealand Association of Occupational Therapists*, Summer.

Llorens, L.A. (1982). Facilitating achievement of higher level behaviors. In J.H. Henry (Ed.), *Readings in clinical education: A resource manual for clinical instructors*. Augusta, GA: Medical College of Georgia.

Llorens, L.A. (1982). *Occupational therapy sequential client care record*. Laurel, MD: Ramsco Publishing.

1983

Llorens, L.A. (1983). The DSM III. Sensory integration and child psychiatry: Implications for treatment and research. *Sensory Integration Special Interest Section Newsletter, 6* (1), 2.

Llorens, L.A. (1983). Educating for professional competence: Accountability theory in practice. *Journal of the New Zealand Association of Occupational Therapists*, Winter.

Llorens, L.A., & Donaldson, K. (1983). Documentation of occupational therapy: A process model. *Canadian Journal of Occupational Therapy, 50*, 171–175.

1984

Llorens, L.A. (1984). Changing balance: Environment and individual. *American Journal of Occupational Therapy, 38*, 29–34.

Llorens, L.A. (1984). Semantic uses of "sensory integration" questioned. *Occupational Therapy Journal of Research, 4* (3), 244–245.

Llorens, L.A. (1984). Theoretical conceptualizations of occupational therapy: 1960–1982. *Occupational Therapy in Mental Health, 4*, 1–13.

Llorens, L.A., Ward, J.M., Still, J.R, & Eyler, R.K. (1984). The role of professional education for occupational therapy. *Occupational Therapy Education Bulletin*, Spring, 6–9.

1985

Llorens, L.A., & Gillette, N.P. (1985). Nationally speaking: The challenge for research in a practice profession. *American Journal of Occupational Therapy, 39*, 143–146.

1986

Llorens, L.A. (1986). Activity analysis: Agreement among factors in a sensory processing model. *American Journal of Occupational Therapy, 40*, 103–110.

Llorens, L.A. (1986). An analysis of occupational therapy theoretical approaches for mental health: Are the profession's major treatment approaches truly occupational therapy? A response. *American Journal of Occupational Therapy, 40*, 103–110.

1987

Llorens, L.A., & Snyder, N.V. (1987). Nationally speaking: Research initiatives for occupational therapy. *American Journal of Occupational Therapy, 41*, 491–493.

Oyster, C.K., Hanten, W.P., & Llorens, L.A. (1987). *Introduction to research: A guide for the health science professional*. Philadelphia: J.B. Lippincott.

1988

Hardison, J., & Llorens, L.A. (1988). Structured craft group activities for adolescent girls. *Occupational Therapy in Mental Health, 8* (3), 101–118.

Llorens, L.A. (Ed.). (1988). *Health care for ethnic elders: The cultural context.* Proceedings of Stanford Geriatric Education Center Conference. (Available from Stanford Geriatric Education Center, 703 Welch Road, Palo Alto, CA 94305.)

1989

Hames-Hahn, C.S., & Llorens, L.A. (1989). Impact of a multisensory occupational therapy program on components of self-feeding behavior in the elderly. *Physical and Occupational Therapy in Geriatrics, 6* (3/4), 63–86.

Kibele, A., & Llorens, L.A. (1989). Going to the source: The use of qualitative methodology in a study of the needs of adults with cerebral palsy. *Occupational therapy in health care. Developmental disabilities: A handbook for occupational therapists.* New York: Haworth Press.

Llorens, L.A. (1989). Health care system models and occupational therapy. *Occupational Therapy in Health Care, 5* (4).

1990

Llorens, L.A. (1990). Research utilization: A personal/professional responsibility. *Occupational Therapy Journal of Research, 10* (1), 3–6.

Ross, H.S., Washington, W.N., & Llorens, L.A. (1990). Health promotion in a multicultural community. *Health Education*, March/April.

1991

Bolding, D.J., & Llorens, L.A. (1991). The effects of habilitative hospital admission on self-care, self-esteem and frequency of physical care. *American Journal of Occupational Therapy, 45*, 796–800.

Llorens, L.A. (1991). Performance tasks and roles throughout the life span. In C. Christiansen & C. Baum (Eds.), *Occupational therapy: Overcoming human performance deficits* (pp. 45–66). Thorofare, NJ: Charles B. Slack.

McCormack, G., Llorens, L., & Glogoski, C. (1991). The culturally diverse elderly. In J. Kiernat (Ed.), *Occupational therapy for the older adult: A clinical manual* (pp. 11–24). Gaithersburg, MD: Aspen Publishers.

1992

Killingsworth, A., Llorens, L.A., Southam, M., Down, J., & Schwartz, K. (1992). *Course reader, OCTH 1131: Human adaptation.* Department of Occupational Therapy, San Jose State University, San Jose, CA.

Llorens, L.A. (1992). Program consultation for children and adults. In E. Jaffe & C.F. Epstein (Eds.), *Occupational therapy consultation: Theory, principles and practice* (pp. 356–363). St Louis, MO: C.V. Mosby.

Llorens, L.A. (1992). Roles for occupational therapist consultation in higher education. In E. Jaffe & C.F. Epstein (Eds.), *Occupational therapy consultation: Theory, principles and practice* (pp. 496–500). St Louis, MO: C.V. Mosby.

Llorens, L.A., Hikoyeda, N., & Yeo, G. (Eds.). (1992). Diabetes among elders: Ethnic considerations. *Proceedings of Stanford Geriatric Education Center Conference.* (Available from Stanford Geriatric Education Center, 703 Welch Road, Palo Alto, CA 94305.)

Shiotsuka, W., Burton, G., Pedretti, L., & Llorens, L.A. (In press). An examination of performance scores on activities of daily living between elders with right and left cerebrovascular accident. *Physical and Occupational Therapy in Geriatrics.*

Chapter Five

A. Jean Ayres

Kay F. Walker

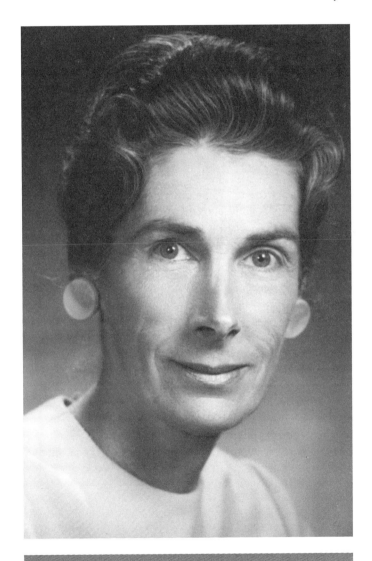

A. Jean Ayres

BIOGRAPHICAL SKETCH

Childhood

Anna Jean Ayres was born in 1923 in California and lived there until her death in 1988. Growing up on a farm in Vasalia, she made friends with the trees and earth. Together with her brother and younger sister, she created pleasurable recreational activities out of whatever was available on the farm. These activities afforded her comfort from the tensions of an unhappy relationship with her mother and older sister.

Throughout childhood, she was not healthy and suffered from what she termed "constitutional inadequacy" (A.J. Ayres, personal communication, June 29, 1981, June 3, 1987). She thought of herself as a bad, difficult, and shameful child who deserved her mother's complaints about her "ugly disposition." Her father was stern and distant, but loving. He embodied the work ethic and instilled in his children the principles of efficiency, economy, hard work, and responsibility for self and others. An educator until he could afford to farm, he placed a high value on education and made many sacrifices in order to send his children to college (A.J. Ayres, personal communication, June 29, 1981, June 3, 1987).

To cope with an emotionally deprived childhood and troubled adolescence, Ayres retreated into herself and followed her mother's advice to use will power to overcome unhappiness. She developed a strong introversion trait that, later in her life, was perceived by others as fortitude in the face of rejection. She stated, "No, I don't think it's courage, I think it's being an introvert and being withdrawn. . . . I've just pulled into myself and I overreacted to the negativism, I just crawl even lower into myself and go my own way. I've had to do it. But I'm suited to doing it" (A.J. Ayres, personal communication, June 29, 1981).

The happiness and love relationships that Ayres lacked in childhood she found in her marriage. She dedicated her first book, *Sensory Integration and Learning Disorders*, to her husband, Franklin Baker. "I will say that I have a nearly perfect, just nearly perfect marriage. Just a real love relationship. A complete pair bond. That's where the love is" (A.J. Ayres, personal communication, June 29, 1981).

Schooling

Ayres attended a country school that was a mile-and-a-half walk from home and had no electric lights or running water. School offered little reprieve from her unhappy home life, and she did not perform well during the first three years of school. She found it hard to express herself and to understand what others were saying, especially if they had an accent. Learning to read gave her her first true understanding of how some words sounded. As an adult, she cited her "damaged left hemisphere" as the cause of her problems, and although she disseminated her life's work through numerous publications and presentations, writing and speaking remained difficult for her (A.J. Ayres, personal communication, June 29, 1981).

She obtained her bachelor's degree in occupational therapy in 1945, her master's degree in occupational therapy in 1954, and her doctorate degree in educational psychology in 1961, all from the University of Southern California (USC). From 1964 to 1966 she engaged in postdoctoral work at the Brain Research Institute at the University of California, Los Angeles (UCLA). This, she says, "was the most fortunate experience I ever had." Although her ideas were not popular at UCLA and she was "low man on the totem pole among all of the scientists" during her two years there (A.J. Ayres, personal communication, June 29, 1981), her work there enabled her to study with neuroscientists and to gain knowledge of the brain.

Work

Ayres took her first occupational therapy job in a Veterans Administration Hospital in 1946. Next she established an OT program at a private psychiatric hospital, where she drafted her first journal article (Ayres, 1949). From there she went to the Kabat Kaiser Institute, where she worked from 1948 to 1953, serving as head occupational therapist. While working toward her master's degree, she gained experience with cerebral palsy patients and with vocational training. She held various positions in the OT and special education programs at USC from 1955 to 1964 and in OT from 1966 to the time of her death.

She felt that her work after her doctorate degree was not supported by her occupational therapy colleagues. She spoke frankly of her experiences:

> It isn't so much to what group I give that which I develop, but what group will accept me. Initially, occupational therapy would not accept me. I could not cope with the resistance and hostility and other negative attitudes. I became so disgusted with occupational therapy in general because I kept wanting to push the field and the field pushed back. I finally became so disgusted and had such a hard time relating to occupational therapists, I said to hell with OT, I'm going to go my way and they can go their way. That's when I left the OT department [at USC] because I just couldn't tolerate the negativism toward me. (A.J. Ayres, personal communication, June 29, 1981)

Ayres saw the rejection of new ideas as not unusual in a university, which she described as potentially a "teeth and claws" place, but stated, "I don't cope well with teeth and claws." She resolved these conflicts by taking the attitude, "I'd just have to be satisfied within myself. I cannot satisfy anyone else. I just wanted to satisfy myself and the committees that grant research funds in Washington, D.C." (A.J. Ayres, personal communication, June 29, 1981).

For eight years after her postdoctoral work, Ayres held a faculty appointment in the special education department of USC. She stated that she found acceptance there because she brought in research funds: "If you bring in research funds and if you produce enough you can keep your desk. If you have a desk and you have an appointment and you have an account number you can make it at a university" (A.J. Ayres, personal communication, June 29, 1981).

After 1971, federal grants were not renewed and there was no funding of any type from the occupational therapy "establishment." Just when it seemed that Ayres' work would go unsupported, an event of great significance to the profession occurred. Two occupational therapists, Lawrence Kovalenko and Patricia Wilbarger, recognized the importance of Ayres' line of inquiry and established a nonprofit foundation (now Sensory Integration International) to serve as a receiving agency for donated funds. Research funds, raised mainly through lecturing, qualified Ayres for additional receipt of a grant from another private foundation. Ayres lectured widely throughout the United States and abroad for two and a half years, bringing gradual grassroots acceptance and financial support for the theory and implementation of principles of sensory integration.

However, Ayres did not perceive her initial lack of financial and professional support as the greatest obstacle she had to overcome. Rather, "The major obstacle is my own brain—my left cerebral hemisphere, in particular. Sensory integrative dysfunction is so complex, so great, that I don't really have the neuronal capacity to handle it as well as I'd like to. That's the biggest obstacle. That, and the problems presented as sensory integrative dysfunction" (A.J. Ayres, personal communication, June 29, 1981, June 3, 1987).

Ayres consistently disseminated her thinking through publications. After her first professional journal article (Ayres, 1949), which was published when she was 29 years of age, she wrote 55 more professional publications, including two books. In addition, she prepared four films and numerous test manuals. Throughout her life, she continued to pose questions, report research findings, and offer theories, thus allowing her work to be utilized and examined.

In 1976, Ayres was appointed adjunct faculty member to the Department of Occupational Therapy at USC. In 1977, she opened the Ayres Clinic, a private facility in Torrance, California. In this carefully designed environment for sensory integrative therapy, she provided therapy for children, conducted research, and developed test instruments and theory. Through her affiliation with USC, she offered postbaccalaureate clinical residencies, training numerous master's students and therapists from throughout the nation and abroad. In 1984, she retired from the Ayres Clinic and turned her energies to the Sensory Integration and Praxis Tests (SIPT) standardization project (American Occupational Therapy Association

[AOTA], 1985). Until the time of her death, she continued her affiliation with USC in an emeritus status and served in an advisory capacity at the Ayres Clinic and for Sensory Integration International.

Development of Theory

Ayres cites the problems of her clients as the central inspiration for her work. "They have certain conditions, responsibility for modification of which I assume; therefore, I must learn what I need to know to ameliorate their condition" (A.J. Ayres, personal communication, June 24, 1981). In the perceptual-motor era of the 1960s, Ayres and such contemporaries as Newell Kephart and Marianne Frostig were exploring the possible perceptual and motor contributions to learning. Ayres realized the need to develop tests of these functions. "I needed to develop tests in order to really get at the problem, and in learning situations, problems are not easily measured, determined, even recognized. When I started out, there weren't any really good tests for looking at dysfunction in children." She developed the motor accuracy test before her doctoral work, but did not standardize it until after she received her degree. In her doctoral program she "wanted to have the kind of instruction, guidance and supervision of test construction that I could see I was going to need later in research" (A.J. Ayres, personal communication, June 29, 1981).

Initially, Ayres focused on developing visual perception tests. "I spent a lot of time and a lot of money developing visual perception tests that never reached the market." Like several of her contemporaries, she wanted to pursue the obvious role of visual perception for reading and other academic tasks. "When Marianne Frostig found out I was developing a test of visual perception she called me on the telephone and asked me not to develop it because she was developing one and I told her I didn't think there would be much conflict" (A.J. Ayres, personal communication, June 29, 1981).

Eventually, however, Ayres began to look beyond visual perception.

> It wasn't a good area to pursue but it took me a long time to figure [that] out. We could see that visual processing problems were central to learning disorders, but we needed to look beyond vision. If you just look at children from a behavioral standpoint and do behavioral type research and modeling, you'll never really discover that a main foundation to visual perception is the vestibular system, with proprioception and other senses also contributing. (A.J. Ayres, personal communication, June 29, 1981)

Ayres consistently relied on the neuroscience and neurobehavioral literature to formulate theory. Her background in neurophysiology and the influence of such clinical theorists as Margaret Rood prompted her to seek alternative answers. "You get that [contribution of vestibular and proprioceptive systems to visual perception] more from studying neurology, and even then you have to make a lot of inferences. You have to go well beyond the printed word to come up with that interpretation" (A.J. Ayres, personal communication, June 29, 1981). Rather than waiting for someone else to extract clinical applications from the literature, Ayres did so, explaining:

> Therapists dash in where scientists fear to tread. It's a dangerous thing to do but it's what builds theory. Theory is not the facts. Theory is putting the facts together so you can use them and in our case to enhance the development of children. This is always my end objective. (A.J. Ayres, personal communication, June 29, 1981)

Ayres received some of the highest accolades in the profession of occupational therapy: the Eleanor Clarke Slagle Lectureship in 1963, the Award of Merit in 1965, the Roster of Fellows in 1973, and appointment as a charter member of the Academy of Research in 1983. In 1987, the American Occupational Therapy Foundation established the A. Jean Ayres Award for outstanding achievement in occupational therapy research, theory, or practice (American Occupational Therapy Association, 1987). Despite the controversy surrounding her work, Ayres nonetheless made a great impact on occupational therapy theory. Yet because of her childhood and the rejection of her work in the past, when told of the thousands who hold her in extremely high esteem, she stated, "And you know, it's hard for me to hear it, but I hear the pediatricians quite clearly when they declare, in print, that sensory integration therapy lacks value" (A.J. Ayres, personal communication, June 29, 1981, June 3, 1987).

On December 16, 1988, Ayres succumbed to a lengthy struggle with cancer. Finding "orthodox treatment of cancer not working well," she engaged in "some nonorthodox approaches" and concentrated her attention on her work with Sensory Integration and Praxis Tests (A.J. Ayres, personal communication, June 3, 1987). Before her death, she was able to see their completion.

In a special tribute to Ayres at the 1989 American Occupational Therapy Conference, President Elnora Gilfoyle stated,

> For all her genius and complexity, she had an acute appreciation of the commonplace rhythms of life. The intricacies of the nervous system, the change of seasons, the instinctive capabilities of animals, the human drive to accomplish. These were the forces which caught her fascination and inspired inquiry. The fact that she dedicated her life to the study of the most basic, yet poorly understood, aspects of human function reflects her essence. (American Occupational Therapy Association, 1989a, p. 4)

As Florence A. Clarke remembers Ayres' influence, "Jean taught me to search for authenticity, strive to achieve the highest academic standards, be vigilantly responsive to the needs of others and to stay on the right course despite resistance in order to help the world" (American Occupational Therapy Association, 1989b, p. 15).

THEORETICAL CONCEPTS

Sensory Integration—The Term

Although the terms "sensation" and "integration" appeared frequently in Ayres' early writings (Ayres, 1958, 1960, 1961b, 1963b), it was not until 1968 that she combined these terms into "sensory integration" (SI) (Ayres 1968a, 1968b). She first used the term "sensory integration" to describe the brain's ability to "filter, organize and integrate the masses of sensory information" (Ayres, 1968a, p. 43). Learning, she argued, was a function of this neuropsychological ability, and reading could be described as "the end product of a long evolutionary course in which the increased capacity of sensory integration, accompanied by the ability to emit an adaptive motor response, has furnished a critical foundation" (Ayres, 1968a, p. 170). "Certain types of learning disability" could therefore "be interpreted partially in terms of dysfunction within the brain's integrative functions" (Ayres, 1968b, p. 43). Although Ayres acknowledged that "exactly how sensory integration occurs in the brain remains elusive," she insisted that lack of knowledge should "not be an excuse for avoiding an issue basic to all learning" (Ayres, 1968b, p. 43). This lack of knowledge, she asserted, "must be faced and dealt with in as adequate manner as possible with full recognition of the limitations involved and with the realization that any conceptual framework is in some respects erroneous and will require constant modification as new knowledge unfolds" (Ayres, 1968b, p. 43). Ayres considered auditory language functions to be part of the total SI process, but stated that they were not the focus of her investigations (Ayres, 1968a, 1968b).

These 1968 articles (Ayres, 1968a, 1968b) were important in that they outlined the parameters of what would become Ayres' life work. In them, Ayres introduced phylogenetic and ontogenetic developmental principles related to SI, linked learning and SI, posed dysfunction in SI as being related to learning disabilities, and identified related evaluation and treatment strategies. She addressed the need for developing a conceptual framework for the brain's integrative processes. She also selected the neural integrative processes she found to be most useful in the therapeutic situation and drew on the neuroscience literature to explain neural mechanisms.

Developmental Bases

Sensory integration theory is a developmental theory based on principles of phylogenetic and ontogenetic development. The source of these principles is in the neuromuscular and neurodevelopmental theories of Fay, Kabat, Knott, the Bobaths, Rood, and Brunnstrom, and the motor development theories of Gesell and others. Ayres showed her knowledge of and interest in these theories in her comprehensive chapter in the third edition of Willard and Spackman's *Occupational Therapy* (Ayres, 1963b). In several other writings, she discussed phylogenetic and ontogenetic principles related to hand function (Ayres, 1954), visual-motor function (Ayres, 1958, 1961a), treatment (Ayres, 1966a), and reading (Ayres, 1968a).

Phylogenetic Development

Ayres applied two phylogenetic principles to SI theory: (1) the importance of sensation, and (2) the interdependence of higher and lower central nervous system (CNS) structures and functions. According to the first principle, vertebrate organisms survived over the course of millions of years because they evolved increasingly complex neural systems that enabled them to interact successfully with their environment. These neural changes resulted either by chance from genetic mutations or through the modification of the CNS via sensory input. SI theory emphasized the latter cause, claiming that "sensory input from the environment actually modified the nervous system because it called for new types of responses" (Ayres, 1963b, p. 364). The evolution of vertebrates coincided with their increase in numbers of sensory nerve fibers and their development of complex systems for processing sensory information. "Enlarging the scope of information supplied to the brain enabled it, in turn, to develop increasingly complex adaptive response" (Ayres, 1972d, p. 23).

The second phylogenetic principle states that as vertebrates evolved, the earlier, simple neural structures were retained and new structures were added. The functions ascribed to the earlier systems remained and were not replaced, but instead were modified and integrated as each new neural level evolved.

> Each structure remained capable of receiving information, integrating it, and organizing an appropriate motor response. While the highest or youngest structure present at any one time in evolution or in any one species today (in humans it is the cerebral cortex) exerted critical influence over all lower structures, the higher centers still maintained a dependence upon lower structures. (Ayres, 1972d, p. 23)

Ontogenetic Development

The ontogenetic principle states that the development of the individual organism recapitulates the development of the species. For example, the motor development of human infants replays the evolutionary progression of vertebrates, which were first capable of swimming movements, then quadrapedal ambulation, and finally bipedal ambulation and dexterous upper extremities. Similarly, motor control progresses from cephalad to caudal, proximal to distal, gross to fine, flexion to extension, adduction to abduction, ulnar to radial, movement in straight planes to rotational movement, and reflexive contraction to voluntary contraction (Ayres, 1963b).

Hypothesized Development of Sensory Integrative Processes

In 1964, Ayres presented a chart, "Hypothesized Sequences in Perceptual Motor Development," which summarized developmental concepts from several other writings (Ayres, 1964a, p. 18) (see Figure 5-1). This chart was expanded in her 1976 book *Interpreting the Southern California Sensory Integration Tests* (Ayres, 1976b, p. 4) and updated in her 1979 book *Sensory Integration and the Child* (Ayres, 1979, p. 60). These charts reflect the increasing refinement of Ayres' conceptualization of SI development.

In 1962 Ayres hypothesized that academic skills and ability to conceptualize in level IV are based on visual-spatial perception and motor skills (level III), which, in turn, evolved from body scheme and motor planning (level II), which began with tactile and visual perception and proprioception (level I). The concepts of body scheme from level II and visual-spatial perception from level III remained essentially the same from one version of the chart to the next, but other elements of the chart underwent considerable revision.

Ayres defined body scheme as "the knowledge we have of the construction and spatial relationships of the different anatomical elements, such as fingers, legs, arms, that make up our body. It involves being able to visualize these elements in movement and in different positional relationships" (1960, p. 308). Body scheme provides a postural model (Ayres, 1961a) or postural frame of reference (Ayres, 1964a) for movement. It develops from the integration of tactual, proprioceptive, and visual sensations. Just as it provides a basis for movement, it is also a result of processing of sensory impulses that are generated through movement. "Motor

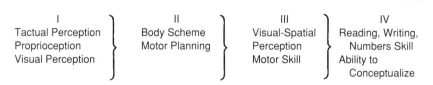

I	II	III	IV
Tactual Perception Proprioception Visual Perception	Body Scheme Motor Planning	Visual-Spatial Perception Motor Skill	Reading, Writing, Numbers Skill Ability to Conceptualize

Figure 5-1 Hypothesized Sequences in Perceptual Motor Development—1962. *Source:* From A.J. Ayres, Perceptual Motor Training for Children. In: *Approaches to the Treatment of Patients with Neuromuscular Dysfunction* (p. 18) by C. Sattley (Ed.), 1964, Dubuque, Iowa: William C. Brown, Publishers. Copyright 1962 by William C. Brown, Publishers.

planning and body scheme are two sides of the same coin. The development of each is dependent upon the other" (Ayres, 1964a, p. 19).

Visual-spatial perception develops in concert with manual manipulation and body scheme and includes perception of form, direction, or position in space and space visualization. As the child handles, explores, and experiments with objects and moves through and experiences space, he or she formulates perceptions and concepts of form and space. The role of vision is to verify what is experienced tactually and kinesthetically. "Visual impressions reinforce and become associated with the manual impressions so that later visual cues can recall the cutaneous and proprioceptive, and the latter can recall the visual" (Ayres, 1958, p. 132). Likewise, the visual stimuli are essential for interpretation of the stimuli arising from manual manipulation. Thus "the same activities which enhance efficiency of motor planning also provided the basis of visual space perception" (Ayres, 1964a, p. 20).

Body scheme is both a basis for movement and derived through movement. Visual-spatial perception guides movement and is derived from the integration of vision, proprioception (including vestibular), and cutaneous sensations as movement occurs. Thus several important ingredients of SI theory are contained in this schematic representation of perceptual motor development.

By 1976, Ayres had developed a model (see Figure 5-2) of SI process to serve as an organizing framework for interpreting the Southern California Sensory Integration Tests (SCSIT) (Ayres, 1976b). Using an expanded version of this model (1979) (Figure 5-3), therapists could trace the school-aged child's problems in behavior, learning, attention, and motor coordination to SI dysfunction in earlier years. Ayres showed how SI contributed to four levels of normal development that

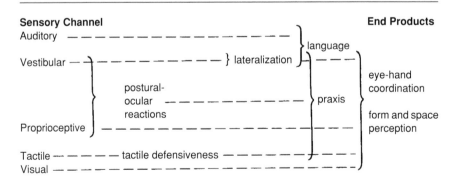

Figure 5-2 Sensory Integration Model—1976. *Source:* Copyright © 1976 by Western Psychological Services. Reprinted with permission of the publisher, Western Psychological Services, 12031 Wilshire Blvd., Los Angeles, CA 90025.

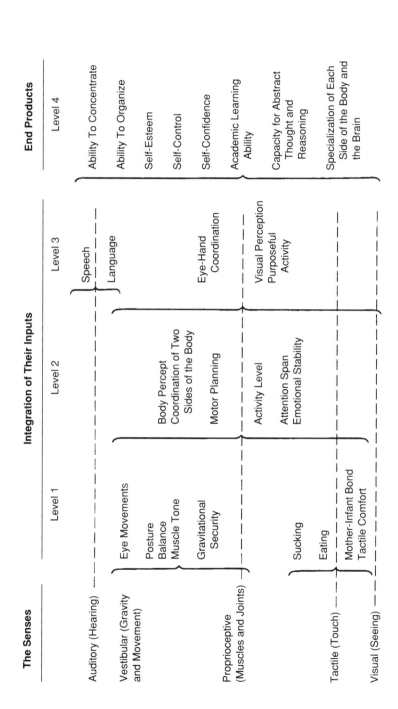

Figure 5-3 The Senses, Integration of Their Inputs, and Their End Products. *Source: A.J. Ayres, Sensory Integration and the Child*, p. 60. Copyright © 1979 by Western Psychological Services. Reprinted with permission of the publisher, Western Psychological Services, 12031 Wilshire Blvd., Los Angeles, CA 90025.

overlapped considerably but were roughly equivalent to the first year of life, the toddler stage, the preschool stage, and the school-age stage (Ayres, 1979).

Ayres hypothesized that the end products (see Figure 5-3) necessary to perform in school and later on a job and to interact successfully with people develop as the result of many years of integration of the sensory systems: auditory, vestibular, proprioceptive, tactile, and visual. In the early months of life (level 1), the tactile system contributes to the survival function of sucking and eating and the psychological function of mother-infant bonding and tactile comfort. Vestibular and proprioceptive sensations provide a basis for eye movements, posture, balance, muscle tone, and gravitational security. In toddlerhood (level 2), vestibular, proprioceptive, and tactile systems converge to contribute to the formation of a body percept and to the coordination of two sides of the body, motor planning, activity level, attention span, and emotional stability. By about age 3 (level 3), the child works to refine skills in eye-hand coordination, visual perception, and speech and language and to engage in purposeful activity. At this level audition and vision join the three basic senses to bring about skill development. Although vision and audition are obviously very important senses, Ayres de-emphasized their role in development and dramatized the contribution of the less obvious senses: vestibular, tactile, and proprioceptive (Ayres, 1979).

The fourth level includes the end products of the integration of sensation occurring during the first six years of life. For formal schooling the child needs a foundation on which to develop the ability to concentrate, organize, and reason abstractly. Self-control, self-esteem, and self-confidence are important for human relationships in the classroom and at home. To provide a neurological basis for academic learning, the specialized functions of the cerebral hemispheres and body sides must be well lateralized. Ayres proposed that these abilities developed through the brain's ability to integrate sensory processes (Ayres, 1979).

Neurological Bases

SI theory is neurologically based in that it is derived from concepts of neural functioning. The four main concepts that it employs are: (1) the integrative process; (2) movement-generated sensation; (3) tactile, vestibular, and proprioceptive basis for visual and auditory functions; and (4) subcortical functions as the foundation for cortical functions.

Integrative Processes of the Central Nervous System

In order to function effectively, the brain must be able to organize sensory input from many sources into a meaningful pattern that can be utilized for movement and learning. It must be able to take information received from an isolated sensory source and compare it to another sensory source for clarification and validation. Because the brain has many more afferents than efferents, it must be able to structure the massive sensory input it receives if it is to perform effectively. The brain's ability to organize, compare, and structure sensory information is referred to as its integrative function.

This integrative process occurs at and among all levels of the CNS, from the spinal cord to the cortex. Within each level, sensory processing from one side of the neuroaxis is integrated with sensory processing from the other side. Thus integrative functions occur both vertically and horizontally in the CNS.

Intersensory or intermodality integration is the capacity of the CNS to associate information from two or more different sensory modalities. The brain gives meaning to the combined input from several sources and then information about another without direct stimulation (Ayres, 1968a). For example, one can identify an orange simply by its scent after one has integrated the sight, touch, taste, and smell of an orange from numerous previous sensory experiences with oranges. Future sensory encounters with an orange through one sense—for example, its scent—will produce associations with its appearance, texture, and taste. In this way, intersensory integration contributes to concept formation.

This ability to make sense of the environment contributes to human beings' adaptive powers. The development of individual adaptive ability parallels the species' phylogenetic development of neural structures that have allowed for increased capacity for processing sensory information.

Convergent neurons provide the neuroanatomical basis for intersensory integration. These multisensory neurons receive input from several sensory modalities. "The most commonly reported modalities showing convergence are visual, auditory, olfactory, somesthetic, and vestibular" (Ayres, 1972d, p. 30). The spinal cord, brainstem, and cerebrum contain nuclei made up of convergent neurons that provide for intersensory integration throughout the neuroaxis (Ayres, 1958, 1968b, 1972d, 1975a).

Movement Processes

Sensation is one of the first components of a motor act.

> Motor acts are initiated either directly or indirectly by some environmental factor that became known to the individual through sensory stimulation. One sees a pencil before one grasps it; one feels too warm and throws off the covers; one hears a horn at the side and changes the direction of the car; one feels the bag of groceries slipping and gives it a firmer hold. (Ayres, 1963b, p. 365)

To produce movement, the CNS must integrate sensation: it must organize incoming sensations, combine them with past sensory processes, and use them to formulate an anticipated motor response. Once the movement is under way, the CNS must monitor it, evaluate it, and alter it as needed for future reference. Although movement is a product of CNS organization, the process of integrating sensation for movement can also be said to have an organizing effect on the CNS. Thus sensory integration for movement is both a result of and a prerequisite for CNS organization. The important role of sensorimotor functions in CNS organization is supported by Ayres' finding that children's scores on the Gesell Developmental Scales, which may be assumed to reflect CNS maturity, are correlated with their scores on perceptual motor tests (Ayres, 1969b).

Movement, as it occurs, generates sensations that provide additional data for CNS processing. These include tactile, kinesthetic, proprioceptive, and vestibular sensations that arise from the body as it moves. These sensations inform the CNS about the movement as it is being produced: the stretch of the skin as it moves over a joint, joint motion and position, relative position of body parts; position of the head in relationship to the body and to the earth's gravitational force; and speed duration and strength of muscle contraction. The CNS must integrate this sensory information with that from other senses to determine whether the intended movement was executed. The analysis of sensory information enables the CNS to adjust the formulation of subsequent motor responses. The integration of the sensations that are generated through movement enables the development of sensorimotor abilities.

The integration of sensation for movement is important not only for sensorimotor functions but also for learning and cognition. Humans became intelligent creatures through the evolution of a motor system that afforded them the opportunity to explore and learn about their environment. Ayres suggested that the sensory integrative aspects that enable one to become a competent sensorimotor being are related to competence in early academic skills and that the brain's ability to integrate sensations for movement underlies the brain's ability to organize sensations for learning. In short, she proposes that "sensory integrative processes subserve some aspects of cognition" (Ayres, 1975a, p. 304).

Tactile, Proprioceptive, and Vestibular Bases for Auditory and Visual Functions

The contribution of vision and hearing to academic performance is readily apparent and has been widely studied by numerous researchers and theorists. In contrast, Ayres focused on the impact of tactile, proprioceptive, and vestibular systems on the neural processes underlying learning.

Drawing on neuroscience literature, Ayres reported that the tactile, proprioceptive, and vestibular systems mature in utero earlier than the visual and auditory systems. "There is quite general agreement that the phyletically older systems (tactile, olfactory, gustatory, vestibular, and proprioceptive) mature before the younger auditory and visual systems" (Ayres, 1975a, p. 314). During fetal life the stimulation of these older systems results first in reflex movements of the neck and mouth and then in reflex movements of the arms, legs, and trunk (tactile); eye movements (vestibular); and muscle contraction (proprioceptive). The functioning of these systems early in life makes possible the life-sustaining abilities to suck, swallow, breathe, and move.

The sensory systems develop in concert with one another and not independently of each other. Through sensory integration, each sensory system influences and is influenced by other sensory systems. Sensory systems that develop earlier have an impact on those that develop later. Likewise, the functioning of the earlier systems influences the functioning of the later developing systems: "the normal development of visual perception requires intersensory integration from other sources, especially somatosensory and vestibular" (Ayres, 1968b, p. 46). Ayres hypothesized that auditory processing is probably enhanced through stimulation of other senses (e.g., vestibular), and that visual perception and auditory processing are to a certain extent dependent upon processing of stimuli from the tactile and vestibular systems (Ayres, 1972c, p. 83).

Dysfunction in development of the early systems may affect the development of the later systems. Thus, SI dysfunction involving tactile, proprioceptive, and/or vestibular systems may contribute to learning problems that are observed in the performance of auditory or visual tasks. The child's learning difficulties may be due not only to problems in auditory or visual processes but also to the SI deficits caused by problems in tactile, proprioceptive, and vestibular processes. Enhancing the brain's ability to learn through auditory and visual modes by ameliorating SI dysfunction involving the tactile, proprioceptive, and vestibular systems is the goal of SI therapy (Ayres, 1958, 1968b, 1972a, 1972c, 1972d, 1975a).

Brainstem Functions

SI theory explains how the CNS integrates sensation for human learning and movement. Unlike theories and research that focus on cortical processes for learning and movement, this theory emphasizes the functions of subcortical structures for human performance. As we will see, Ayres modified this aspect of SI theory in her later formulations regarding praxis. However, a review of hierarchical neural processes remains useful for understanding SI theory.

The cerebral cortex, also called the neo- (or new) cortex, developed last phylogenetically and is responsible for the complex cognitive abilities and skilled manipulation capabilities that characterize humans. But in keeping with the second phylogenetic principle, it did not replace the earlier developing neural structures, nor did it eliminate the functioning of these structures. Instead, it developed additively upon these older structures by integrating and refining the functions of earlier systems. Functions became replicated with increasing complexity as the neuroaxis evolved from spinal cord to brainstem to cerebrum. "Cortical functions, then, are in some respects still dependent upon brainstem functions" (Ayres, 1975a, p. 318).

The brainstem is one of the major structures in which sensory integration occurs (Ayres, 1975a).

> At one time in the evolutionary process, the brainstem, as the highest neural structure, provided sufficient organization and direction to enable the organism to interact adaptively with its environment, albeit at a primitive level. Those functions, although greatly modified, still operate in man today. (Ayres, 1972d, p. 40)

The major nuclei of the brainstem, including the thalamus, are: (1) sensory nuclei for the vestibular, tactile, proprioceptive, auditory, visual, and gustatory systems; (2) motor nuclei for eye, facial, and throat movements; eye and postural reflexes; and muscle tone; (3) limbic nuclei for mood and for stereotypical motions associated with survival functions; (4) autonomic nuclei for cardiovascular, gastrointestinal, and pulmonary functions; and (5) reticular nuclei for arousal, alerting, and attentional functions. The brainstem is in a position to perform major integrative functions and to influence the functioning of the neocortex. Ayres argued that "any major neural structure receiving sensory input from many sources is apt to have widespread influence over the rest of the brain. Multiplicity of input usually means convergence of input and where there is convergence of input there is integration of input" (1972c, p. 82). The brainstem and thalamus are "good examples of structures to which the principle is applicable" (Ayres, 1972d, p. 53).

In addition to the brainstem, the other subcortical structures also have important intersensory integration functions. The cerebellum "receives input from all sensory sources over the afferent neurons and from much but not all of the cerebral cortex, processes it, and then uses it to influence ongoing neuronal activity, especially down the spinal cord, to brainstem nuclei, the thalamus, basal ganglia and cortex" (Ayres, 1972d, p. 47). The cerebellum plays a role in the smoothness and timing of movements, muscle tone, vestibular functions, and limbic functions. The basal ganglia function to provide the "regulation of posture and movements of the body in space and the production of complex motor acts." They appear to be "involved in a type of sensory integration that allows one type of sensory input to influence the integration of another type and to utilize that input for moderately complex postural and other bodily movements" (Ayres, 1972d, p. 49). The limbic system

> is concerned with primitive patterns of behavior necessary for individual and species survival, including vegetative functions, defending the body against attack, and the simple perceptual motor functions needed to fulfill these survival functions. Its function is clarified when it is considered the primary cortical structure in a large proportion of vertebrates. Fish have no neocortex; amphibians, reptiles, and birds have little, yet all of these animals show basic but well integrated behavior including perceptual, motor, and simple learning and memory. (Ayres, 1972d, p. 49)

In summary, SI for sensorimotor functions occurs in all subcortical levels and provides a foundation for cortical functions. SI dysfunction at the subcortical level can contribute to difficulties in cognitive processes. Enhancement of cognitive processing by improving SI functions mediated in subcortical structures is the aim of SI therapy (Ayres, 1967, 1968b, 1972b, 1972c, 1972d, 1975a).

Sensory Integrative Dysfunction

Ayres described sensory integrative dysfunction in children with learning or behavior problems who had no known peripheral or central nervous system deficits. Like her contemporaries in the 1960s, she was intrigued by the question "Why can't Johnny learn?" when Johnny has a normal IQ and neurological exam, normal hearing, vision, and speech, and no disease or disability. Psychologists, special educators, and language pathologists explained learning problems as "processing deficits" although CNS structures were themselves not lesioned and the peripheral nerves conveying information to and from the CNS were intact. While others focused on specific problems with visual perception, speech and language, and reading, Ayres investigated somatosensory, motor, and vestibular processing deficits as indicators of sensory integration dysfunction.

Ayres conducted numerous factor analytic and other studies to construct and refine typologies of sensory integrative dysfunctions. Her first typology was based on a factor analytic study of 100 learning disabled children and 50 normal children. It identified five discrete patterns of dysfunction: (1) developmental apraxia; (2) perceptual dysfunction of form and position in two-dimensional space; (3) tactile defensiveness; (4) deficit of integration of function of the two sides of the body; and (5) perceptual dysfunction of visual figure-ground discrimination. This classification scheme, presented in her Eleanor Clarke Slagle lecture (1963a), provided her with a framework for test development and theory building in sensory integration (Ayres, 1963a, 1965). Because the five syndromes were not found in the normal subjects, it was clear that Ayres had indeed isolated areas of dysfunction that were not characteristic of normal development (Ayres, 1965).

Support for the aberrant nature of these symptom complexes was gained in two studies (Ayres, 1966b, 1966c) of normal children in whom these factors were not clearly shown. In one of these studies, however, praxis (motor planning) and somatosensory scores accounted for most of the variance (Ayres 1966c), whereas in the other study, praxis accounted for least of the variance (Ayres, 1966b). This discrepancy may be explained by differences between the two study samples. In the first study (Ayres, 1966b), 10 percent of the subjects had probable CNS dysfunction, and three children had mild cerebral palsy; in the other study, all subjects were normal. The children with CNS deficits in the first study may have accounted for the praxis factor loadings. If so, those findings would support the apraxia syndrome as a developmental deviation.

Ayres (1989) conducted a cluster analysis of the SIPT to construct diagnostic profiles. The six profiles revealed by the analysis are used in the Western Psychological Services Test Report of the SIPT and displayed in a ChromaGraph (see Figure 5-4). The clusters are named and defined in Exhibit 5-1.

Visual Form and Space Dysfunction

Educators and psychologists have developed numerous tests to assess visual form and space dysfunction. Ayres also spent years developing visual-perceptual tests. These early tests identified areas of visual form and space dysfunction: form constancy (perceiving a form as being the same, regardless of changes in apparent size or color); spatial orientation (perceiving location and position of objects in space); spatial relationships (perceiving the relative positions of objects); and visual figure ground (distinguishing figure from opposing background).

Ayres connected form and space perception deficits to children's learning problems in several factor analytic studies of the SCSIT (Ayres, 1965, 1969a, 1972f, 1977a). Tests that loaded on this factor included tests that were purely visual

---

Exhibit 5-1 Six Comparison Groups on the WPS ChromaGraph

Group	Definition
Generalized Sensory Integration Dysfunction	Tends to have below average integration scores on all SIPT subtests and both practic and somatosensory deficits.
Visuo- and Somatodyspraxia	Low scores on Design Copying, Finger Identification, Graphesthesia, Postural Praxis, Sequencing Praxis, Bilateral Motor Coordination, Standing and Walking Balance, Motor Accuracy, and Kinesthesia. Has the lowest Postrotary Nystagmus score of the six groups.
Dyspraxia on Verbal Command	Severe difficulties with Praxis on Verbal Command and the highest Postrotary Nystagmus test score of the six groups.
Deficit in Bilateral Integration and Sequencing	Low average scores on Standing and Walking Balance, Bilateral Motor Coordination, Oral Praxis, Sequencing Praxis, and Graphesthesia.
Low Average Sensory Integration and Praxis	Tends to have low average scores on all areas of the SIPT.
High Average Sensory Integration and Praxis	Above average functioning in all areas of the SIPT.

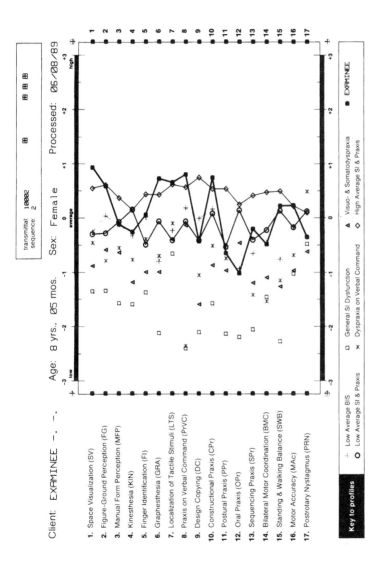

Figure 5-4 ChromaGraph of Diagnostic Profiles Revealed by Cluster Analysis of Sensory Integration and Praxis Tests. *Source: Sensory Integration and Praxis Tests* (1988) by A.J. Ayres. Reprinted by permission of the publisher, © copyright 1988, Western Psychological Services, 12031 Wilshire Blvd., Los Angeles, CA.

(space visualization), tests that tapped visual and motor functions (design copying), and tests that involved visual, motor, tactile and proprioceptive functions (graphesthesia, kinesthesia, manual form perception).

In contrast to the prevailing viewpoint that visual form and space dysfunction could be identified and treated in isolation, Ayres found that it often accompanied praxis, postural, ocular, and somatosensory dysfunction in children with learning and behavior problems. Elaborating on Trevarthen's hypothesized dual modes of vision, she contrasted ambient vision, or perception of the surrounding environment, with focal vision, or perception of near visual stimuli. Ambient vision relies upon a spatial map of the environment that the organism develops through subcortically mediated, postural-ocular experiences with gravity and space as locomotion progresses through prone, sitting, quadraped, and bipedal postures. Focal vision, in contrast, requires precise attention to details of orientation and form in central vision and is a function of the cerebral cortex. According to Ayres, the ability to discriminate the orientation of a letter on a page derived from cortical, focal visual functions and also from the environmental spatial map provided by subcortical structures. Although the ambient/focal vision and cortical/subcortical dichotomies are not as separate as Ayres suggested, these concepts were useful for bringing attention to the possible linkage of somatosensory, proprioceptive, and motor functions to visual perception.

This linkage was further supported by the factor analytic studies of the SIPT (Ayres, 1989). A visuopraxis factor emerged that was composed of three overlapping components: form and space perception, visuomotor coordination, and visual construction (Ayres & Marr, 1991; Fisher & Murray, 1991). The form and space perception component included low scores in tests of Space Visualization, Figure-Ground Perception, Constructional Praxis, Design Copying, and Manual Form Perception. The visuomotor coordination component included low scores in Motor Accuracy and Design Copying tests. Visual construction problems were identified in Design Copying and Constructional Praxis tests. Although this factor was named visuopraxis because of the "common conceptual link between praxis and visual perception" (Ayres & Marr, 1991, p. 210), it was not considered a type of dyspraxia.

Although Ayres identified visual form and space problems in many of her factor analytic studies, she consistently viewed these problems in the context of somatosensory, proprioceptive, and praxis functions rather than seeing them primarily as problems in processing by the visual system. She considered visual form and space perception to be an "end product" of sensory integration. Consequently, she never emphasized visual perceptual training as part of sensory integrative therapy.

Developmental Dyspraxia

Developmental dyspraxia is "a disorder of sensory integration interfering with praxis, e.g., the ability to plan and execute skilled or non-habitual motor tasks"

(Ayres, 1972d, p. 165). Sequencing of movements to produce a coordinated series of actions is faulty. Although the child can learn new tasks, doing so takes longer and is more difficult than it would be for children with normal SI development. Everyday activities such as fastening buttons and riding a bicycle may be laborious and frustrating for the child and may be late to develop. Unlike adult apraxia, which is usually due to left, language-dominant hemisphere lesion, developmental dyspraxia is found in the absence of neurological problems of muscle weakness, tremors, spasticity, or sensory loss.

Having consistently found a relationship between low scores on praxis tests and low scores on tactile tests (Ayres, 1965, 1969a, 1971, 1972f, 1977a), Ayres theorized that the development of praxis was related to tactile (skin) and proprioceptive (muscle, tendon, and joint) somatosensory processing. Cutaneous, muscle, joint, tendon, and deep tissue receptors are constantly activated as the skin moves over a muscle that is contracting. The resultant flow of sensory input to the CNS sustains and provides the basis for development of a body scheme, which in turn provides a dynamic map that the brain uses for organizing, ordering, and timing of movements. If the information which the body receives from its somatosensory receptors is not precise due to faulty sensory integration, "the brain has a poor basis on which to build its scheme of the body; consequently, the capacity to motor plan cannot develop normally" (Ayres, 1972d, p. 170).

Ayres argues that praxis and postural and bilateral integration differ in their patterns of dependence on tactile, proprioceptive, and vestibular sensory systems:

> While postural and bilateral integration appear to be especially and directly dependent upon vestibular input, praxis is especially and directly dependent upon discriminative tactile functions with the vestibular system providing more of a substrate. Both systems are dependent upon proprioceptors, with posture more related to the muscle spindle and praxis to joint receptors. . . . The major substrate of praxis is believed to be diencephalic and cortical while the brain stem is the major integrating site for postural and bilateral integration. (Ayres, 1972d, p. 171)

In the 1980s, Ayres expanded her view of developmental dyspraxia to include conceptual and cognitive processes mediated by the cerebral cortex, especially the left hemisphere. Drawing on others' investigations of clumsy children and research in adult dyspraxia, as well as on her own insights from her clinical practice and research, she proposed three processes in developmental dyspraxia: "ideation or conceptualization; planning a scheme of action; and motor execution" (Ayres, 1985, p. 19).

Ideation is the conceptual process of imagining an interaction between one's body and an object through purposeful movement. Ayres referred to it as a "concept of possible object-person interaction" (Ayres, 1985, p. 20) that was "believed to be largely dependent upon sensory integration and resultant knowledge of available body actions" (Ayres, 1985, p. 21). Such knowledge of available body actions was dependent on the tactile system. She posited that ideation was a "generalized neurophysiological function" (Ayres, 1985, p. 22) that served various functions, including praxis, language, and organized behavior. She noted the need for research to verify the links among praxis, language, and behavior that have been observed clinically when therapy for dyspraxia results in improvements in praxis, language, and organizational abilities.

The motor planning process of praxis is "a consciously formulated internal plan of action that occurs before actual motor execution" (Ayres, 1985, p. 23). The planning process is an intermediate process between ideation and execution of a purposeful act. Thinking about one's actions characterizes the motor planning process and is necessary for learning motor tasks. When thinking and planning are not required, the movement has become automatic.

Two requisites for the motor planning process are somatosensory integration and sequencing ability. Somatosensory integration of tactile, kinesthetic, proprioceptive, and vestibular sensation provides the brain with information about "how the body is designed and how it functions as a mechanical being" (Ayres, 1985, p. 24). The sequencing aspect of motor planning orders a series of joint positions and movements and muscle tensions into an organized action. Providing a plan of transition from one component of the movement to the next is a sequencing function. Sequencing functions are generally thought to be mediated in the left hemisphere.

Execution of the action—that is, the observable motor act itself—is the culmination of ideation and planning. Through execution, one can infer the quality of ideation and planning. Problems in execution due to dyspraxia are distinguishable from those due to neuromotor problems. Neuromotor problems involve spasticity, fluctuating tone, and involuntary motion, whereas dyspraxia may (or may not) involve reduced muscle tone. Thus, in a child who has no neuromotor problems but does have motor execution problems, one could look for difficulty in ideation and planning.

In a study of 182 children with learning or behavior problems, Ayres, Mailloux, and Wendler (1987) sought to identify types of developmental dyspraxia and to determine whether these types would be differentially associated with sensory (i.e., visual, tactile, kinesthetic, proprioceptive, vestibular) or auditory language functions. Types of dyspraxia were not supported, and there was no sufficient evidence of differential associations with sensory systems. However, a linkage between tactile functions and praxis was again shown, as was a linkage between visual processes and praxis. The authors concluded that there was evidence for a somatopractic function and that "two basic elements of the general practic function appear to be tactile processing and ideation or concept formation" (Ayres et al., 1987, p. 105). They related visual perception to ideational processes for praxis since the visual tests that had the strongest associations with praxis were those that required considerable concept formation.

The most recent factor and cluster analysis of the Sensory Integration and Praxis Tests (Ayres, 1989; Ayres & Marr, 1991) revealed three factors related to praxis: somatopraxis, visuopraxis, and praxis on verbal command associated with prolonged postrotary nystagmus.

The somatopraxis factor included low scores on tests of praxis and somatosensory/proprioceptive processing: Postural Praxis; Bilateral Motor Coordination; Sequencing Praxis; Oral Praxis; Graphesthesia; Standing and Walking Balance; and possibly Praxis on Verbal Command. Ayres labeled the somatosensory tests in a separate factor (Ayres & Marr, 1991); however, the coexistence of low praxis scores with low somatosensory scores remains a requisite for diagnosing somatodyspraxia (Cermak, 1991).

The visuopraxis factor included three areas of visual perception: form and space perception (with loadings on tests of Space Visualization, Figure Ground Perception, Constructional Praxis, Design Copying, and Manual Form Perception); visuomotor coordination (with loadings on Motor Accuracy and Design Copying); and visual construction (with loadings on Constructional Praxis and Design Copying). The visuopraxis factor was not considered a disorder of praxis per se but was named visuopraxis because of the "common conceptual component to praxis and visual perception" (Ayres & Marr, 1991, p. 210) that Ayres, Mailloux, and Wendler had already discovered in their 1987 study. Low scores on visuopraxis tests in the absence of tactile or somatosensory dysfunction were considered to indicate hemisphere dysfunction rather than a sensory integration disorder (Fisher & Murray, 1991).

The Praxis on Verbal Command Test assesses the ability to assume postures in response to verbal instructions. Low scores on this test loaded with high scores on Postrotary Nystagmus (i.e., prolonged Postrotary Nystagmus). Other tests that loaded on this factor included Oral Praxis, Sequencing Praxis, Bilateral Motor Coordination, and Standing and Walking Balance. In contrast, the somatosensory and visuopraxis test scores were average or low-average. The Praxis on Verbal Command pattern of SIPT scores was found in a study of children with language disorders, and Ayres interpreted this as suggestive of left hemisphere rather than sensory integrative dysfunction (Ayres & Marr, 1991).

The picture of dyspraxia is further complicated by the cluster that Ayres named "visuo-somatodyspraxia." This is one of the final six clusters used in the computer-scored WPS ChromaGraph of the SIPT. Children identified in this cluster may score low in praxis scores and somatosensory and/or visual tests. However, Ayres notes that the "visuopraxis scores should be delineated instead as form and space perception, visuomotor coordination, or visual construction deficits" (Ayres & Marr, 1991, p. 227).

In summary, Ayres' updated theory of praxis emphasized conceptual processes that are dependent on somatosensory integration. In her later work, Ayres continued to emphasize the importance of tactile, kinesthesic, proprioceptive, and vestibular system functioning as a basis for cortical processes of ideation, planning, and sequencing (Ayres, 1985). She also continued to view dyspraxia as a sensory integrative disorder when it was associated with disorders in the somatosensory system. She claimed that in the absence of other signs of sensory integrative disorder, problems related to visuopraxis and praxis on verbal command were not sensory integrative disorders but rather possible *outcomes* of poor praxis or related to hemisphere dysfunction.

Tactile and Sensory Defensiveness

The disinhibition syndrome of hyperactivity and distractibility has been long recognized as a major problem in many children with learning and behavioral deficits. Ayres expanded this syndrome in 1964 to include tactile defensiveness. Tactile defensiveness is characterized by expressions of "feeling of discomfort and a desire to escape the situation when certain types of tactile stimuli are experienced" (Ayres, 1964c, p. 8). Ayres did not develop tests for tactile defensiveness. Instead, she suggested that the examiner observe the child's negative reactions to tactile stimuli during tactile testing. Questions about when the test would end, comments about not liking the test, withdrawing the hand or moving the body away from the examiner, complaints of a painful stimulus, giggling, or angry comments were all clues that the child found tactile stimuli to be aversive (Ayres, 1964c). Other examples of tactile defensive behavior include avoidance of bathing, haircuts, being touched on the face, sand play, going barefoot, and wearing certain fabrics (Ayres, 1979). Assessments of tactile defensiveness developed by other researchers include Larson's (1982) sensory history and Royeen and Fortune's (1990) Touch Inventory for Elementary School-Aged Children (TIE).

In 1964, Ayres (1964c) proposed that tactile defensiveness was a result of the predominant influence of the protective tactile system, which led to diffuse, alerting, and warning reactions in response to tactile stimuli with concomitant fright, flight, or fight responses. The protective system is older phylogenetically, develops early ontogenetically, and must be inhibited in order for discriminative functions to develop. The discriminative tactile system provides for tactile discrimination of two- and three-dimensional objects and for tactile localization. Predominance of the protective system prevents optimal functioning of the discriminative system.

The presence of tactile defensiveness would seem to contribute to poor performance on tactile discrimination tests that are susceptible to distractibility or that include a light tactile stimulus. In general, however, tests of tactile discrimination have had stronger correlations with praxis tests, whereas somatosensory scores may or may not be depressed in the presence of tactile defensiveness. Thus tactile defensiveness seems to be a problem of disinhibition involving the tactile system rather than a product of a disordered tactile system itself (Ayres, 1976b). Tactile defensiveness and poor tactile discrimination are two separate disorders involving the tactile system, and thus it does not follow that when tactile defensiveness is reduced, improvements in tactile discrimination should be expected (Fisher & Dunn, 1983).

The concept of a continuum of functioning rather than hierarchical, protective versus discriminative tactile functioning has been suggested (Royeen & Lane, 1991). According to this revised model, excessive excitation of the reticular formation through the diffuse thalamic projection system is the neurological correlate for the syndrome of hyperactivity, distractibility, and tactile defensiveness. For unknown reasons, in some individuals, the arousal functions of the reticular activating system predominate and interfere with cortical association and recruitment responses needed for perceptual, attentional, and cognitive processes. Sensory input is inadequately modulated, resulting in heightened responsivity to sensation and difficulty in controlling behavioral responses and focusing attention.

According to Ayres, prolonged nystagmus (Ayres, 1975b) and choreoathetosis (Ayres, 1977c) share an underlying neurological basis with tactile defensiveness, in that all three could be considered indicators of CNS disinhibition or hyperexcitability. Finding that choreoathetosis shared variance with the effect of the asymmetrical tonic neck reflex on equilibrium, Ayres suggested that choreoathetosis was a release phenomenon (1977b) and a problem of insufficient inhibition of motor responses (1977c). Of 54 children with choreoathetoid movements, 31 of whom received SI therapy and 23 of whom received special education only, those receiving therapy made gains in eye-hand coordination after a year of SI therapy (although the gains were not statistically significant). Whether the SI therapy affected the SI substrates of eye-motor coordination or the motor release problem itself was not clarified in this study (Ayres, 1977c).

Recently the term "sensory defensiveness" has been introduced to refer to several types of defensive responses to sensory stimuli (Wilbarger & Wilbarger, 1990). Tactile defensiveness has been viewed as one type of sensory defensiveness that is similar to gravitational insecurity and aversive responses to vestibular-proprioceptive stimuli (Royeen & Lane, 1991). Gravitational insecurity refers to a fearful, defensive reaction to vestibular-proprioceptive stimuli when the body is not in contact with the floor, such as when swinging on suspended equipment (Fisher, 1991). Aversive responses to vestibular-proprioceptive stimuli include autonomic nervous system responses such as nausea, sweating, and dizziness.

Royeen and Lane (1991) consider tactile defensiveness, as well as gravitational insecurity and aversive responses to vestibular stimuli, to be examples of sensory defensiveness, a disorder of sensory modulation that results from an imbalance of descending mechanisms for modulation of sensory stimuli. They have suggested that the limbic system is the neurological correlate of sensory defensiveness.

A study of ten autistic children (Ayres & Tickle, 1980) that investigated level of responsivity to auditory, visual, tactile, vestibular, proprioceptive, olfactory, and gustatory stimuli as a predictor of response to SI therapy showed that SI therapy could be effective in treating sensory defensiveness and tactile defensiveness in particular. Reactions to 14 sensory stimuli were classified as either hyporesponsive, normal, or hyperresponsive. After 1 year, the group was divided into the best and poorest respondents to therapy. Children with hyperresponsivity (e.g., tactile defensiveness, avoidance of movements, gravitational insecurity) and who exhibited an orienting response to an air puff were the best respondents. Ayres and Tickle concluded that those autistic children who were able to register sensory input but could not modulate it benefited more from the organizing effect of SI therapy than did those children who were hyporesponsive to or did not orient to sensory stimuli.

Vestibular Dysfunction

As Ayres' factor analytic studies (1965, 1969a) demonstrate, bilateral integration deficits are linked to postural problems, and both disorders show an association with low academic achievement. As early as 1963, in her Eleanor Clarke Slagle lecture, Ayres speculated that the association between diminished body balance and poor integration of sides of the body might be due to a neurophysiological deficit that was basic to both (Ayres, 1963a). In 1972, Ayres proposed a syndrome of postural and bilateral integration (PBI) with major symptoms including poorly integrated postural and ocular mechanisms, poor bilateral integration, and poor visual perception (Ayres, 1972d). Later research led her to implicate the vestibular system in this syndrome, and eventually to propose that vestibular system dysfunction played a significant role in problems of interhemispheral communication and hemispheric specialization as well. Ayres advanced

> the postulate that the brainstem interhemispheral integrating mechanism is functionally associated with the brainstem postural reflexes and reactions and, furthermore, that inadequate maturation of the brainstem mediated postural reactions interferes with maturation of the brainstem interhemispheral integrative mechanisms. The resultant dysfunction interferes with the development of specialization of function of the cerebral cortex. (Ayres, 1975a, p. 342)

In 1976, Ayres redefined the PBI as a syndrome of vestibular and bilateral integration dysfunction (VBI) that involved poor interhemispheral communication and inadequate cerebral specialization and deficits in the vestibular system (Ayres, 1976a). Inadequate integration of the two body sides, hyporesponsive nystagmus, and deficient postural responses describe its symptomatology. VBI diagnosis depends on the Postrotary Nystagmus and Bilateral Motor Coordination Tests and a variety of clinical observations (i.e., poor eye pursuits across the midline; lack of agreement of eye-hand preference; lack of agreement of ear-hand preference); lack of definite right ear superiority on the Dichotic Listening Test; preferred hand scoring lower on the Motor Accuracy Test; deficit Space Visualization Contralateral Use score; immature righting and equilibrium responses; poorly integrated primitive postural reflexes; lack of flexibility in rotation around the longitudinal axis of the body; reduced postural background movements to orient and adjust the body posturing to a task; muscle hypotonicity; poor co-contraction; and poor discrimination of right and left body sides (Ayres, 1976b).

Ayres' theory of vestibular dysfunction evolved over a period of several years and was based on several studies of the effectiveness of SI therapy, which stimulates the vestibular system and encourages maturation of postural responses in treating learning disabilities. One such study (Ayres, 1972b) evaluated the success of SI therapy in improving the academic performance of children in whom auditory language problems were identified as the cause of their academic difficulties. Five months after the termination of therapy, greater gains in academic scores were made by the experimental group that received SI therapy than by the control group. To explain how this nonacademic therapy could improve academic performance, Ayres proposed that the vestibular and somatosensory input that SI therapy provided enhanced the brain's capacity for intersensory integration of visual, auditory, vestibular, and somatosensory processing, thereby enhancing the brain's capacity for learning. She also hypothesized that "normalization of postural mechanisms organized in the midbrain enable[s] better cortical interhemispheral communication upon which reading must be quite dependent" (Ayres, 1972b, p. 342).

Once Ayres had developed the Postrotary Nystagmus (PRN) Test (Ayres, 1975b), she could assess an ocular reflex reflective of vestibular functioning. A subsequent study (Ayres, 1976a) using PRN test results as a variable thus enabled her to make significant additions to a theory implicating vestibular-based dysfunction in learning disabilities of children. Ayres compared academic gains made by matched groups of children with hypoactive, normal, or prolonged (hyperreactive) postrotary nystagmus who did or did not receive SI therapy in addition to special education. She found that children with hyporesponsive nystagmus who received only special education were less able to profit academically from this regimen than children with hyperreactive or normal nystagmatic responses. However, children with hyporesponsive nystagmus who received SI therapy made academic gains, whereas children with hyporesponsive nystagmus who received only special education showed no change in achievement level. Ayres concluded that hyporesponsive nystagmus identifies a type of vestibular disorder that interferes with academic learning.

The learning disabled children with hyporesponsive nystagmus appeared less dysfunctional and more normal than the children with normal or prolonged nystagmus. The hyporesponsive nystagmus group was more intelligent, was in better physical condition, had better auditory language functions, and showed a higher baseline of academic achievement than the normal or prolonged nystagmus groups. Since children with hyporesponsive nystagmus made up nearly one-half of the sample, whereas their normal incidence is 14 percent, the more capable learning disabled children appeared to suffer from a prevalent vestibular disorder.

Children with prolonged duration nystagmus seemed to have more neurological involvement, and some of them had signs of left cerebral hemisphere dysfunction. This group was less responsive to SI therapy.

As part of the same study, Ayres investigated the predictability of the Dichotic Listening Test for SI dysfunction in learning disabled children. Patterns of associated scores were identified, but were not statistically significant. Children who showed low right-left ear ratios (infrequent use of the left hemisphere) scored poorly on tests of auditory language function (Ayres, 1977b). Two explanations were offered: (1) poor interhemispheral communication leading to poor hemispheric specialization and (2) poor left hemisphere functioning. Because nearly one-half of the sample population had hyporeactive nystagmus, the involvement of the vestibular system was implicated (Ayres, 1976a).

In short, this important 1976 study yielded many useful theoretical, diagnostic, and clinical results. It showed that learning disabled children with vestibular sensory integrative dysfunction could make academic as well as sensory integrative gains when sensory integration therapy was provided in addition to special education. It also laid the groundwork for delineation of the syndrome of vestibular and bilateral integration (Ayres, 1976a). Vestibular disorder, as characterized by hyporesponsive nystagmus, was linked to academic deficits, including auditory language dysfunction (Ayres, 1978).

The association between the vestibular system and auditory language functions was again demonstrated in a 1981 study (Ayres & Mailloux, 1981) of four aphasic children. Using a single case method, Ayres found that rate of growth in language comprehension increased in all of the children and expressive language improved in two of the children after they received SI therapy. Hyporesponsive postrotary nystagmus, indicative of vestibular disorder, was found in the pretesting of the two children who made the greatest gains in expressive language. The therapy emphasized, and all the children sought, experiences in vestibular stimulation.

These results led to the hypothesis that SI therapy promotes auditory processing in those neural systems that are dependent on vestibular and somatosensory processing. Further, Ayres concluded that SI therapy was effective in facilitating language development in aphasic children with somatosensory and vestibular processing disorders, and suggested that the vestibular system was one of a complex of contributing mechanisms underlying expressive speech.

The development of additional tests in the SIPT and subsequent factor and cluster analysis of the SIPT led to further refinement of a disorder of bilateral integration (Ayres, 1989; Ayres & Marr, 1991). A bilateral integration and sequencing (BIS) factor was identified with low scores on Sequencing Praxis, Bilateral Motor Coordination, Graphesthesia, Standing and Walking Balance, Oral Praxis, and Manual Form Perception. In addition, low scores on Postural Praxis were observed in the cluster analysis, but BIS disorder is often seen without low Postural Praxis (Knox, Mack, & Mailloux, 1988). The BIS label is used in the absence of somatopraxis or other explanations of the low scores. When low somatosensory and praxis scores are seen, the bilateral integration and sequencing scores may more appropriately be considered as part of the praxis picture. In addition, when there is evidence of higher level dysfunction, such as with high Postrotary Nystagmus and low Praxis on Verbal Command, the bilateral integration and sequencing problem is not considered a sensory integration problem.

TOOLS FOR THEORY DEVELOPMENT

Ayres developed and tested her theories through literature review, research studies, and clinical practice. Factor analyses and cluster analyses were used in theory development and test construction. Clinical studies investigated the effectiveness of SI therapy for learning disabled and other patient groups.

Literature Review

Ayres consistently used neuroscience, neuropsychology, neurobehavioral, and neurophysiology literature sources to support her assumptions, pose questions, extrapolate findings, and interpret clinical problems. SI theory is a neurologically based theory that seeks to bridge the gap between basic science research and its application to human clinical problems. The neuroscience body of knowledge is a continuing resource for the development of new theory.

Although references to neuroscience literature are found in nearly all of Ayres' writings, her book *Sensory Integration and Learning Disorders* (1972d) provides the most complete discussion of the conceptual neurological bases of her theory. It includes a comprehensive review of principles of brain function, integrative processes, CNS levels, sensory modalities and factors, syndromes, and neural systems as they relate to SI theory. Chapters on specific disorders include sections on neurological, neuroanatomical, and neurophysiological considerations (Ayres, 1972d).

Factor Analytic and Related Studies

Factorial designs are useful for summarizing interrelationships among variables concisely and accurately. The R-technique and Q-technique are the most frequently used types of two- and three-mode factor analysis. The R-technique is used to factor variables (test scores) collected at the same time from a number of individuals. Computation of R involves correlations among various test scores from each subject, thus preserving information about tests but obscuring information about the individual (when pairs of a subject's score are summed, information about that subject is lost). The Q-technique is used to factor an individual's data collected at the same time from a number of variables (test scores). Computation of Q involves correlations among various subjects' scores on a given test, preserving information about subjects but obscuring information about tests. Thus, the R-technique is useful when one wishes to know how test scores are grouped but one is not concerned with the subjects' characteristics. Conversely, the Q-technique is useful when one wishes to group subjects and identify types of individuals but one is not concerned with test characteristics (Gorsuch, 1974).

Cluster analysis is useful for discovering groupings of subjects (Knox, Mack, & Mailloux, 1988). Cluster techniques seek to group subjects into meaningful clusters so that subjects within the group are similar and subjects from different clusters are not alike. Although Ayres used factor analysis for most of her work, she also used cluster analysis for diagnostic groupings on the SIPT.

Having established five syndromes of SI dysfunction in children with learning disabilities and having not observed them in normal children, Ayres proceeded to sharpen the definitions of and provide specific guidelines for, diagnosing types of SI dysfunction and to revise the Southern California Sensory Integration Tests (Ayres, 1972e). Implicating left hemisphere dysfunction in the auditory language factor and right hemisphere dysfunction with the factor "poorer coordination on the left than right side of the body," Ayres (1969a) began to differentiate sensory integration dysfunction from hemisphere dysfunction. This and subsequent studies of academic, language, and sensory integration measures of children with learning problems (Ayres, 1971, 1972f, 1977a) helped Ayres to differentiate the role of sensory integration dysfunction in auditory-language and learning problems and to provide guidelines for test interpretation.

Clinical Practice

Throughout her career, Dr. Ayres was actively involved in clinical practice. In the therapy setting she identified problems, formulated questions, and applied her theoretical approaches. The real world of clinical practice consistently guided her research and theory development efforts. In her clinical research she investigated patterns of perceptual-motor and then SI dysfunction, primarily in the learning disabled, but also in autistic, aphasic, and deaf-blind subjects. She explored effects of SI therapy on a variety of behavior problems, perceptual-motor problems, and skill deficits in children with learning disabilities, neurological disorders, autism, and schizophrenia.

APPLICATION TO OCCUPATIONAL THERAPY PRACTICE

The extent to which a theory is used by persons in the profession is an ultimate criterion for evaluating it. Meleis (1985, p. 158), in her model for theory critique, states, "The final test of any theory is whether or not it is adopted by others." A theory's "circle of contagiousness" indicates where the theory is used geographically; how the theory has been used for research, education, administration, and/or clinical practice; and whether the theory has been used cross-culturally (Meleis, 1985).

The literature on SI published by persons other than Ayres provides a means to assess the circle of contagiousness of SI therapy. This theory has been applied in research and clinical practice and has influenced education in occupational therapy. SI theory is the most widely researched model for practice in occupational therapy. Through the organization Sensory Integration International (SII) and the efforts of interested therapists, SI theory courses have been taught by SII faculty in several countries, including Canada, Japan, and Israel. A review of the literature spawned by SI theory, research, and practice is beyond the scope of this chapter. The reader is referred to *Sensory Integration Theory and Practice* (Fisher, Murray, & Bundy, 1991) for a comprehensive update of theory and therapy based upon new findings in neural-related literature and studies related to the SIPT. The chapter authors in *Sensory Integration Theory and Practice* are themselves accomplished SI researchers who have taken the next step in developing SI theory.

Evaluation and Assessment

Test construction occupied much of Dr. Ayres' efforts. She developed, revised, and reformulated tests for identifying what were termed perceptual-motor problems in the 1960s and what were later referred to as SI dysfunction.

Ayres' first test, the Ayres Space Test, was published in 1962 (Ayres, 1962). It consisted of 60 egg and diamond formboard items. Other early tests included the Southern California Motor Accuracy Test (Ayres, 1964b), the Southern California Kinesthesia and Tactile Perception Tests (Ayres, 1966e), and the Southern California Figure-Ground Visual Perception Test (Ayres, 1966d). The Southern California Perceptual-Motor Tests (Ayres, 1968c) included tests for imitation of postures, bilateral motor coordination, crossing the body midline, standing balance, and right-left discrimination. In 1972, these tests were compiled and republished as the Southern California Sensory Integration Tests (Ayres, 1972e) in order to make testing materials for all 17 tests available in one kit. Changes in the 1972 version included restandardization and reduction of the number of items of the Space Visualization Test (formerly Ayres Space Test), extension of norms for the Figure-Ground Visual Perception Test and the Motor Accuracy Test, and addition of the Position in Space Test and the Design Copying Test (Ayres, 1972e).

The Southern California Postrotary Nystagmus Test, published in 1975, is a procedure for testing the functioning of this vestibularocular reflex (Ayres, 1975b). This test, along with other observations of vestibular-related postural abilities, was important for the interpretation of syndromes related to vestibular functioning.

Revisions of the Southern California Motor Accuracy Test provided norms for three different speeds for right- and left-hand performance. This new procedure allowed children with dysfunction who tend to draw very quickly or very slowly to be more accurately compared to the normative sample (Ayres, 1980a). The Motor Accuracy Test—Revised was the major change in a 1980 edition of the Southern California Sensory Integration Test (Ayres, 1980b).

The Sensory Integration and Praxis Tests (SIPT) (Ayres, 1989) were developed in the 1980s to provide a psychometrically sound test instrument that included tests not available in the Southern California Sensory Integration Tests (SCSIT) (Ayres, Mailloux, & McAtee, 1985). Several tests from the SCSIT were omitted or revised, and four new praxis tests were developed. The normative data for the SIPT were collected on 2,500 children in the United States and Canada, unlike those for the SCSIT, which were collected on children from southern California and which included differing numbers of subjects for the various tests. Computer scoring and interpretation of the SIPT by the test publisher offer accurate, efficient test results for the user and incorporate up-to-date research findings in the test interpretation (Ayres, Mailloux, & McAtee, 1985). A list of the tests included in the SIPT is shown in Exhibit 5-2.

Treatment

Principles

Sensory integrative therapy focuses on control of sensory input that proceeds according to a developmental sequence and requires an adaptive response. The therapist carefully selects therapeutic equipment and activities for the desired somatosensory and vestibular sensation. Developmental sequences are used to recapitulate normal development. Somatosensory and vestibular system development enhances visual and auditory functions. Activities emphasize brainstem, postural responses, and subcortical intersensory integration as precursors of cortical functions. Adaptive responses require organized interaction between the child and the environment and are a natural outcome of accurate and precise sensory input. Thus, adaptive responding is the ability to integrate sensations for motor behavior for effective interaction with the environment. Adaptive responses may be as simple as figuring out how to get one's body in a prone position on a scooter board or as complex as writing one's name. A procedure is considered therapeutic if it helps the child make increasingly mature responses to the therapy environment (Ayres, 1979).

The child's responses are used to guide the treatment. The therapist closely observes the child's spontaneous movements, postural responses, and motor patterns and skills for the desired adaptive behavior. Responses to a given activity or piece of equipment indicate how the child's nervous system interprets the stimuli. Activities that the child enjoys and seeks are generally considered indicative of those things that are integrating to the child's nervous system. Self-initiated activity in a selected environment is thought to be more integrative than imposed activities or tasks. Such an approach offers pleasurable, playful experiences that tap into the child's innate drive toward sensory integration. This invitational approach to therapy is referred to as the "art" of therapy (Ayres, 1979).

The therapist uses activity analysis to analyze the sensations needed for and generated by the activity. The reaction being facilitated or inhibited and the SI requirements for the motor response are carefully observed as the child interacts with the activity (Ayres, 1979).

SI therapy is a movement-based therapy. Movement is used for its sensation-producing effect. Movement generates vestibular, tactile, and proprioceptive sensation that is integrated with visual and auditory sensation. Movement both imposes organization on sensation and is an indicator of the status of that organization (Ayres, 1979).

The treatment sequence begins with improving SI in general through broad stimulation of vestibular and tactile systems. It proceeds with enhancement of the maturation of postural responses and the body's dynamic relationship with the earth's gravitational force. Treatment then emphasizes development of the capacity to motor plan and encouragement of interaction of the two body sides. These steps provide the basis for development of form and space perception and related behavioral, perceptual, and cognitive functions that are important for learning (Ayres, 1975a).

Because of the powerful effects of vestibular and somatosensory stimulation, precautionary measures are mandatory. Therapists should observe for signs of nausea, hyperexcitability, sleepiness or sleeplessness, undesirable increases or decreases in muscle tone, and defensive responses. Adherence to safety factors such as well-padded floors, durable suspension supports, and equipment maintenance procedures is also very important in ensuring a safe therapy environment (Ayres, 1975a, 1979).

Sensory integration therapy is most effective when used in conjunction with services that address other needs of the child and when the child's family is involved (Koomar & Bundy, 1991). The ultimate aim of SI therapy, or any therapy, is to enable the child to function better in his or her occupational roles.

Equipment

Sensory integrative equipment is essential to provision of SI therapy. This equipment enables movement in a variety of planes and requires innumerable

Exhibit 5-2 Brief Description of the 17 Subtests of the Sensory Integration and Praxis Tests

The following is a general and brief description of the 17 SIPT subtests. Consult the SIPT Manual (WPS Catalog No. W-260M) for detailed information about these subtests.
1. Space Visualization (SV). In this puzzle-like test, the child indicates which of two forms will fit a formboard. This test measures visual perception and mental rotation of objects.
2. Figure-Ground Perception (FG). The child points to pictures which are hidden among other pictures. This test measures how well the child visually perceives a figure against a confusing background.
3. Manual Form Perception (MFP). The child identifies unusual shapes held in the hand. This test measures tactile perception and visual perception.
4. Kinesthesia (KIN). The child attempts to put his or her finger at the same place the therapist had previously put it. This test assesses the sense of arm position and movement.
5. Finger Identification (FI). The child points to his or her finger that the therapist touched. This test measures tactile perception.
6. Graphesthesia (GRA). The child draws with a finger the same simple design the therapist drew on the back of the child's hand. This test measures tactile perception and motor planning.
7. Localization of Tactile Stimuli (LTS). The child points to the spot where the therapist had lightly touched the child's arm or hand with a pen. This test measures tactile perception.
8. Praxis on Verbal Command (PrVC). The child executes a series of coordinated movements which have been described verbally. This test assesses ability to translate verbal descriptions into various postures.
9. Design Copying (DC). The child copies a series of increasingly complex line drawings, following detailed instructions. This test measures two-dimensional constructional praxis and visuomotor coordination.
10. Constructional Praxis (CPr). The child builds with blocks, using structures built by the therapist as models. This test measures three-dimensional constructional praxis.
11. Postural Praxis (PPr). In this test, the child imitates unusual body postures demonstrated by the therapist. The ability to conceptualize, plan, and execute movements is assessed.
12. Oral Praxis (OPr). The child imitates movements of the tongue, lips, and jaw. The ability to plan and execute facial movements is assessed.
13. Sequencing Praxis (SPr). The child imitates a series of simple arm and hand movements. This test measures bilateral coordination and the ability to plan and execute sequential movements.
14. Bilateral Motor Coordination (BMC). The child imitates a series of arm and foot movements. This test evaluates the ability to coordinate the two sides of the body.
15. Standing and Walking Balance (SWB). The child holds various standing and walking postures, with eyes open and eyes closed. This test reflects integration of sensation from gravity and proprioceptors.
16. Motor Accuracy (MAc). In this test, the child draws a line on top of a long, curving printed line. Visuomotor coordination and motor planning are measured.
17. Postrotary Nystagmus (PRN). The child is rotated clockwise and counterclockwise on a rotation board. This test measures processing of vestibular sensory input.

Source: Sensory Integration and Praxis Tests by A.J. Ayres. Reprinted by permission of the publisher, © copyright 1988, Western Psychological Services, 12031 Wilshire Blvd., Los Angeles, CA.

combinations of muscular, balance, and coordination responses. Equipment developed in the Ayres Clinic includes the suspended hammock, scooter board ramp, platform swing, carpeted barrel, quadruped balancing board, inner-tube barrel, "helicopter" suspended apparatus, and vibrating table. Scooter boards, large therapy balls, suspended bolsters, and T-stools developed in other sensory motor therapies are used in SI therapy as well (Ayres, 1979).

Therapy Emphasis in Various Forms of Sensory Integrative Dysfunction

Therapy for developmental dyspraxia addresses problems with ideation or concept of the activity, planning a course of action, and executing the plan. For the child with ideational problems, the therapist selects the simplest activity that the child can perform using his or her whole body in relationship to the therapeutic equipment. For severe ideational problems, the therapist helps the child through the activity manually and verbally and through modeling. Because the typical therapy equipment may be too complicated for the child with these conceptual problems, the therapist may need to create simplified activities.

For the child with problems in planning and executing movements, the therapist selects activities eliciting strong motor responses to provide massive sensory flow from somatosensory and proprioceptive systems. These activities, which emphasize total flexion, extension, rotary, and diagonal movements, provide the postural basis for planning and executing movements. Planning and executing movements proceed from simple praxis activities, such as moving effectively from one place to another, to more complex praxis activities involving sequences of movement (Ayres, 1985). Koomar and Bundy (1991) suggest a progression of activities from isolated to combined movements, from movements of the whole body to movements that activate one part of the body and inhibit others, and from feedback-dependent to feedforward-dependent actions. Feedback-dependent activities are those that require the individual to depend upon feedback arising from movement as it occurs; feedforward-dependent activities require the individual to anticipate the sequence of movements that will be needed to perform the activity. The more complex the activity, the greater the demands for adequate processing of sensory information for feedback and feedforward to plan and execute activities in time and space.

Therapy for vestibular-based dysfunction emphasizes motion, rotation, and starting and stopping actions to activate the vestibular system. Extension postures and alternating flexion and extension for co-contraction and bilateral activities are incorporated into the treatment. Righting and equilibrium responses are facilitated in prone, supine, and upright positions. The rate of vestibular stimulation is varied to produce desired calming or excitatory effects. Because of the autonomic reactions associated with vestibular stimulation, the therapist must observe for signs of autonomic distress such as sweating, pallor, respiratory changes, flushing, nausea, seizures, or dizziness.

Problems with modulation of sensory input (overresponsivity, underresponsivity, fluctuating responsivity, or delayed responsivity) manifest as tactile defensiveness, gravitational insecurity, aversive response to vestibular stimulation, and diminished sensory registration. These conditions require the therapist to calibrate sensory input carefully and to monitor the child's responses (Koomar & Bundy, 1991).

CRITIQUE OF SENSORY INTEGRATION THEORY

Theory

Sensory integration is one of the more controversial therapies for learning disabilities. Sieben (1977) criticized this approach citing as faulty its assumption that children with learning disabilities have something wrong with their brainstems. He also criticized the assumptions that controlled stimulation of vestibular and somatosensory systems improves brainstem integration for vision and hearing and that there is carryover from mastery of postural skills to academic skills. In contrast, Lerer (1981) stated that the SI concepts are accurate and are based on 100 years of biomedical research efforts. He argued that SI theory concerning implication of the brainstem in sensory motor dysfunction is "probably valid" and that medical and other professionals recognize similar symptomatology in which the brainstem may be important.

Ottenbacher and Short (1985) identified literature supporting the assumption that subcortical brain areas contribute to complex processes of learning and cognition. They also noted that the "active management of children in meaningful, challenging activities that provide a vast array of multisensory and motor stimulation and feedback" (1985, p. 304), which characterizes SI therapy, is well documented in the literature.

Ayres' attempts to link bilateral integration (and hemispheric communication and hemispheric lateralization) and vestibular functioning have remained speculative since the role of the vestibular system has not been clearly established. Fisher (1991) makes several important points regarding this issue.

First, Ayres used the Postrotary Nystagmus (PRN) Test as an indicator of central vestibular processing, i.e., brainstem central nervous system processing of vestibular information, and assumed intact peripheral structures and functions. Whether the duration of postrotary nystagmus reflects central or peripheral vestibular functioning remains controversial, and doubts on this matter have been used to discredit vestibular-related sensory integration dysfunction. In defense of sensory integration theory, Fisher (1991) urges readers to differentiate between those studies in which indicators of *peripheral* vestibular function are measured (peak slow-phase eye velocity during vestibular nystagmus) and those studies in which indicators of *central* vestibular processing are measured (circularvection, time course of vestibular nystagmus, duration of optokinetic afternystagmus, and postural control under conditions of sensory conflict). (p. 84)

Second, the PRN assesses one aspect of vestibular functioning: compensatory eye movements in relationship to the position and movements of the head. Other ocular and postural responses are tested through clinical observations that do not differentiate roles of the vestibular and proprioceptive systems. Ocular pursuits, tested as part of the postural-ocular deficits, are mediated by the visual system, not the vestibular system.

Third, although Ayres differentiated the roles of proprioceptive, tactile, and vestibular input in her views of praxis or bilateral integration (see Ayres, 1972d, p. 171), she often referred only to discriminative tactile functions and their role in praxis (Cermak, 1991; Fisher, 1991). This lack of clarity was due, in part, to the lack of tests of proprioception and the difficulty with separating proprioception from vestibular and tactile functions. (Also, generally, the term *proprioception* includes vestibular as well as muscle, joint, tendon, and deep pressure receptors.) The postural abilities that we assess through clinical observations call for combined proprioceptive, vestibular, and tactile processing.

Fisher (1991) and Cermak (1991) refine Ayres' views on the relative contribution of tactile, proprioception, and vestibular systems. They hypothesize that dyspraxia is a dysfunction of somatosensory processing and that the bilateral integration and sequencing deficit is a dysfunction of vestibular and proprioceptive processing. Further, bilateral integration dysfunction may be a form of dyspraxia that involves the proprioceptive and vestibular system and is characterized by impaired bilateral, anticipatory responding in sequences of actions. Dyspraxia may be seen alone or in combination with bilateral integration and sequencing dysfunction.

Finally, Ayres' hypothesized brain stem interhemispheral mechanism has not been supported by neurological correlates. However, the importance of proprioception, vestibular, and tactile input to motor cortices for body scheme, motor control, motor planning, anticipatory responding, attention, orientation, and sequencing has been demonstrated (Cermak, 1991; Fisher, 1991). To this author, continuing to view a brainstem-cortical hierarchy is no longer as useful as conceptualizing these structures as aspects of one interactive neural system.

Testing

Ayres' first tests, the Southern California Sensory Integration Tests (SCSIT), were criticized for their incomplete standardization information, sample size variations of 13 to 70 subjects on the subtests, and small sample size of fewer than 100 in each age group. Other concerns included reliability and validity of the SCSIT. The Sensory Integration and Praxis Tests (SIPT) (Ayres, 1989) were developed to replace the SCSIT with a psychometrically sound instrument.

Reliability

Reliability of the 17 SIPT subtests was generally good. Interrater reliability coefficients ranged from .94 to .99 (Ayres, 1989). Test-retest reliability coefficients were .60 or better on all tests except for Postrotary Nystagmus (.48), Kinesthesia (.50), Localization of Tactile Stimuli (.53), and Figure-Ground Perception (.56), and the median for all tests was .74. These reliability coefficients are a considerable improvement over those of the 17 SCSIT subtests. On the SCSIT, test-retest coefficients ranged from .01 to .94, with a median of .53 (Ayres, 1980b) and were below .70 on 73 percent of the tests (Evan & Peham, 1981).

Validity

Construct- and criterion-related validity studies were conducted for the SIPT (Ayres & Marr, 1991). Construct validity was investigated through factor and cluster analysis. Factor analyses were conducted with a normative sample ($n =$ 1750), dysfunctional children ($n = 125$), and a combined group of dysfunctional children ($n = 117$) matched to children in the normative sample ($n = 176$). A cluster analysis was conducted on the latter combined group. The results of these studies further clarified theoretical constructs identified in Ayres' earlier factor analytic studies. Two types of criterion-related validity studies were conducted. First, in the absence of comparable sensory integration tests, SIPT profiles were compared across other diagnostic groups that had prior diagnosis and would be expected to conform to patterns that were in keeping with the diagnosis. Second, SIPT scores were compared to scores on the Kaufman Assessment Battery for Children (K-ABC); the Luria-Nebraska Neuropsychological Battery, Children's Revision; the Bruininks-Oseretsky Test of Motor Proficiency; and the Bender-Gestalt Test.

The validity studies of the SIPT were considerably more comprehensive than were the validity investigations of the SCSIT. The original versions of the SCSIT provided some validity data (Ayres, 1962, 1964b, 1966e) and included the ability of the test to discriminate between normal and dysfunctional groups. Concurrent validity was also shown through correlation with similar published tests. Manuals for the later versions of the SCSIT did not include validity information (Ayres, 1972e, 1980a).

Research Methods

Factor analysis is a research method that can identify both theoretical constructs in a developing theory and the operational characteristics of those constructs. Thus it can be used to examine both construct validation of test instruments and the underlying theory (Gorsuch, 1974). Ayres' factor analytic studies established construct validity of her testing instruments and the theorized syndromes of dysfunction. However, Ayres' earlier studies have been criticized for methodological inadequacies (Clark, Mailloux, & Parham, 1985). A closer look at Ayres' studies in terms of factor analytic criteria does reveal some flaws.

Gorsuch (1974) recommends that factor analytic studies meet the following six conditions for generalizability of factor analysis:

1. The number of subjects should not be less than 100, and the absolute minimum ratio is five individuals to one variable.
2. Split sample analysis should be used, keeping those factors that match across the two samples; a large sample is also necessary.
3. Variables should have a history of good reliability estimates and good correlation with other variables in the analysis.
4. Factors should be highly significant based on the tests for this criterion, although significance tests in factor analysis are poor.
5. A minimum of five to six variable loadings should be used for each factor.
6. Data should be factored by several different analytical procedures, keeping only those factors that appear across the procedures used.

Most of Ayres' factor analytic studies meet Gorsuch's first criterion in that they have 100 or more dysfunctional subjects (Ayres, 1965, 1971, 1972f, 1977a; Ayres et al., 1987; Ayres & Marr, 1991), although one study of dysfunctional children (Ayres, 1969a) and two of normal children (Ayres, 1966b, 1966c) do not meet this criterion. Ayres' 1965 study (Ayres, 1965), which has 25 children in each of four groups, does not meet the criterion of a large split sample. The good reliability of the SIPT (Ayres & Marr, 1991) meets criterion 3, but the poor reliability of the earlier SCSIT compromises criterion 3 (Ayres, 1980b). Significances of factors of .01 and .05 are reported (Ayres, 1965, 1966b, 1966c, 1971, 1972f; Ayres et al., 1987); thus criterion 4 is met to some extent, assuming that .01 is considered highly significant. Ayres identifies factors with six or more variables, thus meeting criterion 5. Finally, Ayres uses Q- and R-technique factor analyses to identify factors. She retained those factors that consistently reappear: developmental dyspraxia, deficit in form and space, dysfunction in bilateral integration, and tactile defensiveness. Thus, criterion 6 is met if applied to several studies together and not to individual studies. However, Cummins (1991) has criticized Ayres' factor analytic studies for their lack of cross-validation. His reappraisal of data in eight studies by Ayres from the period 1986–1987 failed to support the factors identified by Ayres.

SI efficacy research has been criticized as being poorly controlled, having too few subjects, not accounting for the Hawthorne effect, and being interpretive and anecdotal (Arendt, MacLean, & Baumeister, 1988; Bochner, 1978; Committee on Children with Disabilities, 1985; Densem, Nutall, Bushnell, & Horn, 1989; Lerer, 1981; Posthuma, 1983; Schaffer, 1984). An analysis of five SI therapy efficacy studies (Schaffer, 1984) identified a likelihood of Type I and Type II errors.

Meta-analyses of SI efficacy studies have yielded conflicting results. Ottenbacher (1982) reported a meta-analysis of eight studies, including three by Ayres, and concluded that the performance of subjects who received SI therapy was significantly better than that of subjects in the control groups. Eight of the forty-nine studies identified met the operational definition of SI therapy for inclusion in the analysis. Although Ayres' (1972b, 1978) effectiveness studies had emphasized improved academic functioning, Ottenbacher found that the dependent variables most affected by SI therapy were motor or reflex variables. In contrast, Kavale and Mattson (1983) conducted a meta-analysis of 180 studies, including one study by Ayres (1972b), to assess the efficacy of perceptual-motor training for improving academic, cognitive, or perceptual-motor scores. The criterion for inclusion of a study in the analysis was the presence of a control group. These authors concluded that "perceptual motor training is not effective and should be questioned as a feasible intervention technique for exceptional children" (p. 165). They were surprised that not even perceptual motor measures showed improvement. Similarly, Myers and Hammill's (1982) actuarial analysis of 35 studies of Kephart, Barsch, Cratty, Getman, and Ayres found that results of these studies failed to support these approaches.

Several factors contribute to the conflicting and controversial results of SI efficacy research (Walker, 1991). First, SI therapy is difficult to administer in a precise, homogeneous fashion due to natural variability in individualized therapy, unique functional levels and responsivity of the individual child, and expertise of the therapist.

Second, although the characteristics of SI therapy have been well delineated by Ayres and others, the actual type of therapy being rendered has often been ill defined or not defined in studies claiming to use SI therapy. Or the therapy described as SI therapy, such as balance beam work (Densem et al., 1989), has not met accepted definitions of SI therapy. The specialized space, equipment, and training required for SI therapy in some cases has been overmodified to the extent that it no longer approximates SI therapy as Ayres designed it.

Third, SI therapy has been confused with other approaches such as neurodevelopmental intervention (Arendt et al., 1988), neurophysiologic retraining regimens (Sieben, 1977), and perceptual motor training (Kavale & Mattson, 1983; Myers & Hammill, 1982). This point was made clear when AOTA President Robert Bing (personal communication, December 20, 1985) and a Sensory Integration International committee (personal communication, December 20, 1985) responded to a recommendation by the Committee on Children with Disabilities (1985) that pediatricians recommend occupational therapy for severe motor problems but not for the dyspraxic or clumsy child because these problems improve with age and the therapy programs have not been the subject of scientific research. Bing and the SII committee not only cited research that showed long-term effects of dyspraxia; they also differentiated SI therapy from passive patterning therapies and cited research to support its superior effectiveness.

Finally, while not a defense of research flaws nor an excuse for limited research, an argument can be made that Ayres' clinical research had empirical merit during the evolution of a body of SI research and theory (Cermak & Henderson, 1990). In response to critiques of SI research methodology (Lerer, 1981), AOTA President May Hightower-Van Damm said,

> In many instances in medicine, psychology, and education, carefully documented behavioral changes are the most important data we have to evaluate a given approach to a presenting problem, i.e., drug therapies, psychotherapy, behavior modification and self-contained classroom instruction. (Personal communication, March 12, 1981)

She went on to state that funding is scarce for comprehensive research projects, that anecdotal and case study research are increasingly acceptable research formats, and that research efforts by clinicians and educators can yield empirical data that are important educationally. Given these conditions, SI research is no more deserving of criticism than any other research into the perplexing problems of learning disabilities.

Occupational therapists have been criticized for their overzealousness in promoting SI therapy for children and for overextension of research findings to other patient populations. Lerer (1981) suggested that SI therapy not be used outside the experimental research situation, and he criticized therapists for subjecting families, taxpayers, and third-party payers to the expense of this experimental therapy. He remarked that "Ayres, in her carefully conducted inquiries, is cautious about drawing definite conclusions from her theories, concepts and hypotheses" (1981, p. 4). Posthuma (1983) questioned the widespread use of SI therapy by occupational therapists in adult psychiatry and cited cost ineffectiveness, lack of standardized tests for adults, and confusion over SI versus other movement therapies as areas that needed to be addressed. She urged the development of research and specialty training to enable SI therapy to be appropriately applied to adults. In a review of SI studies, Ottenbacher (1982) found no studies in psychiatry, geriatrics, or physical disabilities that met empirical standards of traditional behavioral science research. He cautioned therapists not to apply SI therapy prematurely to populations for which the therapeutic effects have not been established. Similarly, Arendt et al. (1988) concluded that SI therapy for persons with mental retardation has not been empirically or theoretically supported and should only be used for research purposes with this population.

Summary of Critiques

In summary, the theoretical assumptions of SI theory have a basis in the neurosciences. However, highly selective interpretations of the neuroscience literature that support SI theory are subject to criticism. Frequent updatings of neuroscience conceptual bases are requisite for future SI theory development.

Psychometric inadequacies of the SCSIT have been corrected in the Southern California Sensory Integration and Praxis Test. The primary purpose of this standardization project was to develop a valid and reliable instrument for evaluation of SI dysfunction in children with learning disabilities. There continues to be a need to develop instruments for identifying SI dysfunction in other patient populations.

Research has shown extant SI dysfunction in some children with learning disabilities. There is some evidence that SI therapy enhances academic learning. Other gains include improvements in motor performance. Further well-designed research needs to be conducted to delineate the types of patient problems most benefited by SI therapy and to assess long-term effects of therapy.

The work of Ayres has had a large impact on the OT field. Although developed for a specific patient group (i.e., children with learning problems), the theory is one of, if not the most, complete of existing OT theories. Its scope includes clinical problem identification, formulation of theoretical constructs, theory validation research, test instrument development, therapy approaches and equipment, and therapy efficacy studies. SI theory has spawned more research, publication, and educational efforts in occupational therapy than any other OT theory to date. It has helped therapists to view patient problems in the context of sensory functioning and has provided another way of perceiving health and dysfunction.

REFERENCES

American Occupational Therapy Association. (1985). Jean Ayres retires from clinical practice. *Occupational Therapy News, 39* (6), 24.

American Occupational Therapy Association. (1987). Ayres award established. *Occupational Therapy News, 41* (11), 3.

American Occupational Therapy Association. (1989a). A. Jean Ayres, PhD, OTR, FAOTA: Profession remembers eminent clinician and scholar. *Occupational Therapy News, 43* (2), 1, 10, 15.

American Occupational Therapy Association. (1989b). OT leaders Ayres and Robinson receive special tributes in Baltimore. *Occupational Therapy Week, 3* (17), 4.

Arendt, R.E., MacLean, W.E., & Baumeister, A.A. (1988). Critique of sensory integration therapy and its application in mental retardation. *American Journal on Mental Retardation, 92* (5), 401–411.

Ayres, A.J. (1949). An analysis of crafts in the treatment of electroshock patients. *American Journal of Occupational Therapy, 3*, 195–198.

Ayres, A.J. (1954). Ontogenetic principles in the development of arm and hand functions. *American Journal of Occupational Therapy, 3*, 95–99.

Ayres, A.J. (1958). The visual-motor function. *American Journal of Occupational Therapy, 12*, 130–138.

Ayres, A.J. (1960). Occupational therapy for motor disorders resulting from impairment of the central nervous system. *Rehabilitation Literature, 21*, 302–310.

Ayres, A.J. (1961a). Development of the body scheme in children. *American Journal of Occupational Therapy, 15*, 99–102.

Ayres, A.J. (1961b). The role of gross motor activities in the training of children with visual motor retardation. *Journal of the American Optometric Association, 33*, 121–125.

Ayres, A.J. (1962). *Ayres Space Test.* Los Angeles: Western Psychological Services.

Ayres, A.J. (1963a). The development of perceptual-motor abilities: A theoretical basis for treatment of dysfunction. *American Journal of Occupational Therapy, 17*, 221–225.

Ayres, A.J. (1963b). Occupational therapy directed toward neuromuscular integration. In H.S. Willard & C.S. Spackman (Eds.), *Occupational therapy* (3rd ed.) (pp. 358–466). Philadelphia: J.B. Lippincott.

Ayres, A.J. (1964a). Perceptual motor training for children. In C. Slattery (Ed.), *Approaches to the treatment of patients with neuromuscular dysfunction: Study Course VI. Third International Conference of the World Federation of Occupational Therapists, 1962* (pp. 17–22). Dubuque, Iowa: William C. Brown.

Ayres, A.J. (1964b). *Southern California Motor-Accuracy Test.* Los Angeles: Western Psychological Services.

Ayres, A.J. (1964c). Tactile functions: Their relation to hyperactivity and perceptual-motor behavior. *American Journal of Occupational Therapy, 18*, 6–11.

Ayres, A.J. (1965). Patterns of perceptual-motor dysfunction in children: A factor analytic study. *Perceptual and Motor Skills, 20*, 335–368.

Ayres, A.J. (1966a). Interrelation of perception, function, and treatment. *Journal of the American Physical Therapy Association, 46*, 741–744.

Ayres, A.J. (1966b). Interrelations among perceptual-motor abilities in a group of normal children. *American Journal of Occupational Therapy, 20*, 288–292.

Ayres, A.J. (1966c). Interrelationships among perceptual-motor functions in children. *American Journal of Occupational Therapy, 20*, 68–71.

Ayres, A.J. (1966d). *Southern California Figure Ground Visual Perception Tests.* Los Angeles: Western Psychological Services.

Ayres, A.J. (1966e). *Southern California Kinesthesia and Tactile Perception Tests.* Los Angeles: Western Psychological Services.

Ayres, A.J. (1967). Remedial procedures based on neurobehavioral constructs. *Proceedings of the 1967 International Convocation on Children and Young Adults with Learning Disabilities.* Pittsburgh.

Ayres, A.J. (1968a). Reading—A product of sensory integrative process. In A. Henderson et al. (Eds.), *The development of sensory integrative theory and practice* (pp. 167–175). Dubuque, IA: Kendall/ Hunt Publishing.

Ayres, A.J. (1968b). Sensory integrative processes and neuropsychological learning disability. In *Learning Disorders* (Vol. 3, pp. 41–58). Seattle, WA: Special Child Publications.

Ayres, A.J. (1968c). *Southern California Perceptual-Motor Tests.* Los Angeles: Western Psychological Services.

Ayres, A.J. (1969a). Deficits in sensory integration in educationally handicapped children. *Journal of Learning Disabilities, 2,* 160–168.

Ayres, A.J. (1969b). Relation between Gesell development quotients and later perceptual-motor performance. *American Journal of Occupational Therapy, 23,* 11–17.

Ayres, A.J. (1971). Characteristics of types of sensory integrative dysfunction. *American Journal of Occupational Therapy, 25,* 329–334.

Ayres, A.J. (1972a). Basic concepts of occupational therapy for children with perceptual-motor dysfunction. *Proceedings of the Twelfth World Congress of Rehabilitation International.* Sydney, Australia.

Ayres, A.J. (1972b). Improving academic scores through sensory integration. *Journal of Learning Disabilities, 5,* 338–343.

Ayres, A.J. (1972c). An interpretation of the role of the brain stem in intersensory integration. In A. Henderson & J. Coryell (Eds.), *The body senses and perceptual deficit: Proceedings of the Occupational Therapy Symposium on Somatosensory Aspects of Perceptual Deficits* (pp. 81–89). Boston: Boston University.

Ayres, A.J. (1972d). *Sensory integration and learning disorders.* Los Angeles: Western Psychological Services.

Ayres, A.J. (1972e). *Southern California Sensory Integration Tests.* Los Angeles: Western Psychological Services.

Ayres, A.J. (1972f). Types of sensory integrative dysfunction among disabled learners. *American Journal of Occupational Therapy, 26,* 13–18.

Ayres, A.J. (1975a). Sensorimotor foundations of academic ability. In W.M. Cruickshank & D.P. Hallahan (Eds.), *Perceptual and learning disabilities in children* (Vol. 2, pp. 301–358). Syracuse, NY: Syracuse University Press.

Ayres, A.J. (1975b). *Southern California Postrotary Nystagmus Test.* Los Angeles: Western Psychological Services.

Ayres, A.J. (1976a). *The effects of sensory integration therapy on learning disabled children.* Los Angeles: University of Southern California.

Ayres, A.J. (1976b). *Interpreting the Southern California Sensory Integration Tests.* Los Angeles: Western Psychological Services.

Ayres, A.J. (1977a). Cluster analyses of measures of sensory integration. *American Journal of Occupational Therapy, 31,* 362–366.

Ayres, A.J. (1977b). Dichotic listening performance in learning-disabled children. *American Journal of Occupational Therapy, 31,* 441–446.

Ayres, A.J. (1977c). Effect of sensory integrative therapy on the coordination of children with choreoathetoid movements. *American Journal of Occupational Therapy, 31,* 291–293.

Ayres, A.J. (1978). Learning disabilities and the vestibular system. *Journal of Learning Disabilities, 11,* 18–29.

Ayres, A.J. (1979). *Sensory integration and the child.* Los Angeles: Western Psychological Services.

Ayres, A.J. (1980a). *Southern California Motor Accuracy Test—Revised 1980.* Los Angeles: Western Psychological Services.

Ayres, A.J. (1980b). *Southern California Sensory Integration Tests—Revised 1980.* Los Angeles: Western Psychological Services.

Ayres, A.J. (1985). *Developmental dyspraxia and adult onset dyspraxia.* Torrance, CA: Sensory Integration International.

Ayres, A.J. (1988). *Sensory Integration and Praxis Tests.* Los Angeles: Western Psychological Services.

Ayres, A.J., & Mailloux, Z.K. (1981). Influence of sensory integration procedures on language development. *American Journal of Occupational Therapy, 35,* 383–390.

Ayres, A.J., Mailloux, Z.K., & McAtee, S. (1985). An update of the Sensory Integration and Praxis Tests. *Sensory Integration Special Interest Section Newsletter, 8* (3).

Ayres, A.J., Mailloux, Z.K., & Wendler, C.L. (1987). Developmental dyspraxia. Is it a unitary function? *Occupational Therapy Journal of Research, 7* (2), 93–110.

Ayres, A.J., & Marr, D.B. (1991). Sensory Integration and Praxis Test. In A.G. Fisher, E.A. Murray, & A.C. Bundy (Eds.), *Sensory integration theory and practice* (pp. 203–229). Philadelphia: F.A. Davis.

Ayres, A.J., & Tickle, L.S. (1980). Hyper-responsivity to touch and vestibular stimuli predict positive response to sensory integration procedures in autistic children. *American Journal of Occupational Therapy, 34,* 375–381.

Bochner, S. (1978). Ayres, sensory integration and learning disorders: Question of theory and practice. *American Journal of Mental Retardation, 5,* 41–45.

Cermak, S.A. (1991). Somatodyspraxia. In A.G. Fisher, E.A. Murray, & A.C. Bundy (Eds.), *Sensory integration theory and practice* (pp. 137–165). Philadelphia: F.A. Davis.

Cermak, S.A., & Henderson, A. (1990). The efficacy of sensory integration procedures. Part II. *Sensory Integration Quarterly, 18* (1), 1–5, 17.

Clark, E., Mailloux, Z., & Parham, D. (1985). Sensory integration and children with learning disabilities. In P.N. Clark & A.S. Allen (Eds.), *Occupational therapy for children* (pp. 359–405). St. Louis: C.V. Mosby.

Committee on Children with Disabilities. (1985). School aged children with motor disabilities. *Pediatrics, 76,* 648–649.

Cummins, R.A. (1991). Sensory integration and learning disabilities: Ayres' factor analyses reappraised. *Journal of Learning Disabilities, 24* (3), 160–168.

Densem, J.F., Nutall, G.A., Bushnell, J., & Horn, J. (1989). Effectiveness of a sensory integrative therapy program for children with perceptual-motor deficits. *Journal of Learning Disabilities, 22* (4), 221–229.

Evan, P.R., & Peham, M.A. (1981). *Testing and measurements in occupational therapy: A review of current practice with special emphasis on the Southern California Sensory Integration Tests.* Minneapolis: University of Minnesota.

Fisher, A.G. (1991). Vestibular-proprioceptive processing and bilateral integration and sequencing deficits. In A.G. Fisher, E.A. Murray, & A.C. Bundy (Eds.), *Sensory integration theory and practice* (pp. 71–107). Philadelphia: F.A. Davis.

Fisher, A.G., & Dunn, W. (1983). Tactile defensiveness: Historical perspectives, new research. A theory grows. *Sensory Integration Special Interest Section Newsletter, 6* (2), 1–2.

Fisher, A.G., & Murray, E.A. (1991). Introduction to sensory integration theory. In A.G. Fisher, E.A. Murray, & A.C. Bundy (Eds.), *Sensory integration theory and practice* (pp. 3–26). Philadelphia: F.A. Davis.

Fisher, A.G., Murray, E.A., & Bundy, A.C. (Eds.). (1991). *Sensory integration theory and practice.* Philadelphia: F.A. Davis.

Gorsuch, R.L. (1974). *Factor analysis.* Philadelphia: W.B. Saunders.

Kavale, K., & Mattson, P.D. (1983). One jumped off the balance beam: Meta-analysis of perceptual motor training. *Journal of Learning Disabilities, 16* (3), 165–173.

Knox, S., Mack, W., & Mailloux, Z. (1988). *Interpreting the Sensory Integration and Praxis Tests.* Los Angeles: Sensory Integration International.

Koomar, J.A., & Bundy, A.C. (1991). The art and science of creating direct intervention from theory. In A.G. Fisher, E.A. Murray, & A.C. Bundy (Eds.), *Sensory integration theory and practice* (pp. 251–314). Philadelphia: F.A. Davis.

Larson, K.A. (1982). The sensory history of developmentally delayed children with and without sensory defensiveness. *American Journal of Occupational Therapy, 36,* 590–596.

Lerer, R.J. (1981). An open letter to an occupational therapist. *Journal of Learning Disabilities, 14,* 3–4.

Meleis, A.I. (1985). *Theoretical nursing: Development and progress.* Philadelphia: J.B. Lippincott.

Myers, P.I., & Hammill, D.D. (1982). *Learning disabilities: Basic concepts, assessment practices and instructional strategies.* Austin, TX: PRO-ED.

Ottenbacher, K. (1982). Sensory integration therapy: Affect of effect. *American Journal of Occupational Therapy, 36,* 571–578.

Ottenbacher, K., & Short, M.A. (1985). Sensory integrative dysfunction in children: A review of theory and treatment. *Advances in Developmental and Behavioral Pediatrics, 6,* 287–329.

Posthuma, B.W. (1983). Sensory integration: Fact or fad. *American Journal of Occupational Therapy, 37,* 343–345.

Royeen, C.B., & Fortune, J.C. (1990). TIE: Touch Inventory for Elementary School Aged Children. *American Journal of Occupational Therapy, 44,* 165–170.

Royeen, C.B., & Lane, S.J. (1991). Tactile processing and sensory defensiveness. In A.G. Fisher, E.A. Murray, & A.C. Bundy (Eds.), *Sensory integration theory and practice* (pp. 108–133). Philadelphia: F.A. Davis.

Schaffer, R. (1984). Sensory integration therapy with learning disabled children: A critical review. *Canadian Journal of Occupational Therapy, 51* (2), 73–77.

Sieben, R.I. (1977). Controversial medical treatments of learning disabilities. *Academic Therapy, 13,* 133–147.

Walker, K.F. (1991). Sensory integrative therapy in a limited space: An adaptation of the Ayres Clinic design. *Sensory Integration Special Interest Section Newsletter, 14* (3), 1, 2, 4.

Wilbarger, P., & Wilbarger, J.L. (1990). *Defensiveness in children: An intervention guide for parents and other caregivers.* PDP Products, 12015 N. July Ave., Hugo, MN 55038.

BIBLIOGRAPHY

1949

Ayres, A.J. (1949). An analysis of crafts in the treatment of electroshock patients. *American Journal of Occupational Therapy, 3,* 195–198.

1954

Ayres, A.J. (1954). A form used to evaluate the work behavior of patients. *American Journal of Occupational Therapy, 8*, 73–74.

Ayres, A.J. (1954). Ontogenetic principles in the development of arm and hand functions. *American Journal of Occupational Therapy, 8*, 95–99.

1955

Ayres, A.J. (1955). Proprioceptive facilitation elicited through the upper extremities. *American Journal of Occupational Therapy, 9*, 1–9, 57–58, 121–126.

Ayres, A.J. (1955). A pilot study on the relationship between work habits and workshop production. *American Journal of Occupational Therapy, 9*, 264–276.

1957

Ayres, A.J. (1957). A study of the manual dexterity and workshop wages of thirty-nine cerebral palsied trainees. *American Journal of Physical Medicine, 36*, 6–10.

1958

Ayres, A.J. (1958). The visual-motor function. *American Journal of Occupational Therapy, 12*, 130–138.

Ayres, A.J. (1958). Basic concepts of clinical practice in physical disabilities. *American Journal of Occupational Therapy, 12*, 300–302.

1960

Ayres, A.J. (1960). Hemiplegia. In *Occupational therapy reference manual for physicians* (pp. 38–42). Dubuque, IA: William C. Brown..

Ayres, A.J. (1960). Occupational therapy for motor disorders resulting from impairment of the central nervous system. *Rehabilitation Literature, 21*, 302–310.

Ayres, A.J. (1960). Research for therapists. *Proceedings of the American Occupational Therapy Association 1960 Conference* (pp. 79–82). Rockville, MD: American Occupational Therapy Association.

1961

Ayres, A.J. (1961). Development of the body scheme in children. *American Journal of Occupational Therapy, 15*, 99–102.

Ayres, A.J. (1961). The role of gross motor activities in the training of children with visual motor retardation. *Journal of the American Optometric Association, 33*, 121–125.

1962

Ayres, A.J. (1962). Perception of space of adult hemiplegic patients. *Physical Medicine and Rehabilitation, 43*, 552–555.

1963

Ayres, A.J. (1963). The development of perceptual-motor abilities. A theoretical basis for treatment of dysfunction. *American Journal of Occupational Therapy, 17*, 221–225.

Ayres, A.J. (1963). Occupational therapy directed toward neuromuscular integration. In H.S. Willard & C.S. Spackman (Eds.), *Occupational therapy* (3rd ed.) (pp. 358–466). Philadelphia: J.B. Lippincott.

1964

Ayres, A.J. (1964). *Perceptual-motor dysfunction in children.* Monograph from the Greater Cincinnati District, Ohio Occupational Therapy Association, Cincinnati.

Ayres, A.J. (1964). Perceptual-motor training for children. In C. Slattery (Ed.), *Approaches to the treatment of patients with neuromuscular dysfunction: Study Course VI, Third International Conference of the World Federation of Occupational Therapists, 1962* (pp. 17–22). Dubuque, IA: William C. Brown.

Ayres, A.J. (1964). Integration of information. In C. Slattery (Ed.), *Approaches to the treatment of patients with neuromuscular dysfunction: Study Course VI. Third International Conference of the World Federation of Occupational Therapists, 1962* (pp. 49–57). Dubuque, IA: William C. Brown.

Ayres, A.J. (1964). Perspectives on neurological bases of reading. In M.P. Douglass (Ed.), *Claremont Reading Conference, 28th yearbook* (pp. 113–118). Claremont, CA: Claremont Graduate School Curriculum Laboratory.

Ayres, A.J. (1964). Tactile functions: Their relation to hyperactivity and perceptual-motor behavior. *American Journal of Occupational Therapy, 18,* 6–11.

1965

Ayres, A.J. (1965). A method of measurement of degrees of sensorimotor integration. *Archives of Physical Medicine and Rehabilitation, 46,* 433–435.

Ayres, A.J. (1965). Patterns of perceptual-motor dysfunction in children: A factor analytic study. *Perceptual and Motor Skills, 20,* 335–368.

1966

Ayres, A.J. (1966). Interrelation of perception, function, and treatment. *Journal of the American Physical Therapy Association, 46,* 741–744.

Ayres, A.J. (1966). Interrelationships among perceptual-motor abilities in a group of normal children. *American Journal of Occupational Therapy, 20,* 288–292.

Ayres, A.J. (1966). Interrelationships among perceptual-motor functions in children. *American Journal of Occupational Therapy, 20,* 68–71.

Ayres, A.J., & Reid, W. (1966). The self-drawing as an expression of perceptual-motor dysfunction. *Cortex, 2,* 254–265.

1967

Ayres, A.J. (1967). Remedial procedures based on neurobehavioral constructs. *Proceedings of the 1967 International Convocation on Children and Young Adults with Learning Disabilities,* Pittsburgh, PA.

1968

Ayres, A.J. (1968). Sensory integrative processes and neuropsychological learning disability. In *Learning disorders* (Vol. 3, pp. 41–58). Seattle, WA: Special Child Publications.

Ayres, A.J. (1968). Reading—A product of sensory integrative process. In H.K. Smith (Ed.), *Perception and Reading. Proceedings of the Twelfth Annual Convention of the International Reading Association* (Vol. 12, Part 4). Newark, DE.

1969

Ayres, A.J. (1969). Relation between Gesell development quotients and later perceptual-motor performance. *American Journal of Occupational Therapy, 23,* 11–17.

Ayres, A.J. (1969). Deficits in sensory integration in educationally handicapped children. *Journal of Learning Disabilities, 2*, 160–168.

1971

Ayres, A.J. (1971). Characteristics of types of sensory integrative dysfunction. *American Journal of Occupational Therapy, 25*, 329–334.

Ayres, A.J. (1971). The challenge of the brain. Perceptual Motor Conference (sponsored by the Physical Education Division of the American Association for Health, Physical Education, and Recreation). Sparks, NV.

1972

Ayres, A.J. (1972). Types of sensory integrative dysfunction among disabled learners. *American Journal of Occupational Therapy, 26*, 13–18.

Ayres, A.J. (1972, August–September). Basic concepts of occupational therapy for children with perceptual-motor dysfunction. *Proceedings of the Twelfth World Congress of Rehabilitation International.* Sydney, Australia.

Ayres, A.J. (1972). *Sensory integration and learning disorders.* Los Angeles: Western Psychological Services.

Ayres, A.J. (1972). Sensory integration process: Implications of deaf-blind from learning disability children. In W.A. Blea (Ed.), *Proceedings of the National Symposium for Deaf-Blind* (pp. 81–89). Pacific Grove, CA.

Ayres, A.J. (1972). Improving academic scores through sensory integration. *Journal of Learning Disabilities, 5*, 338–343.

Ayres, A.J., & Heskett, W.M. (1972). Sensory integrative dysfunction in a young schizophrenic girl. *Journal of Autism and Childhood Schizophrenia, 2*, 174–181.

Ayres, A.J. (1972). An interpretation of the role of the brain stem in intersensory integration. In A. Henderson & J. Coryell (Eds.), *The body senses and perceptual deficit. Proceedings of the Occupational Therapy Symposium on Somatosensory Aspects of Perceptual Deficits* (pp. 81–89). Boston: Boston University.

1975

Ayres, A.J. (1975). Sensorimotor foundations of academic ability. In W.M. Cruickshank & D.P. Hallahan (Eds.), *Perceptual and learning disabilities in children* (Vol. 2, pp. 301–358). Syracuse, NY: Syracuse University Press.

1977

Ayres, A.J. (1977). Effect of sensory integrative therapy on the coordination of children with choreoathetoid movements. *American Journal of Occupational Therapy, 31*, 291–293.

Ayres, A.J. (1977). Cluster analyses of measures of sensory integration. *American Journal of Occupational Therapy, 31*, 362–366.

Ayres, A.J. (1977). Dichotic listening performance in learning-disabled children. *American Journal of Occupational Therapy, 31*, 441–446.

Ayres, A.J. (1977). A response of defensive medicine. *Academic Therapy, 13*, 149–152.

1978

Ayres, A.J. (1978). Learning disabilities and the vestibular system. *Journal of Learning Disabilities, 11*, 18–29.

1979

Ayres, A.J. (1979). The sensory registration function in autistic and aphasic/apraxic children. In *Piagetian theory and its implication for the helping professions: Proceedings of the Ninth Interdisciplinary Conference*. Los Angeles: University of Southern California.

Ayres, A.J. (1979). *Sensory integration and the child*. Los Angeles: Western Psychological Services.

1980

Ayres, A.J., & Tickle, L.S. (1980). Hyper-responsivity to touch and vestibular stimuli predict positive response to sensory integration procedures in autistic children. *American Journal of Occupational Therapy, 34*, 375–381.

1981

Ayres, A.J., & Mailloux, Z. (1981). Influence of sensory integration procedures on language development. *American Journal of Occupational Therapy, 35*, 383–390.

1983

Ayres, A.J., & Mailloux, Z. (1983). Possible pubertal effects on therapeutic gains in an autistic girl. *American Journal of Occupational Therapy, 37*, 535–540.

1984

Ayres, A.J., & Cermak, S.A. (1984). Crossing the body midline in learning-disabled and normal children. *American Journal of Occupational Therapy, 38*, 35–39.

Slavik, B.A., Kitsuwa-Lowe, J., Danner, P.T., Green, J., & Ayres, A.J. (1984). Vestibular stimulation and eye contact in autistic children. *Neuropediatrics, 15*, 33–36.

1985

Ayres, A.J. *Developmental dyspraxia and adult onset dyspraxia*. Torrance, CA: Sensory Integration International.

Ayres, A.J., Mailloux, Z., & McAtee, S. (1985). An update of the Sensory Integration and Praxis Tests. *Sensory Integration Special Interest Section Newsletter, 8* (3).

1987

Ayres, A.J., Mailloux, Z.K., & Wendler, C.L. (1987). Developmental dyspraxia. Is it a unitary function? *Occupational Therapy Journal of Research, 7* (2), 93–110.

1989

Ayres, A.J. (1989). Forward. In L.J. Miller (Ed.), Developing norm-referenced standardized tests [Special issue]. *Physical and Occupational Therapy in Pediatrics, 9* (1), xi–xii.

1991

Ayres, A.J., & Marr, D.B. (1991). Sensory Integration and Praxis Test. In A.G. Fisher, E.A. Murray, & A.C. Bundy (Eds.), *Sensory integration theory and practice* (pp. 203–229). Philadelphia: F.A. Davis.

PSYCHOLOGICAL TESTS

1962

Ayres, A.J. *Ayres Space Test.* Los Angeles: Western Psychological Services.

1964

Ayres, A.J. (1964). *Southern California Motor-Accuracy Test.* Los Angeles: Western Psychological Services.

1966

Ayres, A.J. (1966). *Southern California Figure Ground Visual Perception Tests.* Los Angeles: Western Psychological Services.

Ayres, A.J. (1966). *Southern California Kinesthesia and Tactile Perception Tests.* Los Angeles: Western Psychological Services.

1968

Ayres, A.J. (1968). *Southern California Perceptual-Motor Tests.* Los Angeles: Western Psychological Services.

1972

Ayres, A.J. (1972). *Southern California Sensory Integration Tests.* Los Angeles: Western Psychological Services.

1975

Ayres, A.J. (1975). *Southern California Postrotary Nystagmus Test.* Los Angeles: Western Psychological Services.

1980

Ayres, A.J. (1980). *Southern California Motor Accuracy Test—Revised 1980.* Los Angeles: Western Psychological Services.

Ayres, A.J. (1980). *Southern California Sensory Integration Tests—Revised 1980.* Los Angeles: Western Psychological Services.

1989

Ayres, A.J. (1989). *Sensory Integration and Praxis Tests.* Los Angeles: Western Psychological Services.

REPUBLISHED ARTICLES

1959

Ayres, A.J. (1959). Proprioceptive erleichterungsmethoden. *Krankengymnastic, 11,* 191–195, 196–200, 220–225.

1967

Ayres, A.J. (1967). Types of perceptual motor deficits in children with learning difficulties. In A. Bilovsky, Attwell, & Jamison (Eds.), *Readings in learning disability.* New York: Selected Academic Readings.

1971

Ayres, A.J. (1971). Interrelations among perceptual-motor abilities in a group of normal children. In C. Kopp (Ed.), *Readings in early development for occupational and physical therapy students*. Springfield, IL: Charles C Thomas.

1973

Ayres, A.J. (1973). The development of perceptual-motor abilities: A theoretical basis for treatment of dysfunction. In American Occupational Therapy Association, Inc. (Ed.), *The Eleanor Clarke Slagle lectures, 1955–1972* (pp. 127–135). Dubuque, IA: Kendall/Hunt.

1974

Henderson, A., Llorens, L., Gilfoyle, E., Myers, C., & Prevel, S. (Eds.). (1974). *The development of sensory integrative theory and practice: A collection of the works of A. Jean Ayres*. Dubuque, IA: Kendall/Hunt.

PROFESSIONAL FILMS

1966

Ayres, A.J. (1966). *Perceptual-motor evaluation of a perceptually normal child*. Los Angeles: UCLA.

Ayres, A.J. (1966). *Perceptual-motor evaluation of a child with dysfunction*. Los Angeles: UCLA.

1969

Ayres, A.J., & Heskett, W.M. (1969). *Clinical observations of dysfunctions in postural and bilateral integration*.

Ayres, A.J., & Heskett, W.M. (1969). *A therapeutic activity for perceptual-motor dysfunction*.

Chapter Six

Mary Reilly

Julia Van Deusen

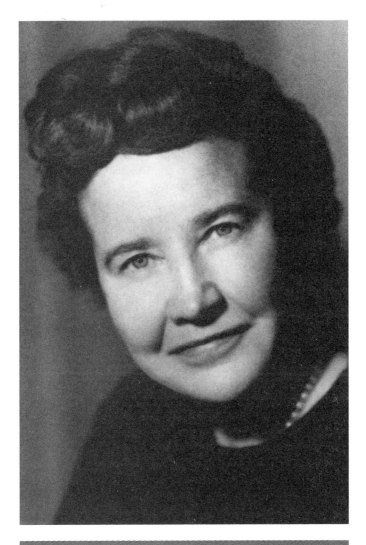

Mary Reilly

Source: Courtesy of the American Occupational Therapy Association, Inc., Rockville, Maryland.

BIOGRAPHICAL SKETCH

Mary Reilly was born in Boston in 1916. A major early influence shaping her scholarly career was her experience at Girls' Latin High School (W. West, personal communication, July 7, 1987). She became interested in occupational therapy while working as a camp counselor earning money for college tuition. There she became fascinated by stories of patients related by a fellow employee, an occupational therapist. Somehow, arts and crafts as media were never mentioned, so that it was with much surprise, on beginning OT training, that Reilly encountered her first craft lessons (W. West, personal communication, July 7, 1987). She did, however, obtain her certificate in occupational therapy from the Boston School of Occupational Therapy in 1940 and for her first job chose to work with cerebral palsied patients at a Crippled Children's Program in Michigan (Occupational Therapy Yearbook, 1957). Experience with these patients, as well as with the brain-injured soldiers at Letterman Army Hospital (Reilly 1956b), led to her early studies on the central nervous system's relevance to occupational therapy. Her sophisticated knowledge of neurodevelopmental principles and their application to occupational therapy is apparent even at this early stage.

During her years with the U.S. Army Medical Department (1941–1955), Reilly came to realize that a focus only on the CNS ignored the necessary emphasis on the development of patient skills and competence. Reilly's work with the army began when she was appointed Chief Occupational Therapist at Lovell General and Convalescent Hospital, Fort Devens, Massachusetts. From 1944 to 1946, she was OT Consultant to the Service Command Surgeon's Office, Fourth Service Command, Atlanta, Georgia. In this position, she supervised occupational therapy at two convalescent, eleven general, and six regional and station hospitals. At this time, she also provided technical assistance for a War Department Technical Manual, a medical supply catalogue, and an apprentice training course of study. For this "outstanding devotion to duty and superior achievement" she was granted the Meritorious Civilian Service Award (Meritorious, 1947).

In 1951 and 1955 Reilly obtained, respectively, a BS degree from the University of Southern California (USC) and an MA degree from San Francisco State College in California. In 1959 she earned her EdD degree from the University of California at Los Angeles (UCLA), where she wrote her dissertation on a theoreti-

Note: Some years ago Dr. Reilly, who was distressed over the direction in which the profession was moving, determined that she needed to take an ethical position of withdrawal from active involvement in occupational therapy. When the authors communicated with her about this book, she wished them success in the venture but chose not to make any active contribution out of concern that to do so would be construed as capitulation.

cal basis of planned change in professional education. Following her doctoral work she was made chief of the Rehabilitation Department of the Neuropsychiatric Institute at UCLA (Reilly, 1966b; Yearbook, 1972).

At UCLA Reilly came into contact with a person who had a major influence on her scholarly work, the social scientist M. Brewster Smith. Basic ideas relevant to Reilly's work were Smith's views on intrinsic motivation and competence. He proposed that attitudes of self-respect and hopefulness are highly relevant to competence and that human beings are capable of actively constructing their lives in a dignified manner (Smith, 1974). In his foreword to Reilly's book *Play As Exploratory Learning* (1974c), Smith concurs with her underlying premises and expresses hope that "the efforts of Dr. Reilly and her collaborators will turn out to be a part of a new stream of interest in play as a scientific problem, and as a therapeutic and educational strategy" (Smith, 1974, p. 16). Although claiming the social psychology perspective of Smith as her primary influence, Reilly readily credits the contributions of other psychologists, such as Bruner, White, and McClelland; vocational theorists, such as Super and Roe; and the founders of occupational therapy, such as Adolph Meyer (M. Reilly, comments on unpublished student paper, August 9, 1986).

Reilly began her association with USC students while she was still at UCLA. After she assumed a full-time position as director of graduate programs in the OT department at USC, she influenced the work of her graduate students, which was to have a major impact on the field of occupational therapy.

Over the years, Reilly has received a number of honors for her creative scholarly activities. She is a fellow of the American Occupational Therapy Association (AOTA) and was awarded the Eleanor Clarke Slagle Lectureship for 1961. She was named a charter member of the Academy of Research of the American Occupational Therapy Foundation (AOTF) in 1983, being cited for her exemplary contributions to "the development of a generic paradigm for practice" (American Occupational Therapy Foundation [AOTF], 1983). When she retired in 1977 she became a professor emeritus of USC. She also found an intellectual "home" at Oxford University in England, where she occasionally studied, lectured, and consulted (W. West, personal communication, July 7, 1987).

In her retirement years, Reilly has lost faith in the field of occupational therapy because she feels it has placed the interests of the profession over those of the chronic patient—that patient most in need of OT services (Reilly, 1984). Without benefit of the occupational behavior (OB) approach, the chronic patient is at high risk of becoming "a member of the hard core unemployable poor" (To Treat, 1968). In fact, although Reilly has continued her interest in scholarly activity, she has abandoned the field because she perceives the reductionistic point of view as still inappropriately dominating occupational therapy (W. West, personal communication, July 7, 1987).

An early contributor to the professional literature (Licht & Reilly, 1943; Reilly & Barton, 1944), Reilly has been a colorful and creative figure in the field of occupational therapy. Her development of the paradigm of occupational behavior is one of the most significant influences on the evolution of the OT profession. When introducing a number of proposals for "modernizing" the field into congruence with OB thinking, Reilly stated: "To the rational who value the continuity of civilization, tradition means pouring the old wine of knowledge into the new bottles of contemporary issues and problems" (Reilly, 1971, p. 243). Reilly has succeeded in doing just that!

THEORETICAL CONCEPTS

Foundations

The "occupation" in occupational therapy has been emphasized by Reilly from the time of her earliest scholarly work. In 1943, she wrote that the essential difference between occupational therapy and physical therapy was not that occupational therapy treatment is active and physical therapy treatment is passive, but rather that occupational therapy's purpose is to help the patient integrate the fundamental motions elicited by physical therapy into total activities (Licht & Reilly, 1943).

This core concept of occupational functioning as the goal of treatment underlies all of Reilly's research. Addressing occupational therapists' use of splinting, she wrote, "I shall attempt to explore what I believe my role should be. This I shall do via a process of rational thinking based upon some soul searching" (Reilly, 1956a, p. 118). Drawing on occupational therapy's unique perspective based on observations of patient functioning, she then concluded that appropriate orthopedic devices enabled patients to assume "their rightful place in life" (Reilly, 1956a, p. 132), that is, their occupational roles.

In her early writings Reilly explored occupational therapy for the physically disabled (Licht & Reilly, 1943; Reilly, 1956a, 1956b). Her knowledge of neurophysiology made her realize that for the newly brain injured, participation in activities of daily living must be delayed. Yet she never abandoned the central concept that patients must eventually perform movements voluntarily in occupational behavior (Reilly, 1956b).

Believing that the domain of occupational therapy is promotion of life satisfaction through occupational (work) and recreational roles, Reilly proposed to OT educators criteria for a curriculum designed to foster practice in performance of these roles (Reilly, 1958). Disease and injury can profoundly disrupt the self-actualization that one ordinarily obtains as worker and recreator, and occupational therapy restores the patient to these roles (Reilly, 1958). A curriculum to support

OT practice would use qualitative, quantitative, and historical perspectives to promote the critical thinking of students. Course content would include growth and development, neurophysiology, and psychology (Reilly, 1958).

Research as well as educational programming must address the central domain of occupational therapy. In 1960, when Reilly first addressed the role of research, OT research was in its infancy. She argued that it should focus on such variables as achievement, creativity, and patterns of aptitudes, interests, and abilities relating to activities as a whole, rather than dealing with a specific modality, such as arts and crafts (Reilly, 1960).

Having long advocated the individual's need for productive and creative occupation as the core concept of occupational therapy, Reilly was presented the opportunity to refine this concept as the Eleanor Clarke Slagle lecturer at the 1961 AOTA conference. Drawing on historical literature in the field, she formulated the central founding belief of occupational therapy as the oft-quoted hypothesis: "that man, through the use of his hands as they are energized by mind and will, can influence the state of his own health" (Reilly, 1962, p. 2). The major implication of this hypothesis is that the individual can manually and creatively "deploy his thinking, feelings, and purposes to make himself at home in the world and to make the world his home" (Reilly, 1962, p. 2).

In her lecture, Reilly considered the value of this hypothesis and whether 20th-century America was the time and place for its testing through occupational therapy practice. She argued that human beings have an intrinsic need to master and improve their environment through skills acquired in their various life roles, and that they suffer dysfunction and dissatisfaction if this need is blocked by disease or injury (Reilly, 1962). Reilly proposed that the unique content of the OT body of knowledge was the nature of productive and creative occupation, particularly from a developmental perspective. The treatment process should focus on work satisfaction and "the ability to experience pleasure in achievement, to tolerate the frustrations of struggle, to sustain the burden of routine tasks, and to maintain the level of aspiration within the reality level of work skills" (Reilly, 1962, p. 7). The goal of the OT process is for patients to engage actively with their life role tasks. Treatment techniques should address the dysfunctions and difficulties people experience on coping with play, work, and school situations (Reilly, 1962). Reilly (1962) closed her Slagle lecture by reiterating the grand purpose of occupational therapy—to help patients influence the state of their own health—but she did not predict whether the field could or would be able to fulfill this mandate.

Published in the *American Journal of Occupational Therapy* (Reilly, 1962) and reprinted in Canada (Reilly, 1963), Reilly's Slagle lecture had a profound impact on the field. As her paradigm of occupational behavior evolved, it was fleshed out by her graduate students and cited and used throughout the United States and Canada (Madigan & Parent, 1985; Matsutsuyu, 1983; Woodside, 1976). Because of her position at USC, Reilly was also able to develop an OT graduate curriculum based on her occupational behavior point of view (Reilly, 1969a, 1969b).

Parameters of the Paradigm

Reilly (1969a) considers four concepts central to her paradigm: (1) the human need to be competent and to achieve; (2) the developmental aspects of work and play; (3) the nature of occupational role; and (4) the relationship of health and human adaptation. Although Reilly's work was not organized according to these concepts, they are clearly discernible in both her writings and those of her graduate students.

 The basic premise underlying the OB paradigm is that human beings have a vital need to produce, to create, to master, and to improve their environment; that is, to be competent and to achieve in their daily occupation. And because human beings need to be competent, they also need to function in occupational roles, which are the vehicles for competency (Reilly, 1962).

In the process of meeting their need for achievement, human beings acquire interests, abilities, skills, and habits of cooperation or competition that support their various occupational roles throughout the life span. Reilly broadly defined occupational roles to include preschooler, student, housewife, and retiree as well as the paid worker (Reilly, 1969a). Occupational choice is a key point in the occupational role developmental process, providing a bridge between the skills and habits of the child and the mature roles of the adult (Matsutsuyu, 1983).

It was Reilly's plan in building the OB paradigm to describe the aptitudes, abilities, interests, and motivational states supporting occupational roles at each stage of the developmental process (Reilly, 1969a). Only when normal roles could be understood at each stage would it be possible to identify and address occupational role dysfunction (Reilly, 1969b).

Reilly views the health of human beings in terms of level of adaptation to their environment rather than in freedom from pathology. Occupational role dysfunction is the domain of occupational therapy. It is the responsibility of the occupational therapist to evaluate and facilitate the adaptive skills of occupationally dysfunctional patients. This responsibility entails maximizing the healthy behaviors of patients (Reilly, 1966b). A major hypothesis of the OB paradigm is that children's play, social recreation, and even chores are critical to the development of the adaptive skills necessary for competence in the complex work and daily living roles of adults. Play is a safe area for the handicapped child or dysfunctional adult to accumulate successful graded experiences for adaptation to life roles (Reilly, 1966a, 1966b).

Whether the patient is an adult or child, it is the goal of occupational therapy to assess the developmental level of the patient's occupational roles and to foster appropriate growth. Emphasis is placed on environmental support for achievement and an appropriate balance of daily activity. The occupational therapist becomes the advocate for patients to practice a healthy balance of work, rest, and play within the OT clinic, the institution as a whole, and eventually within the larger community environment (Reilly, 1966a, 1966b).

Reilly has found the constructs of open systems theory and hierarchy useful in guiding her paradigm development because of their interdisciplinary nature and complexity (Reilly, 1969a, 1974b). Viewing occupational behavior from these perspectives allows for both longitudinal and cross-sectional approaches to investigation.

Florey (1981) has succinctly reviewed the constructs of open systems theory and hierarchy as they relate to the OB paradigm. The human being can be conceived of as an open system that evolves and undergoes different forms of growth and development. As an open system, the human being maintains itself in relation to its environment via a process of input, throughput, and output of energy or matter. Growth or change, as applied to human skills, may occur in terms of amount of skill or complexity of skill.

The concept of hierarchy relates to the process of change over time. This process is orderly but dynamic: behavior changes from simple to complex and from less to more autonomous. Higher levels of behavior direct lower levels. However, lower levels serve to constrain the higher ones in such a way that a change at any level of the hierarchy will affect all levels. Thus newer skills can emerge from the recombination, reorganization, and transformation of more primitive skills (Florey, 1981).

Work-Play Continuum

According to Reilly, "Play serves the function of adaptation by facilitating man's manipulatory and social skills and serves society by socializing the aggression of its members" (Reilly, 1974a, p. 113). An action and an attitude are both involved in play. The action must be voluntary, and the attitude is one of amusement, fun, and pleasure (Takata, 1969). The label given to play changes as the person ages: "play" becomes "recreation" for adults and "leisure" for the retired. Examples of activity that may be play are music, dramatics, games, and crafts (Reilly, 1974a, p. 60).

Because Reilly proposed play as the instrument by which dysfunctional patients could experience achievement and learn healthy adaptation to their environment, her major work concerned the investigation of play (Reilly, 1974a, 1974b). Analyzing play from the perspectives of the evolutionary biologists, psychologists, anthropologists, and sociologists, she concluded that play is "a behavior in search of an explanation" (Reilly, 1974a, p. 115).

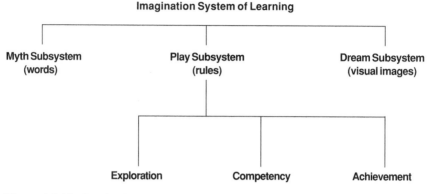

Figure 6-1 The Imagination System of Learning

Reilly sees play as one of three subsystems of the imagination system of learning (see Figure 6-1). The other two subsystems are myth and dream. Although the other subsystems use words or visual images, play uses rules as symbols to represent reality. Through "doing" in play, human beings learn the rules of the hows and whys of objects in their environments. The result is the development of skills leading to competency and the mastery of the real world (Reilly, 1974b).

Within the play subsystem of the imagination, Reilly posed a hierarchy of three subsystems: exploration, competency, and achievement. Intrinsically motivated play that is undertaken for the pure pleasure of doing it is termed exploratory. It is associated with sensory, esthetic, and novel experiences. Developmentally, it is the early childhood stage of play. Although Reilly initially described the attitude developed by exploratory play as trust (Reilly, 1974b), her later studies led to her present position that this stage of play generates an attitude of curiosity (M. Reilly, comments on unpublished student paper, August 9, 1986).

The competency stage of play comes developmentally later than exploration. It involves persistence and practice for task mastery. Although Reilly originally believed that it led to an attitude of self-confidence (Reilly, 1974b), she currently considers it to engender hope (M. Reilly, comments on unpublished student paper, August 9, 1986).

The third phase of play behavior is termed achievement because it focuses on competitive performance and has a standard of excellence. Competition may be with self or with others (Reilly, 1974b). Reilly presently believes that achievement behavior leads to an attitude of altruism (M. Reilly, comments on unpublished student paper, August 9, 1986). At this stage the human being has gained control over his or her environment. "The man who has played his way gradually and safely towards the skillful mastery of his world" is now free to show concern for others (Reilly, 1974b, p. 148).

The results of Reilly's intensive interest in play were twofold: (1) she derived a number of "rules of thumb" about play to encourage others to pursue this line of investigation, and (2) a number of her graduate students chose to study play as their thesis projects. Before Reilly's major publication several students had already explored this area and thus contributed to the volume on play edited by her (Hurff, 1974; Knox, 1974; Michelman, 1974; Shannon, 1974; Takata, 1974).

ELABORATION OF THEORY BY REILLY'S STUDENTS

Because the OB paradigm was only in an early stage of development, the studies of Reilly's students made major contributions to it. These studies were exploratory; they drew up principles of relevance to occupational therapy and described clinical applications in the areas of work-play, motivation and environment, and temporal adaptation.

Work-Play Continuum

Takata's research on play (1969, 1971, 1974, 1980) extended Reilly's research in this area. His six principles on play (Takata, 1971) guided the studies of other graduate students working under the direction of Reilly (Florey, 1981).

1. Play is spontaneous, pleasurable, complex behavior.
2. Play involves sensory, motor, mental, or a combination of all three processes.
3. Play can involve exploration, experimentation, imitation, and repetition.
4. Play integrates the child's internal and external worlds.
5. Play has temporal and spatial limits.
6. Play follows a developmental sequence. (p. 283)

Robinson (1977) developed the concept of the construct of rule. Rules organize information from the environment. Play is the arena where this learning can occur—where information on space, time, and interpersonal relations can be processed for daily living skills. Concepts of curiosity and conflict are key to understanding rule learning through play.

Michelman (1969, 1971, 1974) was interested in the relationship between art experiences and symbolic and creative development. From an extensive review of the literature, Michelman identified a six-step symbolic developmental sequence starting with scribbling and culminating in representational works.

Florey (1969, 1971) identified four principles from her study of childhood play as the critical arena for the development of intrinsic motivation:

1. Play is spare-time learning.
2. Play involves action on human and nonhuman objects.
3. Environmental conditions affect play. For example, anxiety inhibits and novelty facilitates play.
4. Constitutional deficits may interfere with play satisfactions.

Drawing on Reilly's ideas about the developmental nature of work and play, Florey also discussed variables critical for fostering intrinsic motivation in the older child and adult.

Florey's major contributions to the OB literature were a review of Reilly's position on play for an OT textbook (Florey, 1985) and an analysis of the studies on play done under Reilly's guidance (Florey, 1981). Florey categorized these studies according to the principles identified by Takata and provided information on their relevance to OT practice.

Other studies of play include those of Zorn (1969), who studied games as an arena for the development and practice of cognitive skills, and DeRenne-Stephan (1980), who used a systems approach to analyze imitation as a critical mechanism of play.

Because play is the antecedent to work, occupational behavior addresses the entire developmental continuum of play and work (Reilly, 1969a). Reilly urged the study of work-play phenomena in their environmental context. Although Reilly herself did not investigate the work part of the continuum as intensely as she addressed play, several of her graduate students focused on the aspects of OB more directly related to work.

Shannon (1970, 1972b, 1977) and Matsutsuyu (1971) shared and disseminated Reilly's view of the importance of the work-play phenomena for occupational therapy. Occupational choice, occupational role, and socialization are important concepts because human beings become socialized into their occupational roles (Matsutsuyu, 1971).

Shannon's work-play model (Shannon, 1970, 1972b) emphasized the kinds of work-play-social skills necessary for the adaptation of disabled persons to their environments. These work-play-social skills should be central to occupational therapy whether programming involves prevention, maintenance, or restoration. Shannon's model was based on six premises.

1. The human being is activity-oriented, and this activity consists of work and time free from work (maintenance activities and play).
2. A balance of rest, play, and work appropriate to each individual's needs is required for positive physical and mental health.

3. A deficiency in learning how to work or to play creates the potential for maladaptive behavior.
4. Inability to work or play leads to mental illness.
5. The hospital environment can contribute to the deterioration of work-play skills.
6. The primary objective for the hospitalized patient is restoration of function for resumption of daily living. (p. 112)

Although acknowledging the nature of the work-play continuum, Shannon showed particular interest in work adjustment programming for young men in the military (Shannon, 1970, 1972a, 1974). He identified the developmental tasks of adolescence, concluding that a common element was that of choice. Occupational choice involves a series of developmental stages spanning childhood play and adult work roles and ends in selection of an occupation. Shannon cited Ginzberg's stages of the development of occupational choice (Shannon, 1972a). Briefly, these stages are a pretend, fantasy period based only on interests, a tentative stage in which alternative vocational possibilities are weighed, and a final stage when a single, realistic choice is made.

True to the open systems perspective, Shannon also reviewed the environmental influences on occupational choice. Occupational therapy can facilitate the adolescent choice process by providing activities that foster self-discovery and decision making, that enable experimentation in work roles and the development of occupational skills, and that promote constructive use of time free from work.

Pezzuti (1979) centered her discussion of occupational choice on the female adolescent. She concurred with Shannon on the developmental nature of the process from the exploratory play of early childhood through the final phase of occupational choice. She argued, however, that women's dual role options—homemaker and paid worker—complicate their occupational choice process. The development of occupational choice includes three elements: (1) opportunity for a genuine choice; (2) exposure to appropriate work role models and role playing; and (3) participation in play activity for development of skills, values, interests, and cognitive realization.

Pezzuti found that the attitudes and skills that contribute to a sound occupational choice growth process at various life stages are trust (infancy), a sense of competence within immediate surroundings and motor development (early childhood), identification with role models and mastery of self-help skills (childhood), and rudiments of organizational, social, and work skill competencies (school age). By adolescence, a sense of competence in roles, independence from parents, and occupational choice should occur (Matsutsuyu, 1971).

A second work concept receiving the attention of Reilly's students was that of occupational role. Moorhead (1969) made a major contribution in this area, identifying the common elements among the various occupational roles, such as worker, homemaker, and retiree. These roles all serve as vehicles for self-identification and for identification within society. Early occupational roles—player, student, and others—influence adult occupational behavior.

Moorhead (1969) provided a list of variables critical to occupational role performance. Autonomy and independence variables include a realistic perception of one's own strengths and weaknesses and an ability to make firm decisions and manage time. Motivation and orientation to one's interests and satisfactions and appreciation of alternatives are implementation variables. Maintenance variables include standards and stability of work task behavior, performance under stress, interpersonal competence, work-play-rest balance, and ability to handle role conflicts. Moorhead (1969) also developed four categories for analyzing occupational role development: (1) learning and socialization in childhood roles, (2) issues around occupational choice, (3) influences of environment on patterns of achievement and failure, and (4) course of adult occupational mobility or solidification.

Matsutsuyu (1971) cited Schmaltz's thesis project on the place of the socialization process in learning occupational role. The OT setting should facilitate role maintenance, learning, and relearning. Maintenance focuses on keeping intact daily living skills active. If a patient is assessed as able to learn new roles, occupational role development should be emphasized. If occupational role dysfunction is present, relearning may be the goal.

Motivation and Environment

A crucial concept of the OB paradigm is human motivation. Because of its importance this concept was addressed early by Reilly's students (Florey, 1969) and continues to be discussed (Bell, 1975; Burke, 1977; Sharrott & Cooper-Fraps, 1986). Motivation cannot be understood apart from environment.

Florey (1969) proposed that intrinsic motivation was the kind of motivation most relevant to occupational therapy. "Intrinsic motivation builds toward self-reward in independent action that underlies competent behavior" (Florey, 1969, p. 320). Satisfaction in completion of the activity itself is intrinsically motivating.

Because competence breeds competence, Florey (1969) described in detail the environmental conditions that foster competence in children and adults. Childhood play is vital to the development of intrinsic motivation. Environmental factors critical to play are the presence of humans and of novel nonhuman objects among familiar objects. The environment should allow for exploration, repetition, and for imitation of competent role models and should be free of such stresses as hunger, fear, and pain. For the older child the environment should provide tools, instruction for useful productivity, and opportunity to relate to peers and to adult models of sportsmanship and craftsmanship. In adulthood, intrinsic motivation is related to achievement. Tasks should present challenges within the adult's range of abilities. The environment should foster responsibility for outcome and present feedback on results.

For some individuals, when there is a standard for excellence, competition fosters achievement (Bell, 1975). Therefore, competitive behavior needs a task-related, self-related, or other-related standard of excellence (Florey, 1969; Bell, 1975). Bell (1975) utilized the interrelationship between risk taking and competition to identify individuals for whom competition would be motivating.

Under Reilly's guidance, Burke's graduate thesis (Burke, 1977) elaborated the concept of personal causation—that human beings are motivated to interact effectively with their environment—as a means of understanding human motivation. This internal motivation is directed primarily toward producing environmental change. Feedback on the effectiveness of current behavior provides guidance for future behavior. Thus adaptation to life's endless challenges can occur and humanity survives.

Four theoretical statements by Burke (1977) underlie the concept of personal causation:

1. Success leads to feelings of success, which lead to more success.
2. Individuals who perceive they have control over their environments show active behaviors.
3. A belief that one has skills to address obstacles generates a sense of control.
4. A feeling of worth accompanies use of one's own resources to change one's environment. (p. 256)

Sharrott and Cooper-Fraps (1986) associated lack of intrinsic motivation with dysfunction in occupational behavior and presented two criteria—lack of satisfaction to self and lack of satisfaction to society—for determining such dysfunction. People can become dysfunctional if they do not derive satisfaction from their occupational roles, or if their role performance does not meet society's standards.

Reilly (1966a) was probably the first vocal environmental manager in the field of occupational therapy. Addressing the 1965 AOTA conference, she stated,

> We should be the first to realize that a hospital environment should be a place where the patient's daily living skill could be improved because of the environment and not despite it; and that the homes and the jobs or schools are progressive extensions of the same concepts. (1966a, p. 224)

Although little of the work addressing the OB paradigm could avoid the environmental context, several of Reilly's students chose to address this topic directly.

Gray (1972) describes conditions or practices within a hospital environment that can negatively affect such daily living (work-play) skills as self-care skills, social skills, and general or specific work skills. She also describes those practices affecting loss of time, leisure time, and decision-making skills. Some practices cited are failure of staff to serve as appropriate role models, lack of patient evaluation in the specified skill area, and lack of encouragement for patients to practice skills in the hospital setting.

Parent (1978) reviewed the literature on the effects of sensory and perceptual deprivation and of immobilization and social isolation. The demonstrated impact of deprivation and isolation on the hospitalized patient provides support for the OT position that meaningful occupation is essential to maintain hospitalized patients' functioning.

Klavins (1972) emphasized the importance of cultural influences on patient behaviors in occupational therapy. "As part of the human environment, culture is that special way of life which characterizes it" (Klavins, 1972, p. 176). Work-play behaviors are influenced by the values held by one's cultural group. Therapists must know, accept, and work within the value and belief structures of patients from a variety of cultural backgrounds.

Drawing on the research from the field of environmental psychology, Dunning (1972) developed a classification system for study of environments through analysis of their components: space, people, and tasks. She analyzes the space component in terms of territoriality, privacy, crowding, and objects in the environment; the people component in terms of social role relationships and social distance; and the task component in terms of potential use of objects and space, given their presence, availability, desirability, and feasibility. Dunning designed a grid showing the givens, possibility for change, and preference for change. She applied her analysis to psychiatric outpatients.

Temporal Adaptation

Although time is not a part of the physical environment, it is "the inescapable boundary for human existence and activity" (Kielhofner, 1977, p. 237), so that it is, in a sense, one's surroundings. Kielhofner (1977) treated the concept of temporal adaptation in depth as part of his master's work with Reilly. He derived seven propositions relevant to occupational therapy as a preliminary framework for the generation of treatment strategies and demonstrated their utility through discussion of case histories (1977).

The first proposition describes the cultural basis of every person's perspective toward time. The second proposition states that the formal learning of the cultural notions of time is only part of the temporal training begun in childhood. Kielhofner argues that there are three levels of learning through which each person acquires a unique temporal frame of reference: the formal, the technical, and the informal.

The third proposition incorporates Reilly's notion of life spaces and a temporal order to daily living. Time is organized around the life spaces of existence (self-maintenance), subsistence (work), and discretionary time (recreation/leisure). Health in relation to this aspect of time means a balance of life spaces consistent with the values, interests, and goals of an individual and of his or her society.

Proposition four states that time for each individual is organized around his or her social roles, although these roles should not be considered as unchanging. Proposition five defines time use as a function of a person's internalized interests, values, and goals.

Habits are intimately linked with temporal functioning. According to proposition six, habits are the basic structures that order daily behavior in time.

Finally, in proposition seven, Kielhofner proposes that the temporal dysfunction of patients may be a more difficult problem to address than pathology per se. The goal of achieving temporal adaptation is applicable to all dysfunctional categories of patients.

APPLICATION TO OCCUPATIONAL THERAPY PRACTICE

Educational Needs

In order for occupational therapists to base service on the occupational behavior paradigm, their educational training must be based on the OB perspective. The master's entry-level curriculum at USC, which Reilly developed, was based on that perspective (Reilly, 1969a).

The USC curriculum included content from the biological system of medical science, the personality system of the psychological sciences, and the social system of the social sciences. The medical sciences were part of the curriculum but because of the fundamental difference between medicine's goal of reducing illness and occupational therapy's goal of reducing the incapacities resulting from illness, medicine was not a major focus. Emphasis was placed on the behavioral sciences because occupational therapy's major concern is the identification and treatment of occupational role dysfunction. Reilly made the behavioral science content relevant by selecting from many disciplines—anthropology, psychology, sociology, social geography, psychiatry, economics, political science, and law—those portions dealing with human behavior (Reilly, 1969a). Social psychology, particularly the developmental aspects of human achievement, was a core curricular area because the development of healthy adaptive behavior is a basic part of the occupational behavior paradigm (Reilly, 1969b).

Clinical Application

Without clinical application a paradigm can have no value for a profession concerned with patient treatment. Reilly's OB paradigm has evolved along with OT service over the years. The best illustration of this symbiosis is Reilly's original psychiatric program at the Neuropsychiatric Institute (NPI) at UCLA (Reilly, 1966b).

The NPI program was designed both to serve as a teaching model and to provide OT service to 100 psychiatric patients.

> The NPI model assumed as its foundation and first specification the need (1) to examine the life roles of patients relative to community adaptation; (2) to identify the various skills which support them; and (3) to create an environment where the relevant rehabilitative behavior could be evoked and practiced. (Reilly, 1966b, p. 62)

Occupational therapists functioned in clinician, administrator, and teacher roles. Evaluation of the NPI program showed that occupational therapy was an important service in the restoration of healthy adaptive behavior.

The NPI program was structured according to five principles.

1. Occupational behavior is developmentally acquired.
2. Patient programming should be graded from craft work in the OT clinic to work in the larger institutional environment to work in the community.
3. Occupational therapy must provide realistic decision-making arenas for the patients.
4. Because basic needs of patients in areas of food, shelter, and safety are met by other services in the hospital, occupational therapy should emphasize programming to meet cognitive, esthetic, and self-realization needs of patients.
5. Occupational therapy should engineer a normal daily pattern of work, play, and rest for the lives of the patients and tailor programs to their abilities, interests, ages, and occupational roles.

APPLICATION OF THE PARADIGM BY OTHERS

Assessment

From its inception the OB paradigm has been intimately linked to OT practice through the development of assessment tools for clinical use. The case method was the clinical problem-solving vehicle that was considered consistent with the

OB paradigm (Line, 1969). Line evaluated the case methods of several disciplines and selected that of business administration as the model for occupational therapy. This method allows the professional to gain an understanding of the problem and develop a plan to solve it that maximizes patient assets and minimizes weaknesses. The case method as a problem-solving vehicle for OT was piloted by the OT graduate students at USC. The frame of reference was human adaptation to role expectations in work and play roles. Data were collected by direct observation, tests, interviews, and history taking and were classified according to structure, function, expectancies, patterns of success and failure, and prior learnings and learning style. The data thus collected were organized into social, activities of daily living (ADL), and disease adaptation categories. Analysis of data led to problem definition and development of a plan of action. That plan seemed to be the weakest component in the pilot study for application of the OB method to occupational therapy.

The case method approach confirmed the need for assessment tools relevant to the OB point of view. Many of Reilly's graduate students conducted extensive literature searches to support the development of such tools. The purpose of their work was not to create rigorous psychometric instruments, but rather to develop tools to guide the data collection phase of clinical problem solving by a professional person knowledgeable about OB. Thus the descriptions of the assessment tools were often illustrated with applications to patient case material. The flexibility of this approach to assessment allowed emphasis to be placed on the individual differences observable in human occupational behavioral dysfunction.

Fifteen approaches to assessment are briefly described below. The reader is referred to the references for the detailed information necessary for clinical application.

Takata (1969) developed the Play History to identify the quality and quantity of play in multihandicapped children. It can be used to obtain a play deficit diagnosis.

Matsutsuyu (1969) based her 80-item Interest Checklist on six propositions gleaned from a literature review. Interests (1) are family influenced; (2) evoke affective responses; (3) are choice states; (4) can be manifested in effective action; (5) can sustain action; and (6) reflect self-perception. Matsutsuyu's assessment tool also included a special interest section and a leisure-time history.

After an extensive review of the literature on interests, Borys (1974) investigated an indirect approach to interest study. She compared values of subjects showing a low interest in daily living (minimal activity participation, low curiosity, and low risk taking) to those with high interest. Low-interest subjects gave greater value to security, whereas high-interest subjects gave greater value to self-development and contributing to others. Thus, one of the measures of values evaluated in this study (the Buhler Life Goals Inventory) had utility for occupational therapy in terms of daily living interests.

Michelman (1969) developed a sequential growth gradient as a means of evaluating symbolic and creative development. She developed a brief checklist for assessing creative growth.

Knox's Play Scale (1974), which was based on normal behaviors of the child from birth to six years, assessed the developmental level of space management, material management, imitation, and participation.

Hurff's Play Skills Inventory (Hurff, 1980) assessed the individual's readiness to move into adolescence in sensory, motor, perceptual, and intellectual areas.

Pezzuti's self-evaluative tool (Pezzuti, 1979) provided information on the developmental task level of female adolescents.

Occupational choice and role were concerns of other assessments. Shannon designed the Inventory of Occupational Choice Skills (1974) with a companion rating scale. Black's Adolescent Role Assessment (Black, 1976) identified deficiencies in the occupational choice process by examining such issues as childhood-play, adolescence-socialization, school, peers, adolescence-occupational choice, and adulthood-work.

Moorhead (1969) developed an occupational history format centered around an analysis of childhood roles, the issue of occupational choice, patterns of achievement and failure, and occupational role mobility. Related to this assessment was a screening tool, the Occupational Role History (Florey & Michelman, 1982). This semistructured interview format contained questions about worker-homemaker roles and school. Role status could be classified as functional, temporarily impaired, or dysfunctional. Vause-Earland included these in her study of the "Perceptions of Role Assessment Tools in the Physical Disability Setting" (1991).

Zorn (1969) provided guidelines to determine cognitive level. Bell's five-question interview (1975) asked the participant to select low-risk, intermediate-risk, and high-risk items. An intermediate-risk score indicated that competition would motivate competent performance.

Dunning (1972) and Gray (1972) developed tools emphasizing the environment. Dunning's tool assessed the interaction between the patient and environment based on her environmental grid. Gray identified the presence of depersonalizing conditions in the hospital environment.

Treatment

The breadth of the clinical applicability of the OB paradigm has been demonstrated by its application to other cultures and to diagnostic groups other than psychiatric inpatients. The Canadian inpatient psychiatric service at the McMaster University Medical Center organized its OT program to be consistent with Reilly's OB paradigm (Woodside, 1976).

According to the OB paradigm, deficits in OB result from genetic or environmentally elicited gaps in occupational skill development and from the effects of illness or institutionalization. It is the task of occupational therapy to fill the gaps or counteract the effects of illness.

Treatment goals include maintenance, correction, or new learning of occupational behaviors. Through assessment, development, and patterns of work-play skills, OB strengths and weaknesses and current and potential environments can be identified. Therapist attitudes that foster occupational behaviors include respect for the patient and faith in the patient's ability to succeed and live his or her own life. The occupational therapist needs to be the patient's advocate in changing the environment to support OB.

Woodside (1976) suggested five treatment guidelines.

1. Select and use activities that are interesting and challenging for each patient.
2. Use activity that reflects the developmental stages from playing with the activity to learning under a teacher to independent performance.
3. Provide the patient with guidance and feedback.
4. Teach general, transferable work skills such as relating to authority figures, rather than specific work skills.
5. Make the OT clinic a laboratory for human productivity. (p. 13)

Although originating with psychiatric patients, the OB paradigm has been clinically applied to several other occupationally dysfunctional populations. With young men considered to be juvenile delinquents (Paulson, 1980), occupational therapy focused on goal-oriented tasks in the problem areas of daily living skills, occupational social behaviors, and prevocational skills. The success rate as indicated by active participation in vocational training was 80 percent.

The OB approach also was found to be applicable to the young adult with mild mental retardation (Webster, 1980). Webster described a 20-year-old female who was assessed for her interests, abilities, skills, and values. Her assets and weaknesses were identified in terms of developmental level in the occupational choice process. In order to further development, treatment goals addressed her weaknesses, such as deficient money management skills.

Heard (1977) discussed the application of OB concepts to the chronically physically disabled adolescent. She identified three critical points for the use of concepts of role in treating OT patients in the clinic. Roles cannot be fulfilled without the skill mastery that leads to automatic routines or habits. Role progression organizes daily living, and the ease of occupational role acquisition depends on the adaptive nature of the individual. Heard's assessment of a 17-year-old female with cerebral palsy revealed her strengths and deficits. Through OT programming this patient was able to acquire the worker role of salesperson.

CONCLUSION

Reilly has had a powerful influence on the development of the profession of occupational therapy. Her work has generated numerous studies by students who have refined her theories, applied them clinically, and developed assessment tools for clinical use. Perhaps the most far-reaching consequence of Reilly's work has been the model of human occupation developed by two of her students, Kielhofner and Burke (1980). The next chapter includes this model.

REFERENCES

American Occupational Therapy Foundation. (1983). Ayres, Reilly, Yerxa named to Academy of Research. *Occupational Therapy Journal of Research, 3*, 185–187.

Bell, C.H. (1975). Competition as a motivational incentive. *American Journal of Occupational Therapy, 29*, 277–279.

Black, M.M. (1976). Adolescent role assessment. *American Journal of Occupational Therapy, 30*, 73–79.

Borys, S.S. (1974). Implications of interest theory for occupational therapy. *American Journal of Occupational Therapy, 28*, 35–38.

Burke, J.P. (1977). A clinical perspective on motivation: Pawn versus origin. *American Journal of Occupational Therapy, 31*, 254–258.

DeRenne-Stephan, C. (1980). Imitation: A mechanism of play behavior. *American Journal of Occupational Therapy, 34*, 95–102.

Dunning, H. (1972). Environmental occupational therapy. *American Journal of Occupational Therapy, 26*, 292–298.

Florey, L.L. (1969). Intrinsic motivation: The dynamics of occupational therapy theory. *American Journal of Occupational Therapy, 23*, 319–322.

Florey, L.L. (1971). An approach to play and play development. *American Journal of Occupational Therapy, 25*, 275–280.

Florey, L.L. (1981). Studies of play: Implications for growth, development and for clinical practice. *American Journal of Occupational Therapy, 35*, 519–524.

Florey, L.L. (1985). Major theoretical approaches to pediatric occupational therapy. Reilly: An explanation of play. In P.N. Clark & A.S. Allen (Eds.), *Occupational therapy for children* (pp. 36–38). St. Louis: C.V. Mosby.

Florey, L.L., & Michelman, S.M. (1982). Occupational role history: A screening tool for psychiatric occupational therapy. *American Journal of Occupational Therapy, 36*, 301–308.

Gray, M. (1972). Effects of hospitalization on work-play behavior. *American Journal of Occupational Therapy, 26*, 180–185.

Heard, C. (1977). Occupational role acquisition: A perspective on the chronically disabled. *American Journal of Occupational Therapy, 31*, 243–247.

Hurff, J.M. (1974). A play skills inventory. In M. Reilly (Ed.), *Play as exploratory learning* (pp. 267–283). Beverly Hills, CA: Sage Publications.

Hurff, J.M. (1980). A play skills inventory: A competency monitoring tool for the 10 year old. *American Journal of Occupational Therapy, 34*, 651–656.

Kielhofner, G. (1977). Temporal adaptation: A conceptual framework for occupational therapy. *American Journal of Occupational Therapy, 31*, 235–242.

Kielhofner, G., & Burke, J.P. (1977). Occupational therapy after 60 years: An account of changing identity and knowledge. *American Journal of Occupational Therapy, 31*, 675–689.

Kielhofner, G., & Burke, J.P. (1980). A model of human occupation. Part I, Conceptual framework and content. *American Journal of Occupational Therapy, 34*, 572–581.

Klavins, R. (1972). Work-play behavior: Cultural influences. *American Journal of Occupational Therapy, 26*, 176–179.

Knox, S.H. (1974). A play scale. In M. Reilly (Ed.), *Play as exploratory learning* (pp. 247–266). Beverly Hills, CA: Sage Publications.

Licht, S., & Reilly, M. (1943). The correlation of physical therapy and occupational therapy. *Occupational Therapy and Rehabilitation, 22*, 171–175.

Line, J. (1969). Case method as a scientific form of clinical thinking. *American Journal of Occupational Therapy, 23*, 308–313.

Madigan, M.J., & Parent, L.H. (1985). Preface. In G. Kielhofner (Ed.), *A model of human occupation: Theory and application* (pp. vii–x). Baltimore: Williams & Wilkins.

Matsutsuyu, J.S. (1969). The interest checklist. *American Journal of Occupational Therapy, 23*, 323–328.

Matsutsuyu, J.S. (1971). Occupational behavior: A perspective on work and play. *American Journal of Occupational Therapy, 25*, 291–294.

Matsutsuyu, J.S. (1983). Occupational behavior approach. In H.L. Hopkins & H.D. Smith (Eds.), *Willard and Spackman's occupational therapy* (6th ed.) (pp. 129–134). New York: J.B. Lippincott.

Meritorious Civilian Service Awards. (1947). *American Journal of Occupational Therapy, 1*, 33.

Michelman, S. (1969). Research in symbol formation and creative growth. In W.L. West (Ed.), *Occupational therapy functions in interdisciplinary programs for children. Proceedings of the Conference, The Training Function of Occupational Therapy in University-Affiliated Centers* (pp. 88–110). Rockville, MD: Department of Health, Education, and Welfare.

Michelman, S. (1971). The importance of creative play. *American Journal of Occupational Therapy, 25*, 285–290.

Michelman, S. (1974). Play and the deficit child. In M. Reilly (Ed.), *Play as exploratory learning* (pp. 157–207). Beverly Hills, CA: Sage Publications.

Moorhead, L. (1969). The occupational history. *American Journal of Occupational Therapy, 23*, 329–334.

Occupational therapy yearbook. (1957). New York: American Occupational Therapy Association.

Parent, L.H. (1978). Effects of a low-stimulus environment on behavior. *American Journal of Occupational Therapy, 32*, 19–25.

Paulson, C.P. (1980). Juvenile delinquency and occupational choice. *American Journal of Occupational Therapy, 34*, 565–581.

Pezzuti, L. (1979). An exploration of adolescent feminine and occupational behavior development. *American Journal of Occupational Therapy, 33*, 84–91.

Reilly, M. (1956a). The role of the therapist in protective and functional devices. *American Journal of Occupational Therapy, 10*, 118–132, 133.

Reilly, M. (1956b). Therapeutically influenced recovery. *American Journal of Occupational Therapy, 10*, 229–232.

Reilly, M. (1958). An occupational therapy curriculum for 1965. *American Journal of Occupational Therapy, 12*, 293–299.

Reilly, M. (1960). Research potentiality of occupational therapy. *American Journal of Occupational Therapy, 14*, 206–209.

Reilly, M. (1962). Occupational therapy can be one of the great ideas of 20th century medicine. The Eleanor Clarke Slagle lecture. *American Journal of Occupational Therapy, 16*, 1–9.

Reilly, M. (1963). The Eleanor Clarke Slagle lecture. *Canadian Journal of Occupational Therapy, 30*, 5–19.

Reilly, M. (1966a). The challenge of the future to an occupational therapist. *American Journal of Occupational Therapy, 20*, 221–225.

Reilly, M. (1966b). A psychiatric occupational therapy program as a teaching model. *American Journal of Occupational Therapy, 20*, 61–67.

Reilly, M. (1969a). The educational process. *American Journal of Occupational Therapy, 23*, 299–307.

Reilly, M. (1969b). Selecting human development knowledge for occupational therapy. In W.L. West (Ed.), *Occupational therapy functions in interdisciplinary programs for children. Proceedings of the Conference, The Training Function of Occupational Therapy in University-Affiliated Centers* (pp. 64–75). Rockville, MD: Department of Health, Education, and Welfare.

Reilly, M. (1971). The modernization of occupational therapy. *American Journal of Occupational Therapy, 25*, 243–246.

Reilly, M. (1974a). Defining a cobweb. In M. Reilly (Ed.), *Play as exploratory learning* (pp. 57–116). Beverly Hills, CA: Sage Publications.

Reilly, M. (1974b). An explanation of play. In M. Reilly (Ed.), *Play as exploratory learning* (pp. 117–149). Beverly Hills, CA: Sage Publications.

Reilly, M. (Ed.). (1974c). *Play as exploratory learning.* Beverly Hills, CA: Sage Publications.

Reilly, M. (1984). The issue is—The importance of the client versus patient issue for occupational therapy. *American Journal of Occupational Therapy, 38*, 404–406.

Reilly, M., & Barton, W.E. (1944). Do's and don'ts in military occupational therapy. *Occupational Therapy and Rehabilitation, 23*, 121–123.

Robinson, A.L. (1977). Play: The arena for acquisition of rules for competent behavior. *American Journal of Occupational Therapy, 31*, 248–253.

Shannon, P.D. (1970). Work adjustment and the adolescent soldier. *American Journal of Occupational Therapy, 24*, 111–115.

Shannon, P.D. (1972a). The adolescent experience. *American Journal of Occupational Therapy, 26*, 284–287.

Shannon, P.D. (1972b). Work-play theory and the occupational therapy process. *American Journal of Occupational Therapy, 26*, 169–172.

Shannon, P.D. (1974). Occupational choice: Decision-making play. In M. Reilly (Ed.), *Play as exploratory learning* (pp. 285–314). Beverly Hills, CA: Sage Publications.

Shannon, P.D. (1977). The derailment of occupational therapy. *American Journal of Occupational Therapy, 31*, 229–234.

Sharrott, G.W., & Cooper-Fraps, C. (1986). The theories of motivation in occupational therapy: An overview. *American Journal of Occupational Therapy, 40*, 249–257.

Smith, M.B. (1974). Foreword. In M. Reilly (Ed.), *Play as exploratory learning* (pp. 5–8). Beverly Hills, CA: Sage Publications.

Takata, N. (1969). The play history. *American Journal of Occupational Therapy, 23,* 314–318.

Takata, N. (1971). The play milieu: a preliminary appraisal. *American Journal of Occupational Therapy, 25,* 281–284.

Takata, N. (1974). Play as a prescription. In M. Reilly (Ed.), *Play as exploratory learning* (pp. 209–246). Beverly Hills, CA: Sage Publications.

Takata, N. (1980). Introduction to a series: Occupational behavior research for pediatric practice. *American Journal of Occupational Therapy, 34,* 11–12.

To treat not only the injury, but also the man . . . (1968). *Tufts Alumni Review, 14,* 22–23.

Vause-Earland, T. (1991). Perceptions of role assessment tools in the physical disability setting. *American Journal of Occupational Therapy, 45,* 26–31.

Webster, P.S. (1980). Occupational role development in the young adult with mild mental retardation. *American Journal of Occupational Therapy, 34,* 13–18.

Woodside, H. (1976). Dimensions of the occupational behavior model. *Canadian Journal of Occupational Therapy, 43,* 11–14.

Yearbook. (1972). New York: American Occupational Therapy Association.

Zorn, J.A. (1969). Research in cognitive assessment. In W.L. West (Ed.), *Occupational therapy functions in interdisciplinary programs for children. Proceedings of the Conference, The Training Function of Occupational Therapy in University-Affiliated Centers* (pp. 111–120). Rockville, MD: Department of Health, Education, and Welfare.

BIBLIOGRAPHY

1943

Licht, S., & Reilly, M. (1943). The correlation of physical therapy and occupational therapy. *Occupational Therapy and Rehabilitation, 22,* 171–175.

1944

Reilly, M., & Barton, W.E. (1944). Do's and don'ts in military occupational therapy. *Occupational Therapy and Rehabilitation, 23,* 121–123.

1956

Reilly, M. (1956). The role of the therapist in protective and functional devices. *American Journal of Occupational Therapy, 10,* 118–132, 133.

Reilly, M. (1956). Therapeutically influenced recovery. *American Journal of Occupational Therapy, 10,* 229–232.

1958

Reilly, M. (1958). An occupational therapy curriculum for 1965. *American Journal of Occupational Therapy, 12,* 293–299.

1960

Reilly, M. (1960). Research potentiality of occupational therapy. *American Journal of Occupational Therapy, 14,* 206–209.

1962

Reilly, M. (1962). Occupational therapy can be one of the great ideas of 20th century medicine. The Eleanor Clarke Slagle lecture. *American Journal of Occupational Therapy, 16*, 1–9.

1963

Reilly, M. (1963). The Eleanor Clarke Slagle lecture. *Canadian Journal of Occupational Therapy, 30*, 5–19.

1966

Reilly, M. (1966). The challenge of the future to an occupational therapist. *American Journal of Occupational Therapy, 20*, 221–225.

Reilly, M. (1966). A psychiatric occupational therapy program as a teaching model. *American Journal of Occupational Therapy, 22*, 61–67.

1969

Reilly, M. (1969). The educational process. *American Journal of Occupational Therapy, 23*, 299–307.

Reilly, M. (1969). Selecting human development knowledge for occupational therapy. In W.L. West (Ed.), *Occupational therapy functions in interdisciplinary programs for children. Proceedings of the Conference, The Training Function of Occupational Therapy in University-Affiliated Centers* (pp. 64–75). Rockville, MD: Department of Health, Education, and Welfare.

1971

Reilly, M. (1971). The modernization of occupational therapy. *American Journal of Occupational Therapy, 25*, 243–246.

1974

Reilly, M. (1974). Defining a cobweb. In M. Reilly (Ed.), *Play as exploratory learning* (pp. 57–116). Beverly Hills, CA: Sage Publications.

Reilly, M. (1974). An explanation of play. In M. Reilly (Ed.), *Play as exploratory learning* (pp. 117–149). Beverly Hills, CA: Sage Publications.

Reilly, M. (Ed.). (1974). *Play as exploratory learning.* Beverly Hills, CA: Sage Publications.

1977

Reilly, M. (1977). A response to: Defining occupational therapy: The meaning of therapy and the virtues of occupation. *American Journal of Occupational Therapy, 31*, 673.

1984

Reilly, M. (1984). The issue is—The importance of the client versus patient issue for occupational therapy. *American Journal of Occupational Therapy, 38*, 404–406.

Chapter Seven

Gary Kielhofner

Rosalie J. Miller

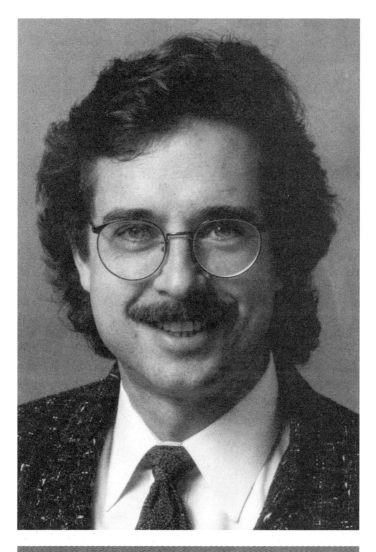

Gary Kielhofner

BIOGRAPHICAL SKETCH

Gary Kielhofner was born in 1949 in Oran, Missouri, a rural area on the northern edge of the Ozarks. He grew up on a 200-acre farm that his great-grandmother and great-grandfather (who came from Alsace-Lorraine) cleared from homestead woods. The local community was quite homogeneous and predominantly Catholic, with strong French and German ties. Kielhofner lived with his four sisters, paternal grandparents, mother and father, and an aunt. He worked on the farm before and after school and, like his father and grandfather before him, was expected to take over the farm.

When he was about ten, an incident happened that had a significant influence on him and his choice of career. His grandparents were in a very serious automobile accident. His grandmother, a vibrant, active woman in her fifties, sustained multiple fractures in one leg. She was then in and out of the hospital for 27 months and stayed in a hospital bed in the family living room each time she was discharged. At the end of that long period, her leg was amputated, leaving about a 10-inch stump. She received only a few sessions of training with a prosthesis from a staff whose attitude was that "here was this mechanical thing she could try out. She fell a couple of times and that was it" (G.W. Kielhofner, personal communication, March 6, 1987). She spent the rest of her life in a wheelchair.

The experience of spending several years of his older childhood seeing his grandmother in a hospital bed and wheelchair, and seeing the failure of her rehabilitation, not only had a powerful impact on Kielhofner's life, but influenced his later thinking about OT theory. He came to realize that the context of the prosthesis was not defined in meaningful terms for his grandmother, as in "You've got to struggle with this situation and if you hang in there, ultimately you will be able to walk and go back to a lifestyle you had before and do all the things you've always done" (G.W. Kielhofner, personal communication, March 6, 1987).

Also around the age of ten, Kielhofner felt a calling to become a Catholic priest. At 14 he went to live at St. Vincent's College, a high school seminary run by the Vincentian Order. He spent the next four years studying in the demanding classical tradition and living a very disciplined life. He graduated in 1967 and entered the novitiate in Santa Barbara, California. Two years later, after a long period of inner turmoil and searching, he left the seminary. He finished his college studies at St. Louis University in 1971 and graduated with a classical bachelor's degree in psychology. While in college at St. Louis, he was active in the peace movement and did volunteer work with rehabilitation patients at the Jewish Hospital. In his senior year he was drafted. He applied for, and after considerable investment of time and effort was granted, conscientious objector status (G.W. Kielhofner, personal communication, March 6, 1987). As his alternative service commitment, he arranged to work full time for half-time pay as director of recreation and an aide in occupational therapy at the Jewish Hospital in St. Louis. As he describes this first job:

> Now, mind you, I had no idea of what occupational therapy was, and I still had plans to go on and be a clinical psychologist. What the occupational therapists learned quickly was that I was good with my hands, so they started having me do things such as cutting out splint materials and working with patients in woodworking and leatherwork. There was no other male in the department, and we had a lot of young male spinal cord injured patients from rural Missouri. They were farm kids. They related to me, and the occupational therapists had me do a lot of work with them. (G.W. Kielhofner, personal communication, March 6, 1987)

Kielhofner was excited about the combination of using his hands to do things and working with patients. The head of that occupational therapy department, Sandy Liemer (now Malone), started encouraging him to become an occupational therapist. In 1972 he entered the OT program at Washington University in St. Louis while still working at the hospital on evenings and weekends. At the end of his first year of the program he went to the 1973 conference of the American Occupational Therapy Association (AOTA) in Los Angeles. He was so impressed with Mary Reilly, the University of Southern California (USC) faculty and graduate students, and the USC philosophy that was a strong influence at that conference that he applied to the basic master's program at USC and began again his entire OT education.

> In the course of those two years Mary Reilly persuaded me to her essential theme, which was that occupational therapy needs to define what its business is, and that its business is dealing with people's everyday occupational problems and using occupation as a therapeutic media, and all that that means. (G.W. Kielhofner, personal communication, March 6, 1987)

Reilly had a tremendous influence on Kielhofner, as she had on many of her students. She helped him identify his strengths and weaknesses, and she demanded more of him than anyone had before. While writing his thesis, Kielhofner felt pushed to his limits, doing seemingly endless rewrites.

> I remember times when I was so discouraged that I would think about "what else can I do besides being an occupational therapist because I am never going to make it, it's impossible." But all the time I really admired her. She probably is the most brilliant person with whom I have ever worked so closely. I lived and breathed her ideas. . . . In many ways I have often thought of myself as sort of an apologia for her because it

was difficult to understand her, and she did not write a lot of what she said and what she taught. For a long time that is sort of how I perceived my work. Although now I think I am beginning to see that I am doing something unique and different. Obviously I stand on her shoulders as the foundation of what I believe, and I could not have ever thought or done anything that I did without her training me, although I think I can now say I disagree with her on some points. (G.W. Kielhofner, personal communication, March 6, 1987)

Kielhofner's master's thesis (1975) presented a history of occupational therapy and the beginnings of the model of human occupation, which he conceptualized as being in harmony with that history. Janice Burke was a postprofessional master's student at USC while Kielhofner was a basic master's student there. They became friends and enjoyed lengthy discussions about Reilly's theories and ideas with which they were both working. After graduating in 1975 they worked together to write an article for the *American Journal of Occupational Therapy (AJOT)* that evolved from the perspective of history encouraged in their graduate study. It was published in 1977 as "Occupational Therapy After 60 Years: An Account of Changing Identity and Knowledge."

In practice at the NeuroPsychiatric Institute (NPI) in Los Angeles, Kielhofner found that he had to work very hard to find creative ways to apply the concepts of occupational behavior (OB). He and Burke "started moving to do this intermediate theory that was between Reilly's occupational behavior paradigm, and what we called a model of practice" (G.W. Kielhofner, personal communication, March 6, 1987). He feels that some people misunderstood their efforts and thought they were trying to replace Reilly's generic OB theoretical formula with this model. However, many of Reilly's students before them had made significant strides in translating OB concepts to make them more applicable to practice. Kielhofner and Burke took that work, integrated it with their own, and figured out a way to organize the results into a workable model. After rejections for both presentation and publication, the model was finally published in *AJOT* in a series of four articles in September, October, November, and December 1980.

Kielhofner worked at the NeuroPsychiatric Institute of UCLA as a staff occupational therapist and coordinator of training from 1975 to 1979. From 1977 to 1979 he was also an assistant clinical professor in the Department of Occupational Therapy at USC. His last three years at NPI he worked on a doctorate in public health. The title of his dissertation was "Evaluating Deinstitutionalization: An Ethnographic Study of Social Policy" (1980a).

In July 1977, Kielhofner married Nancy Croatt, who was head nurse on the adolescent psychiatry ward at NPI. According to Kielhofner, Nancy has influenced him more than anyone else. She has helped him be less concerned about appearances and more caring toward other people. "She is also a magnificent clinician and has an impressive ability to understand people. She is my constant teacher and mentor" (G.W. Kielhofner, personal communication, April 7, 1987). In 1979 they moved to Richmond, Virginia, where he took the position of associate professor and later director of graduate studies in the Department of Occupational Therapy at Virginia Commonwealth University (VCU). In 1982 the Kielhofner's daughter, Kimberly, was born, and in 1984, they had a son, Kristian.

Kielhofner worked at VCU for five years until 1984. During that time he gave over 40 scholarly presentations and workshops, edited one book and co-authored a second, and published over 15 articles on which he was author or co-author. In addition, in 1981 he received the National Merit Award for Outstanding Achievement from the American Public Health Association; in 1983 he was made a Fellow of the AOTA and received the OTR Award of Merit from the Virginia Occupational Therapy Association. In 1984 he was inducted as a charter member of the Academy of Research of the American Occupational Therapy Foundation (AOTF). During this time he also served on several national committees of the AOTA.

In 1984, the Kielhofner family moved to Boston, where Gary Kielhofner served for two years as associate professor in the Department of Occupational Therapy at Sargent College of Boston University. During that time he continued his extensive publications and workshop presentations.

Although he was not considering the position of chairperson of an academic department as a possible career move, he was approached by a trusted colleague about an opening at the University of Illinois at Chicago (UIC). The opportunity to work in a setting with unusually rich resources and to influence persons as a mentor was attractive. He also wanted the challenge of trying to provide leadership as a scholar, in addition to being a manager. Finally, the position offered the opportunity to be in charge of both academic and clinical settings because, as head of the department, he would also be responsible for OT clinical services in the University of Illinois Hospital. The challenge of bringing academic and clinical pursuits closer was very enticing, especially because they are often seen as incompatible or antagonistic in occupational therapy. So, in the fall of 1986, he became a tenured associate professor and head of the Department of Occupational Therapy in the College of Associated Health Professions of the University of Illinois at Chicago. He continues as chair and is now both a full professor of occupational therapy and a professor of community health sciences in the School of Public Health at UIC.

In 1988 Kielhofner received the A. Jean Ayres Award from the AOTF for contributions to theory development. And in 1991 he was the first occupational therapist to be awarded a fellowship from the Japanese Society for the Promotion of Science. It funded him to keynote the 25th anniversary conference of the Japanese Occupational Therapy Association and to consult throughout Japan.

When asked about personal changes since 1988 he stated:

> My kids are older; my wife and I are wiser. And we all religiously leave
> Chicago for the hinterlands on weekends and holidays. We have pur-
> chased and are renovating a 70 year old cottage on the shores of Lake
> Geneva in Wisconsin. It is our base for hikes, bike riding, fishing, wild-
> flower picking, and such. (G.W. Kielhofner, personal communication,
> June 30, 1992)

He sees the Model of Human Occupation as the centerpiece of his theoretical
work (G.W. Kielhofner, personal communication, June 30, 1992).

> I think the model sort of evolved and matured the way a lot of deductive
> theories have. We started with a set of ideas that we inherited from a
> tradition and tried to put them into coherent statements of relationships.
> Now we're in the process of trying to link it to the empirical
> world . . . through research and testing. (G.W. Kielhofner, personal
> communication, March 6, 1987)

Kielhofner sees this work becoming a tradition of research that is responsible
for revising, changing, and correcting the model. He hopes that by the time he
leaves the field this tradition will have contributed an empirically sound practice
model to the profession.

But he also considers that the model is only a *portion* of his work. As he states,
"My work has been varied and multifaceted. . . . I have been concerned with both
the broad sweep of occupational therapy knowledge development and with the
development of one specific model" (G.W. Kielhofner, personal communication,
June 30, 1992).

Kielhofner is a prolific writer who devotes much time to writing in addition to
his 40-hour work week. He attributes his productivity to a passion for writing.

> I find it extremely exciting to formulate ideas and organize them into a
> written record. I also feel compelled to write because so much of occu-
> pational therapy wisdom exists in an oral tradition and has never been
> labeled and organized. (G.W. Kielhofner, personal communication,
> June 3, 1987)

Gerry Sharrot, OTR, who died in 1986, was a friend and colleague who shared
Kielhofner's strong sense of playfulness about ideas. Sharrot was important to
Kielhofner because he analyzed Kielhofner's work critically, helping him become
aware of subtle issues underlying his thinking. "I felt safer knowing he would help
scout out flaws in my ideas, and he understood my insistence on the absolute right
to disagree with myself after I had written something. His death is not only a loss

to me personally but also to the profession" (G.W. Kielhofner, personal communication, June 3, 1987).

From the beginning of his career, most of Kielhofner's publications have been written jointly with other authors. He states that he enjoys working with other people when he writes. To date, of the 55 articles in occupational therapy on which his name appears, 39 are co-authored. Two of his books are co-authored with Barris and Watts, and he was editor of two others, each of which involved collaboration with many contributors. He is sole author of his most recent book.

He has also made numerous oral presentations around the world. In the past three years he has lectured and consulted in Japan, has spent much time in Scandinavia, and is currently dissertation advisor to students in doctoral programs in Sweden.

Kielhofner acknowledges that in his early years in the field he put forth his ideas fairly dogmatically. In recent years, however, he has sought to become more open and flexible in his thinking, drawing both from research findings and from dialogue and debate with others in the field, such as Sharrot. As he says, "I'm realizing more and more that there are very few black and white things in life" (G.W. Kielhofner, personal communication, March 6, 1987).

THEORETICAL CONCEPTS

Temporal Adaptation

In 1977 Kielhofner won the Cordelia Meyers Award for "New Writer of the Year" from *AJOT* for his article "Temporal Adaptation: A Conceptual Framework for Occupational Therapy." In this article he described the concept of time and its meaning in organizing human activity. He presented a temporal frame of reference as a culturally determined perspective that is modified in action by each individual's own values, interests, and goals, which are naturally inclined toward a rhythm of self-maintenance, work, and play. Habits are the structures for organizing time in daily behavior, and social roles determine to a large degree what habits will be formed.

Kielhofner no longer sees temporal adaptation as a separate concept, but has incorporated it into the model of human occupation. He considers this concept to be a stepping stone in his own thinking and a part of the history and development of the model (G.W. Kielhofner, personal communication, March 6, 1987).

General Systems Theory

In 1978, Kielhofner published an article in *AJOT*, "General Systems Theory: Implications for Theory and Action in Occupational Therapy," that laid down the foundation for the model of human occupation. As Reilly had taught him, Kielhofner drew on the works of established theorists, such as von Bertelanffy, Boulding, and Feibleman, to explain the concept of systems theory and the laws governing it. In this article, Kielhofner describes the paradigm of general systems theory (GST) and compares and contrasts it with the paradigm of reductionism, which he considers to underlie much of current OT practice. He stresses the need to bring together the skills and techniques from the reductionist paradigm with the perspective of the GST paradigm.

Reductionism, a perspective popularized in science in the late 1700s, holds that one can reduce phenomena into units that can then be studied, measured, and looked at in relationship with other units through the concept of cause and effect. Its underlying assumption is that the parts can then be pulled together again to provide an understanding of the whole. The medical model is based on this paradigm.

However, reductionism has major flaws as a perspective for occupational therapy. First, putting the pieces together again does not give a complete picture and explanation of the whole. Second, when applied to humans, this view oversimplifies individual and social behavior:

> In occupational therapy, the various units of concern under the reductionist paradigm were joint range of motion, muscle strength, anxiety, reflex, defense mechanism, and others. . . . When all these disassembled components are combined in clinical thinking, the net result is less than the "gestalt" to which GST addresses itself. The larger units of reality for occupational therapy under a systems framework are the human career, the social role, and the ecology, competency, and fitness for social participation. (Kielhofner, 1978, p. 638)

To conceptualize according to a systems perspective is to look at patterns, rather than units. These patterns are governed by laws different from the laws of cause and effect. Rather than measures of central tendency and dispersion, which form the statistical method of description used in reductionist inquiry, GST uses model or network descriptions. Table 7-1 illustrates basic differences between the statistical questions asked in reductionist descriptions and the systems model questions asked in GST descriptions. Kielhofner states:

> This is not to preclude the usefulness of statistical data, but to recognize their limitations. Qualitative data that focus on system and environmental conditions are more operational and more likely to yield effective intervention. For example, information about the degree of intelligence of a retarded patient is not nearly as useful as information about the person's interests, values, habits, skills, and the demands for perform-

Table 7-1 Contrasting Statistical and System Descriptions

Statistical Questions	*Systems Models Questions*
Types of Data:	*Types of Data:*
Nominal. To what class of things does this object belong?	*Network or Conditional.* What is the overall pattern of the system?
Ordinal. What is the rank order position of this object along a single dimension continuum?	*Historical.* How has the system performed over time and what have been its experiences?
Interval. How much of a given characteristic does this object have in relation to other objects? (e.g., 2 times or ¹/₂ time)	*Contextual.* What are conditions in the environment and how are they brought to bear on the system?
Ratio. How much of a given characteristic does this object have when zero equals none of the characteristics?	*Dynamic.* What is the status of this system's ongoing interaction with the environment?

Source: From "General Systems Theory: Implications for Theory and Action in Occupational Therapy" by G. Kielhofner, 1978, *American Journal of Occupational Therapy, 32*, p. 640. Copyright 1978 by American Occupational Therapy Association, Inc. Reprinted by permission.

---

ance under the larger spheres of human experience. Human mechanics, neurological circuitry, and affect are constructs of a lower order, about which decisions would be made in the larger context of patients' day-to-day and lifelong human experiences. This means that activities of daily living and the human career would become a central, rather than a peripheral, concern in occupational therapy.

For instance, it is known that exercise can provide strength and that a dynamic splint provides increased function and that both might contribute to increased capacity for self-care. However, self-care must be organized under a social role, a view of self, and a continuum of life experience. The contribution of increased physical function to overall adaptation depends on many higher-level functions within the patient. What is being suggested here is a hierarchy of function. The manner in which lower levels of functioning are related to higher levels is largely unconsidered in any theory of occupational therapy. (Kielhofner, 1978, p. 640)

Kielhofner acknowledges that much of the information learned under the reductionist paradigm in occupational therapy is useful and helpful. He recommends that occupational therapists use a process of critical analysis to discriminate the accurate information from the errors in reductionist theories and then integrate the accurate information and use it within a GST perspective.

Kielhofner concludes the 1978 article on general systems theory with a description of the laws and characteristics that govern GST. These are "hierarchical arrangement of subparts; openness or self-maintenance in the midst of an interchange of matter and information with an environment; and continuity in the midst of ongoing change" (Kielhofner, 1978, p. 644).

Kielhofner draws on the work of Feibleman (1969) to describe further each of these characteristics of GST and the laws that govern them. A general understanding of GST is necessary to fully comprehend the model of human occupation. Examples from everyday experience are given to illustrate these concepts.

The first concept is that subsystems (gestalt wholes in themselves) are arranged hierarchically within an overall system. Feibleman delineates five laws, three of which govern the relationship between these subsystems and two of which concern change.

1. "Higher levels direct or organize lower levels." Example: The goals one has set for the day can motivate the body to make the necessary movements to get up out of bed.

2. "Higher levels are dependent upon or constrained by the lower levels." Example: If one has a bad case of the flu, one's body may strongly resist getting up out of bed, no matter how motivated one is by goals for accomplishment.

3. "At any level, the mechanism of the level can be found at the level below, and the purpose of the level, at the level above." Example: The mechanism is moving the body; the purpose is to pursue the day's goals.

4. "Less time is required for change at higher levels than at lower levels." Example: One can alter one's goals for the day more quickly than one can get over the flu.

5. "A disturbance or change at one level resonates throughout the other levels." Example: Having the flu affects not only one's body but also one's ability to carry out habits and move toward goals. (Kielhofner, 1978, p. 644)

The second concept is that systems are open and self-maintaining in dynamic interaction with the environment. This interaction involves: "(1) the input of information and material from the environment, (2) a throughput process that transforms the input into some new project [sic], and (3) the output that acts on the environment (which then generates feedback)" (Kielhofner, 1978, p. 644).

A third concept is that evolution and change in the system over time are guided by the feedback loop just described. The system begins as an undifferentiated, spontaneous whole that, through the process of interaction with the environment, becomes increasingly organized, skilled, and differentiated. In humans this process results in the development of habits and in the "establishment of leading parts that dominate the behavior of the system and centralize the system's function" (Kielhofner, 1978, p. 645). These processes enable the system to evolve and become increasingly complex.

It is within the context of these characteristics and laws of general systems theory that Kielhofner and Burke built their theoretical framework—the model of human occupation.

Model of Human Occupation

In September 1980, Kielhofner and Burke published the first of four consecutive articles describing the model of human occupation in *AJOT*. At the outset they state:

> The model presented here is preliminary and exploratory and thus incomplete. It will require substantial empirical validation and conceptual refinement. It is presented to stimulate, rather than confine, thinking in OT. (Kielhofner & Burke, 1980, p. 573)

Kielhofner and Burke originally developed their model to provide a link between Reilly's theory of OB and daily practice in the OT clinic (G.W. Kielhofner, personal communication, March 6, 1987). One of its basic assumptions, which Kielhofner and Burke attribute to Reilly and through her to such writers as Boulding, White, and Dewey, is that:

> All human occupation arises out of an innate, spontaneous tendency of the human system—the urge to explore and master the environment. The model is based on the assumption that occupation is a central aspect of the human experience. It is Man's innate urge toward exploration and mastery and his consequent ability to symbolize that makes him unique among animals. (Kielhofner & Burke, 1980, p. 573)

This interaction of the person with the environment is occupational behavior.

Arrangement in Subsystems

Taking the work that had been done at USC and was part of the OB knowledge that evolved, Kielhofner and Burke pulled it together in new ways and made it "user friendly." They conceived the human occupation system as made up of three subsystems, which they called volitional, habituation, and performance. These subsystems are hierarchically arranged in accordance with GST laws, with volition the highest and performance the lowest. The volitional subsystem is motivated by the innate urge toward exploration and mastery. The function of this system is to initiate action (Kielhofner & Burke, 1980).

The volitional subsystem is made up of three aspects: (1) a sense of personal causation, which is the sense one has of one's ability to affect and influence one's environment, the inner symbolic model of the self as an actor in the world, and the degree to which one feels an ability to direct one's own life; (2) interests, which are those things one enjoys and prefers doing; and (3) values, which are those things one feels are important or right (Kielhofner & Burke, 1980, p. 576).

The habituation subsystem arranges behavior into patterns and roles. Its function is to organize patterns of action that are output by the system; "thus, it maintains order in the output" (Kielhofner & Burke, 1980, p. 574). This subsystem is governed by the volitional subsystem.

The habituation subsystem comprises habits, those activities that have become routine and automatic through practice and repetition, and roles, consisting of internalized expectations for the ways one will behave within certain relationships to people or situations.

The performance subsystem is made up of skills, which are the basic abilities for action. It is governed by the other two subsystems, and its function is to enact the behaviors that they call for (Kielhofner & Burke, 1980). This subsystem is made up of motor, process, and communication skills. These skills have symbolic, neurological, and musculoskeletal components.

In the 1985 book *A Model of Human Occupation: Theory and Application*, which Kielhofner edited, he and Burke elaborated on these subsystem components that had been defined earlier. Basing their discussion on findings from research and observation done from 1980 to 1984, they described belief in skill, belief in efficacy of skill, expectancy of success/failure, and internal/external locus of control as aspects of the volitional component of sense of personal causation. They broke down the volitional component of values into temporal orientation, meaningfulness of activity, occupational goals, and personal standards. They defined interests in relation to discrimination, pattern, and potency (meaning frequency of interests being acted on).

They postulated that the habituation subsystem component of roles is influenced by perceived incumbency (meaning awareness of oneself as in a role); internalized expectations (one's image of others' expectations for oneself in that role); and role balance (a satisfactory integration of a number of roles). Habits are more or less adaptive and satisfying depending on the qualities of "degree of organization, social appropriateness, and flexibility/rigidity" (Kielhofner & Burke, 1985, p. 28).

Development of Subsystems

The human infant enters the world as a totally undifferentiated open system (except at the cellular and organ levels). The first activity of this new human system is exploration. As the baby explores it begins to develop skills. As these skills are repeated/practiced and the child develops competency and mastery (e.g., ability to place blocks on top of one another, ability to grasp spoon), combinations of skills are put together and routinized into habits (e.g., brushing teeth, feeding self, dressing, walking, riding a bicycle). The child begins to develop an understanding of expectations for his or her behavior in certain roles (e.g., family member, sibling, friend, student). Finally, as the child is exploring and developing skills and habits, things are discovered that he or she likes to do or does not enjoy, and so interests develop. Through the interaction that the child has with the environment (human and nonhuman) during exploration and development of competence and mastery, a sense of personal causation or a self-perception of how effective he or she is within the environment is developed. Through interaction with the environment—including family, community, and culture—the child develops values.

Once values, interests, and a sense of personal causation have developed, these qualities exert a controlling and motivating influence on habits, roles, and performance. Kielhofner and Burke maintain that occupational therapy's major focus has been on the lowest level in this hierarchy—on performance and its component skills. Although performance is a crucial aspect of function, Kielhofner and Burke suggest that occupational therapy needs to take what has been learned about the various performance components (much of that information coming from the use of a reductionist perspective) and put it within the larger context of the system. Occupational therapists need to see those components of performance at the lowest level as they are motivated and directed by the higher levels of habits and roles (habituation) and by values, interests, and sense of personal causation (volition) (Kielhofner & Burke, 1980).

> These three subsystems organize and regulate the output of the system. Each contributes to the output in a different way. The volition subsystem has the greatest degree of freedom; it is the level at which action is freely and consciously chosen. The habituation subsystem represents automatic and routine behavior. It regulates the output of the system into regular and predictable patterns. The performance subsystem organizes output at the lowest level, governing small patterns of skilled action. (Kielhofner & Burke, 1980, p. 574)

Consistent with the rules of general systems, however, the lower levels constrain the higher ones. For instance, although one might be motivated to water ski (be interested in doing so, see that activity as fitting into one's value system, and feel that one could do so), if one had never skied before, one would not have developed the necessary skills and patterns of behavior and so would be unsuccessful. However, if one were to experiment, play, and practice, one would (hypothetically) eventually develop the skills and patterns of behavior necessary to ski successfully.

However, for the person who is a paraplegic, the lower subsystem would constrain the higher ones, no matter how motivated he or she was to practice and learn how to water ski. That is because, of course, the motor performance component would be unable to function in the necessary ways. However, because the higher subsystems direct and organize the lower ones and because change can happen more quickly at higher levels than at lower ones, he or she could decide to adapt the activity and learn to use a water sled.

System Interaction with the Environment

Kielhofner and Burke first presented their theory on the way the system interacts with the environment in 1980. In 1985, Kielhofner and others elaborated on this basic conceptualization. The environment consists of objects, people, and events with which the system (the person) interacts, influenced by the culture of which that person is a part. "The open system interacts with the environment by way of a process of input, output, throughput, and feedback. The system represents Man, and the interaction of the system with the environment is human occupation" (Kielhofner & Burke, 1980, pp. 573–574).

The system receives input from the environment. This input enters the system and is processed by each of the three subsystems—volitional, habituation, and performance—as appropriate, in a process called throughput. In this throughput stage, output is organized. The output comprises both information and action, which:

> are combined by the system to achieve results (in the use of skills), to meet expectations for performance (as organized by habits and roles), and to satisfy the system's own purposes (as contained in the volition subsystem). The output of information and action to achieve purposeful ends is occupational behavior. (Kielhofner & Burke, 1980, p. 580)

This behavior generates feedback, the last part of the loop. Feedback about the consequences of one's actions joins with the input that begins a new cycle. "In the feedback process actual performance is compared to expected outcomes. This process allows the system to make adjustments in this performance that, in turn, influence the organization of the system itself" (Kielhofner & Burke, 1980, p. 580).

Input received directly from the environment also can reorganize the system. An example is the expectations for performance made by others—parents, teachers, and the larger culture. Because both feedback and input work to bring about change and adjustment in the system, the open system is said to be self-transforming.

> The system both changes and is changed by the environment; each shapes the other. Man creates his physical and symbolic environment at the time he learns to act competently in it. As the open system explores and masters the environment, it transforms both itself and the environment. (Kielhofner & Burke, 1980, p. 574)

Barris has elaborated on this system-environment interaction (Barris, 1982; Barris, Kielhofner, Levine, & Neville, 1985). Figure 7-1 illustrates the open system concept of the model of human occupation.

Example of the Model of Human Occupation Applied to Normal Development

As a young girl learns to ride a bicycle, she gets input directly from the environment: the texture, temperature, and color of the bicycle; the feel of it to her hands,

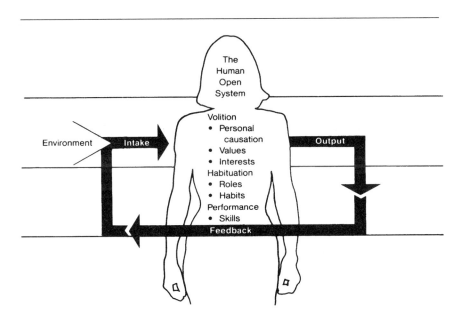

Figure 7-1 Open System Representing Human Occupation. *Source:* From *A Model of Human Occupation: Theory and Application* (p. 35) by G. Kielhofner (Ed.), 1985. Baltimore, Md.: Williams & Wilkins Company. Copyright 1985 by Williams & Wilkins Company. Adapted by permission.

feet, and buttocks; and the instructions of her mother, who is standing beside her. As the child sits on the bicycle seat while her mother holds the bike, this input is processed (throughput). She is very motivated to learn to ride because it is a value and an interest and because she feels she can succeed (volition). She remembers being a whiz on her tricycle and has the clear motor pattern of peddling "down pat" (habituation). She has mastered a good degree of balance by walking on the curbstone, and she has developed normally in her motor skills (performance).

Now, her mother tells her to start peddling, assuring her that she will hold onto the bike. As the girl starts to propel the bike, she begins to get feedback from her vestibular system, from her eyes, and kinesthetically from her body. Meanwhile, her mother is giving her verbal input about how she is doing. This feedback and new input are processed in throughput by the volitional subsystem ("Oh, this isn't as easy as I thought, but Mom is encouraging me, bolstering my motivation"), the habituation subsystem ("It's like riding my tricycle only different"), and the performance subsystem ("You're falling left"). This throughput is organized into output action ("Lean a bit left, turn the wheel slightly left, sit back"). As this process continues, the system is changed. Through practice the girl develops skill in performing the necessary actions. As she masters them they become habits. And once she can ride the bike successfully (once the basic performance requirements have become habits), her concept of herself is changed (increased sense of competence, increased self-esteem), she has a new role (as bicycle rider), and her goals change. And so it goes. The environment is transformed also, by the addition of this girl as a bicycle rider.

Evolution and Change in the System

In "A Model of Human Occupation: Part Two," Kielhofner describes change and development, which he calls ontogenesis, from the perspective of temporal adaptation. Hierarchical change in an open system is influenced by the system's own internal tendencies and by the demands of the environment—two factors that come together in the throughput-output-input feedback cycle (1980b).

> The central problem of change in occupation is to explain how a system with a global tendency toward exploring and mastering its environment is transformed into a socially functioning, productive and self-satisfying entity. The hierarchical change of occupation proceeds from this undifferentiated, innate tendency toward exploration and mastery to individual competence in occupational roles. (Kielhofner, 1980b, p. 657)

Kielhofner presents Reilly's three stages of motivation—exploration to competency to achievement—as the aspects of the volitional subsystem that internally drive the other two subsystems to change. Through exploration one develops skills, through pursuing competence one organizes habits, and through striving for achievement, one develops competent role behaviors (Kielhofner, 1980b).

So one explores and develops skills. Then, driven by the internal desire for competency that one measures to external standards, one develops habits. And finally, motivated by the internal desire to attain a role in the social group—to achieve—together with the external demands of that group for certain behavior, one develops role behavior.

Kielhofner also suggests that as the system changes and develops, these three motivations drive the balance of work and play through the lifetime. In the 1985 book *A Model of Human Occupation*, Kielhofner states that this process is explained through "blending of the occupational behavior and development perspectives in occupational therapy" (Kielhofner, 1985, p. 77). He illustrates this concept, shown in Figure 7-2, and calls it an "occupational life-span theory" (Kielhofner, 1980b).

Kielhofner devotes five chapters in the 1985 book to this concept of occupational development. Two principles affect the development of each subsystem and govern the interrelationship of the subsystems in development. First, development in one subsystem influences the others. (Developing the skills to ride a bicycle influences habits and sense of self.) Second:

> The period for development of each subsystem lengthens as one ascends the hierarchy. The child has mastered a wide range of perceptual motor skills before he or she takes on several differentiated roles and long before a personal system of complex values is shaped. (Kielhofner, 1985, p. 79)

In other words, the input-throughput-output feedback cycle is functioning so as to propel the system toward greater achievement and satisfaction (Kielhofner, 1980c).

As the system matures in an adaptive way, through interaction with the environment and through the characteristics of the subsystems that influence its output, it becomes increasingly more complex and differentiated. This evolution in turn allows it to interact more and more flexibly with the environment. This adaptive development implies that the system is both satisfying its own internal urge to explore and master, and fulfilling the demands of the environment—not all the time, because failure is sometimes a consequence of action, but more often than not. This two-steps-forward-and-one-step-back progression toward increasing adaptation Kielhofner (1980c) originally called "a benign cycle." He currently uses the labels "adaptive" and "maladaptive" cycles for what in 1980 he termed "benign" and "vicious" cycles. A maladaptive cycle develops when a pattern emerges in which either the system is unsatisfied or environmental demands are unmet, or both occur (Kielhofner, 1980c).

Levels of Organization of the Occupational Behavior Career

	Childhood	Adolescence	Adulthood	Old Age
Waking Hours Occupied by Work and Play	Time spent in play		Time spent in work	
Play Yields	Reality is explored via curiosity for rules of competent action.	Competent behavior is learned and experienced in games, personal hobbies, and social events.	Relaxation and recreation support the worker role. Exploration of novel situations allows new roles to be taken on.	Play allows the exploration of past achieve-ments and the unknown future, and maintenance of competence through leisure pursuit of interests.
Relationship of Play and Work	*Exploration* Skills for productivity are acquired and work roles explored through imitation and imagination	*Competency* Personal and interpersonal competency are developed in a matrix of cooperation yielding habits of sportsmanship and crafts-manship.	*Achievement* Play supports the worker roles by providing an arena of retreat and rejuvenation. Exploration in novel situations allows the ongoing development of new competency for work.	*Exploration* Retirement leisure signals that the productive obligation to society has been fulfilled. Past work has earned for the person the right to leisure. Leisure replaces work as the major source of life satisfaction.
Work Yields	Productive behaviors are practiced through chores and in school.	The work role is practiced and the commitment process of occupational choice takes place.	There is entry into worker roles with the requirement of establishing and maintaining a productive and self-satisfying career.	Retirement brings reduced expectations for productivity and personal capacities for productive action are waning.

Figure 7-2 Balance and Interrelationship of Work and Play during the Life-Span. *Source:* From "A Model of Human Occupation, Part Two, Ontogenesis from the Perspective of Temporal Adaptation" by G. Kielhofner, 1980. *American Journal of Occupational Therapy, 34,* p. 661. Copyright 1980 by American Occupational Therapy Association, Inc. Reprinted by permission.

[Maladaptive] cycles may begin from birth, precipitated by some incurred disability. These cycles may also develop slowly as a result of interactions with the environment. . . . They may be precipitated by interactions with the social environment that produce demands beyond the capacity of the system to adapt. They may also be the result of demands being decreased to such a degree that the system is no longer challenged to perform, and the volition subsystem's urge to mastery cannot find expression. Vicious cycles exist wherever the requirements of the system to fulfill the urge to explore and master the world cannot be fulfilled and/or where the environment's demands are not met. (Kielhofner, 1980c, p. 734)

Function/Dysfunction Continuum

Adaptive cycles result in a state of occupational function, whereas maladaptive cycles result in occupational dysfunction. Persons are occupationally functional when they meet both society's need for productive and playful participation and their own need for exploration and mastery, which in turn enhances volition, habituation, and performance. A person is occupationally dysfunctional when any of the above needs are not met (Kielhofner, 1985).

As occupation is enacted through the input-throughput-output feedback cycle, any problems in function may have their origin at any part of the cycle. Occupational dysfunction is recognized at the interface of the person with the environment as a decrease, cessation, ineffectiveness, inappropriateness, or imbalance of output. Environmental factors must therefore be acknowledged in evaluating occupational dysfunction (Kielhofner, 1985).

The three levels of occupational function—exploration, competency, and mastery—are derived from Reilly's theory and "represent states of optimal arousal and involvement with the environment" (Kielhofner, 1985, p. 64). The states of occupational dysfunction that Kielhofner delineates represent stress and a lack of productive involvement with environment.

Kielhofner conceptualizes states of increasing occupational dysfunction, starting with inefficiency, which results "when there is an interference with performing meaningful activity accompanied by dissatisfaction with performance. Sources of inefficiency may be environmental constraints, disease processes, or imbalanced lifestyles" (Kielhofner, 1985, p. 69).

The second state of occupational dysfunction is incompetence, which is characterized by:

a major loss or limitation of skills, a failure or disruption of self-confidence and satisfaction, and inability to routinely and adequately perform the tasks of everyday living associated with occupational roles. It

> may result from marginal learning due to poor environments, from dis-
> ease or from a life-style which erodes system organization. (Kielhofner,
> 1985, p. 71)

Helplessness is the third stage of occupational dysfunction. Kielhofner describes this as:

> total or nearly total disruption of occupational performance coupled
> with extreme feelings of ineffectiveness, anxiety and/or depression. A
> state of helplessness may result from some traumatic episode which
> suddenly renders a healthy person totally dependent or from a lifelong
> series of negative experiences. (Kielhofner, 1985, p. 72)

The process of therapy is one of "providing opportunities for occupational function until individuals can maintain an adaptive open system cycle of their own"
(Kielhofner, 1985, p. 74). In addressing how this goal can be achieved, Kielhofner
states:

> Any changes in the system must begin with the volition subsystem. This
> system, which enacts output, is critical for initiating cycles that can re-
> sult in restoration of a positive trajectory. The environmental conditions
> are also of critical importance. The implications for occupational
> therapy at this point are twofold. The first is that therapy should serve as
> an environment that can begin to present demands for performance and
> elicit the enactment of responses that can result in positive feedback.
> The occupational therapy clinic is an important source of input to the
> system and a critical environment in which [adaptive] cycles can de-
> velop. (Kielhofner, 1980c, p. 736)

It is critical to determine at which level behaviors are disrupted and to begin
with the lowest level of motivation. One must then manage the total environment
of therapy so that the person is encouraged to explore.

> The patient or client is not only the focus but also the instrument of
> therapy. Through engaging in directed occupations, the person begins to
> change the entire cycle, to organize or reorganize the internal compo-
> nents of the system and to increase the potential for adaptive output in
> the future. (Kielhofner, 1985, p. 74)

Once the patient's curiosity has been engaged and exploration has begun, it is
important to change the environment so that competence can be elicited. Then,
once the patient has achieved a point of mastery the demands of the environment
must be "integrated with existing skills and habits to reach achievement of valued
goals" (Kielhofner, 1980c, p. 737).

APPLICATION TO OCCUPATIONAL THERAPY PRACTICE

Three assumptions underlie the application of this model in practice. As Kielhofner states:

> Reilly points out that occupational therapy is directed toward enabling man to fulfill his innate need for "occupation and . . . the rich and varied stimuli that solving life problems provides him." According to this primary assumption, humans are occupational creatures who cannot be healthy in the absence of meaningful occupation.
>
> Reilly has also stated the second assumption: "Man, through the use of his hands as they are energized by mind and will, can influence the state of his own health." According to this assertion, occupation can shape the health of a person, and can thus serve as a means to health. The first two assumptions assert that occupation is both a basic human activity essential to health and a healing process.
>
> A third assumption is that for occupational therapy to be instrumental as a means to an end, it must embody the characteristics of the end itself. This means that occupational therapy must be true "occupation." Therapy must embody the characteristics of purposefulness, challenge, accomplishment, and satisfaction that make up every occupation. Therefore, a theory of occupation is critical to practice.
>
> The idea that, by engaging in occupation designed as therapy, man can restore, increase, and maintain his ability as an occupational creature is the foundation of occupational therapy. A theory of human occupation serves to justify the field's commitment to occupation as a worthy goal for therapy. It also demonstrates how therapy should be organized and carried out. (Kielhofner, Burke, & Igi, 1980, pp. 777–778)

The model of human occupation helps the occupational therapist find an explanation for the pattern of occupational function and dysfunction presented by the patient by (1) indicating the variables on which one should gather information, (2) pointing out the relationships among those variables through the schema of the subsystems and their hierarchical relationships, (3) indicating the relationship between subsystem components and the environment and the effect of this relationship on the whole system, (4) providing an outline of changes that can be expected at different levels of occupational development, and (5) presenting an occupational function-dysfunction continuum from which one can determine a patient's level of performance (Rogers & Kielhofner, 1985).

Thus, in the model of human occupation, assessment is conducted to provide information about the status of the volitional, the habituation, and the performance subsystems; the feedback loop; the development of organization of occupation throughout the life cycle; and the environment. From this information the occupational therapist develops a picture of the patient's level of occupational function or dysfunction (degree of organization or disorganization) and a list of treatment options (Rogers & Kielhofner, 1985).

The choice of how one treats the various areas of dysfunction identified through this assessment is outside the domain of this model. Kielhofner sees evaluation, treatment planning, and treatment implementation as an hourglass (G.W. Kielhofner, personal communication, March 6, 1987). His model is the top half, which is used to conceptualize the individual in her or his occupational wholeness and to assess the level of occupational dysfunction. From this assessment is developed a treatment plan, with goals related to that person's occupational performance needs. Treatment must address all areas assessed: the three subsystems, age, the environment, and the feedback loop. The bottom half of the hourglass he sees as filled with whatever theories, modalities, and facilitative activities will best meet these treatment goals for that individual. In making choices for treatment, the therapist is guided by his or her own training and personal frame of reference, and of course by the understanding of:

> the importance of making the patient's own concerns and values the guiding principle in clinical decision-making. It is the patient and not the therapist who is the agent of change. As open systems, patients organize or reorganize themselves through engagement in occupation. The choice to effectively occupy oneself comes from a sense of personal freedom. The patient must ultimately will the action which is undertaken as part of the clinical process or else true change cannot result. (Rogers & Kielhofner, 1985, p. 145)

The model of human occupation is being applied in practice settings throughout the United States and abroad. Applications of the model to practice in psychosocial settings is described in Barris, Kielhofner, and Watts' books *Psychosocial Occupational Therapy* (1983) and *Occupational Therapy in Psychosocial Practice* (1988).

More than one-third of Kielhofner's 1985 book *A Model of Human Occupation* is devoted to applications of the model to evaluation and treatment in practice settings. This section of the book is divided into five chapters, each of which is concerned with a particular target population: the physically disabled, those with primary psychosocial dysfunction, children, elders, and the mentally retarded. In each chapter the general areas of dysfunction of the target group are reviewed according to the model of human occupation, with recommendations for assessment and intervention. Also included in each chapter are specific case examples illustrating use of the model to assess areas of function and dysfunction and develop treatment plans for individual patients. Much of this material was contributed by therapists who are currently working in direct practice with patients.

Many therapists have published articles describing their use of the model in clinical practice. The model has been used as a framework for assessing and intervening in the occupational functioning of patients with a diagnosis of borderline personality disorder (Salz, 1983), hospice patients (Tigges & Sherman, 1983), patients in chronic pain (Gusich, 1984), native Canadians (Wieringa & McColl, 1987), adolescents with diabetes (Curtin, 1991), young adults in psychiatry (Kielhofner & Brinson, 1989), co-dependent adults (Neville-Jan, Bradley, Bunn, & Gehri, 1991), adults with alcoholism (Scaffa, 1991), adults in a day hospital (Gusich & Silverman, 1991), adults with HIV infection and AIDS (Pizzi, 1990), immigrant women in Canada (Khoo & Renwick, 1989), elders (Burton, 1989a, 1989b), and persons with Alzheimer's disease (Borell, Sandman, & Kielhofner, 1991; Oakley, 1987). The model has also been used to look at adolescents' development (Blakeney, 1985), adults' anger (Grogan, 1991a, 1991b), child psychiatry (Baron, 1991; Sholle-Martin, 1987; Sholle-Martin & Alessi, 1990), adolescent psychiatry (Lancaster & Mitchell, 1991; Sholle-Martin, 1987), and early intervention (Schaaf & Mulrooney, 1989).

Documentation of Postulates through Research

In a 1984 article that appeared in the *Canadian Journal of Occupational Therapy (CJOT)*, Kielhofner states:

> From the model there have been derived basic postulates which state relationships between variables. These have, in turn, been investigated through research. Four major postulates are as follows:
>
> 1. A disturbance of any part of the system reverberates throughout the system. Lower levels can constrain higher levels whereas higher levels can lead to disorganization of lower levels.
>
> 2. The output of the system (i.e., OB) and the status of the system's internal organization are interrelated.
>
> 3. Feedback to the system is influenced by the overall system dynamic including the relationship of volition or choice with output.
>
> 4. The output (i.e., OB) of the system is influenced by the environment of the system and its match to system's characteristics. (Kielhofner, 1984, p. 60)

Kielhofner and others have tested these postulates through reviews of the literature, research studies, and clinical practice.

> In addition to studies which are specifically designed to test proposi-
> tions from the model and clinical research which has attempted to
> operationalize model concepts into assessment instruments of proce-
> dures, there has been descriptive research which elaborates the model.
> (Kielhofner, 1984, p. 60)

As Kielhofner himself has frequently stated, the development of this model has
been influenced by many people. Most of the research has been done as a collaborative effort with colleagues or graduate students. Also a significant body of research has been conducted without Kielhofner's direct involvement.

Kielhofner sees the model as beginning with a set of ideas based in literature
that are inherited from the tradition of occupational behavior. This literature is
from sociology, including systems theory; from psychology, including the science
of human adaptation; and from human development. Kielhofner and others have
tried to frame these ideas into coherent statements of relationships. Presently they
are working to link the model to the practical world through testing and research
(G.W. Kielhofner, personal communication, March 6, 1987).

> A lot of my research has been, and continues to be, development of
> assessments. I like to do this because it has a strong clinical focus. An-
> other source of research is descriptive research that asks whether rela-
> tionships that we hypothesize or theorize are, in fact, borne out in the
> empirical world. And we are also doing qualitative research that asks
> what do we know about the volitional traits or the habituation traits or
> whatever, of people with different types of disabilities. Then the final
> piece of research is testing treatment based on the model. (G.W.
> Kielhofner, personal communication, March 6, 1987)

Kielhofner sees this research as a major part of his work, and intends that
through it, and the revising, changing, and correcting of the model that will result,
he will "leave the field with a practice model that it can use and for which there is
empirical support" (G.W. Kielhofner, personal communication, March 6, 1987).

Development of Assessments

A vitally important area of research is determining the reliability and validity of
tests or assessment instruments used to measure model variables. This determination is a long-term process since many studies need to be done with any one instrument before it can be used with confidence. The work has begun, and a number of
such studies have been reported that have tested wholly new instruments and/or
revised, adapted, and refined existing instruments to fit the needs of the model of
human occupation. Kielhofner's edited book *A Model of Human Occupation*

(1985) contains an appendix entitled "Instrument Library," which includes 64 assessment tools that have been used by the book's contributors to measure different aspects of the human occupation model. The majority of the tools listed were developed for other purposes and before the model of human occupation was formulated. Thus although they can be used to assess various individual aspects of the model (i.e., self-esteem, interests), care must be taken in interpreting results in the context of model concepts until such time as extensive studies show their validity for those purposes. Therefore, instrument development studies are a critical part of the research effort for the model of human occupation.

The following assessment tools have been the focus of initial research concerning their validity and reliability for use with the model of human occupation: the Occupational Picture Interest Sort for Use with Retarded Adults (Scott, 1982; Shakun, 1982), the Role Checklist (Oakley, Kielhofner, Barris, & Reichler, 1986; Sepiol & Froehlich, 1990), the Occupational Role History (Kielhofner, Harlan, Bauer, & Maurer, 1986), the Assessment of Occupational Functioning (Watts, Kielhofner, Bauer, Gregory, & Valentine, 1986), a Short-Term Psychiatric Interview and Rating Scale (Kaplan, 1984), the Bentz Measure of Personal Causation for Retarded Adults (Bentz, 1984), an Assessment of Process Skills (Doble, 1985), the Preschool Play Scale (Harrison & Kielhofner, 1986), the Occupational Questionnaire (Smith, Kielhofner, & Watts, 1986), and the Occupational Performance History Interview (Kielhofner & Henry, 1988 [critiqued by Donohue and McCreedy in 1989] and Kielhofner, Henry, Walens, & Rogers, 1991).

Descriptive Research

Descriptive research on the model has been of two basic types: comparative and correlational. Each is used to test the reality of relationships hypothesized by the model. Comparative studies look at different groups of individuals to ascertain whether they really do differ on selected variables as the model would predict. Correlational studies look at different model variables and test whether they are indeed related in the way that the model suggests. Such studies test the relationship between the human system and the environment.

Comparative Studies

In 1980, Mailloux looked at children with visual-motor integration problems to see whether that disturbance in the performance subsystem would be reflected in a decreased sense of personal causation, a component of the higher-level volitional system. She also tested how self-esteem and visual-motor integration (i.e., aspects of two of the three throughput subsystems) would correlate with student role performance (output). She tested 40 children in a learning disabilities classroom in a public school and found no significant correlations.

In 1981, Scaffa studied differences between 25 alcoholics and 25 nonalcoholics between 18 and 30 years of age to see whether behavioral output of the alcoholics would reflect disorganization in habituation and volitional subsystems. Based on her results, she was able to show significant differences in the habituation subsystem behaviors of the two groups and some meaningful differences in the volitional traits of interest.

In 1983, Lyons found no significant differences in selected volitional traits of 10 employed and 18 unemployed mentally retarded young adults.

In 1985, Lederer, Kielhofner, and Watts looked at 15 delinquent and 15 nondelinquent adolescents to see whether they differed on locus of control, values, and perceptual motor skills. Results showed no statistically significant difference between groups; however, the delinquents placed less value on the roles of student, volunteer, worker, homemaker, and caregiver.

Also in 1985, Smyntek, Barris, and Kielhofner compared volitional and habituation traits of 37 adolescents who were patients in several acute care psychiatric facilities and 36 adolescents who were high school students. Differences in locus of control and in self-esteem were significant, as were potency of interests and value placed on roles and number of present roles. Also, the hospitalized adolescents spent significantly less time in daily living tasks.

In 1986, a study compared personal causation, values, interests, roles, and habitual use of time in three groups: ten high school students, ten adolescents hospitalized for psychosocial problems in conjunction with a primary medical diagnosis, and ten adolescents hospitalized with a primary psychosocial diagnosis. Significant differences were found in locus of control, and nearly significant differences were identified in number of strong interests in the past 10 years. No other differences were found in occupational functioning (Barris et al., 1986).

In 1988, Katz, Josman, and Steinmetz looked at the correlation between cognitive disability theory and the model of human occupation in the ability to differentiate between a psychiatric and a nonpsychiatric group of adolescents.

Correlational Studies

In her research Mailloux (1980) also posed some correlational questions, such as whether there is a relationship among self-esteem and praxis, visual-motor integration, and student role performance. Although she did not find a relationship among these variables, she did find that the self-esteem of learning disabled children in her sample was significantly lower than that of a normative group.

In 1983, Gregory published the results of a study in which he looked at correlations between meaningfulness of activities and life satisfaction of 79 elder adults. He found that amount, enjoyability, meaningfulness, and autonomy of activity and occupational behavior were all correlated with life satisfaction. Age and length of retirement showed no significant correlation.

Knapp (1983) studied 129 elders living independently in Florida. She found no significant correlations between value, interests, and personal causation and life satisfaction for these people, although she did find that "valuing leisure" had some impact.

Also in 1983, Lyons studied the correlation between volitional traits and satisfaction in a group of retarded persons. He found a correlation only between locus of control and satisfaction.

Some correlation was found by Elliott and Barris (1987) between life satisfaction and number and value of roles performed by noninstitutionalized elders.

Oakley, Kielhofner, and Barris' 1985 study of adult hospitalized psychiatric patients was an effort to test assessment based on human occupation theory by determining the correlation between patients' adaptive functioning and their organizational status as measured by their skills, habits, roles, interests, occupational values, and feelings of competence. Results were highly correlated and found to be significantly more predictive than was symptomatology or diagnosis.

Hand-injured adults were the subjects of Fronczek's 1985 study that considered the correlation between compliance and the composite of interests, locus of control, and roles. Some correlation was found between roles and compliance and between interests and compliance.

Duellman, Barris, and Kielhofner (1986) studied subjects from three nursing homes to assess the correlation between availability of activities and number of present and future roles. A positive correlation was found on both variables.

In 1986, Smith, Kielhofner, and Watts published a study that looked at the "relationships between the volition subsystem, activity pattern, and life satisfaction" of 60 older adults (p. 278). They found that in relationship to occupation and life satisfaction there were positive correlations among degree of interests, value, and personal causation. They also found that life satisfaction was more influenced by time spent in work and leisure than by time spent in activities of daily living and rest.

DeForest, Watts, and Madigan (1991) published the results of a pilot study in which they examined the issue of resonance (change in one part of the system affects other parts) by testing whether development of new performance subsystem skills would impact positively on the volitional system. Their subjects did experience positive changes in volition system belief in skills, apparently through their successful performance in craft activities.

Critique of Descriptive Studies

The limited findings of the studies just cited can be attributed to several factors. First, and most important, the assessment tools used in most of those studies have not yet been proven to be valid and reliable. Indeed, a number of them were developed for the study in which they were used. Second, tools used that were developed outside the tradition of the model of human occupation may not measure the appropriate variables within the model. Third, a number of these studies were master's research projects in which the control for variables, number of subjects, and subject selection process procedures may have been inadequate. Certainly there has been too little testing of postulates with too few subjects and with inadequately developed testing instruments to draw any conclusions about the efficacy of the model from the work done thus far.

Qualitative Research

In 1982, Kielhofner (1982a, 1982b) published two articles in which he described the process and importance of qualitative research in occupational therapy and gave examples from ethnography. Work on qualitative research to test assumptions of the model of human occupation (i.e., does development of adjustment to disability actually occur the way the model would suggest?) and to look at interrelationships of variables has just begun. An example of recent qualitative research is Yelton and Nielson's (1991) study, which used a semi-structured interview and an activity configuration with three different Appalachian subjects to explore assumptions of the model regarding the volitional system.

PARADIGM FOR THE PROFESSION

In the preface to his most recent book, Kielhofner wrote: "I have struggled throughout my professional life with the problem of how we might properly think about the range of knowledge within occupational therapy" (1992, p. viii). He explains that this has been such a strong concern of his because it directly impacts on professional identity.

> Professional identity is gained from education, experiences as a therapist, and formal and informal encounters with one's colleagues. While each professional's identity comes from a unique set of personal experiences, it is ultimately shaped by the paradigm—the shared collective culture of the profession.

> Members of a profession without a clear paradigm bear an undue burden in attempting to make sense of their life work. Occupational therapists have had the added problem that their approach is often different than, and misunderstood by, those who practice according to traditional biomedical principles. (1992, pp. 243–244)

Until recently, Keilhofner asserted that occupational therapy's paradigm, this unifying base, should be structured according to Kuhn's conceptualizations as put forth in *The Structure of Scientific Revolutions* (1962). Kielhofner and Burke first presented this idea in a 1977 *AJOT* article. In 1983, *Health through Occupation* (edited by Kielhofner) elaborated on the application of the Kuhnian paradigm to occupational therapy. And in 1986, Keilhofner and Barris further spelled out how knowledge in the field would be organized using Kuhn's concepts as its base. This article in the *Occupational Therapy Journal of Research* was followed by a critique by Labovitz and Miller (1986) that pointed out some of the inconsistencies and problems in Kielhofner's and Barris' proposals.

Because Kielhofner had written about his concern for a unifying base and his recommendations regarding it at the same time as he and Burke developed their model, there was some confusion about the difference between the base and the model and some misunderstanding that he was suggesting the model as the unifying base for the profession. Adding to this confusion was the fact that in his earlier work Kielhofner sometimes used such labels as model, theory, and paradigm interchangeably or at least without clear definition and delineation. (This criticism can, of course, be applied to other writers as well.)

In the mid- to late 1980s, Kielhofner was less certain about how this unifying base should be structured. He acknowledged that, as a practice profession, OT's paradigm could not be exactly what Kuhn conceptualized. He remained convinced, however, that the profession needed to arrive at some consensus about its foundational concepts and philosophical assumptions. As he said:

> I think there are two valid points about what the field needs; the field needs diversity in its views, and the field needs organization and consistency in its views. I think that the challenge for an occupational therapy paradigm is how to manage the tension between these two. (G.W. Kielhofner, personal communication, March 6, 1987)

In 1992, Kielhofner suggested that the paradigm, or "shared collective culture," of the profession, composed of the "basic assumptions and perspectives that unify the field," is made up of three parts: the core assumptions of the field, the focal viewpoint of the profession, and the values central to occupational therapy (1992, p. 13).

From the occupational therapy literature and analysis of models of practice he pulled together the following as the *core assumptions* of the profession:

1. Human beings have an occupational nature.
2. Human beings may experience occupational dysfunction.
3. Occupation can be used as a therapeutic agent. (1992, p. 42)

Kielhofner proposed that the *focal viewpoint* is the particular perspective from which occupational therapists look at the areas of their concern. He asserted that each occupational therapist's viewpoint is grounded in beliefs in holism, in the hierarchical order of phenomena, and in the open interaction between systems and their environment. (1992, p. 64)

He synthesized the *central values* of this paradigm, which he saw as guiding action and directing growth, from extensive review of the available literature. He concluded that occupational therapy *values*: (1) dignity and worth of persons; (2) participation in occupations; (3) self-determination, freedom, and independence; (4) latent capacity; (5) caring and the interpersonal elements of therapy; (6) human uniqueness and subjectivity; and (7) mutual cooperation in therapy (1992).

Kielhofner conceptualized this paradigm as the central core of the profession's knowledge. "It influences what problems the therapist addresses, how those problems are conceived, and what methods the therapist employs to resolve the problems" (1992, p. 246).

He conceived of the rest of the field's knowledge as being wrapped around this common core. Surrounding this paradigm, in his view, is a "band of conceptual practice models" (1992, p. 13). Whereas the paradigm is general and gives coherence to the whole profession in all its diversity, practice models "articulate occupational therapy theory that provides rationale for therapy and guides therapists in practice" (1992, p. 13).

Kielhofner proposed that the profession's theory could be organized into eight "conceptual practice models," and he devoted a chapter to each in his 1992 book. Some of these models were identified with one or two persons, others were syntheses of the works of many. They were the biomechanical model, the cognitive disabilities model, the cognitive-perceptual model, the group work model, the model of human occupation, the motor control model, the sensory integration model, and the model of spatiotemporal adaptation.

Finally, Kielhofner labeled the outside band of this three-layered conceptual sphere the "related knowledge of the field." It consists of the collected "concepts, facts, and techniques from other fields that are used in occupational therapy practice" (1992, p. 13).

Thus Kielhofner proposed that a productive way to organize the vast array of knowledge in the field was to visualize it as a three-layered sphere. The central core is the paradigm—the assumptions, point of view, and values shared by all occupational therapists. Surrounding that is the layer made up of all our conceptual practice models (sometimes called theories or frames of reference). Different therapists use different ones of these at different times. "The relationship between the paradigm and the models is one of mutual influence. The paradigm is a global vision, and the models are practical attempts to implement that vision in practice" (p. 21). And wrapped around the outside is the layer of related knowledge, knowledge that is used by occupational therapists and is important, but that is not unique to occupational therapy.

FUTURE CHALLENGES FOR OCCUPATIONAL THERAPY

Kielhofner sees the biggest challenge to the profession today as the need to develop an academic discipline through research and theory development. He feels this needs to be done soon if occupational therapy education is to continue to be offered at the college and university level.

> We've got to be able to argue to the academic community that we have an academic discipline or we will not remain in universities . . . we will only be in community colleges. To me, the survival of the occupational therapy university system is more critical right now than, for example, whether we survive in acute care practice or whether we survive in schools as practitioners. Those things will evolve and change over time. If we have an academic discipline and the professional status of being in the university we will always be able to go out and make our way in practice arenas. (G.W. Kielhofner, personal communication, March 6, 1987)

His most recent thinking about this issue is powerfully stated as follows:

> Occupation pervades life, is necessary for the maintenance of the human collective, and determines the course of individual lives. As such, it is a powerful force in human existence and a unique part of what it means to be human. In this regard, I share the enthusiasm of the proponents of occupational science for the possibility of the emergence of a distinct discipline organized around the study of occupation in human life. (1992, p. 288)

Kielhofner feels, however, that occupational therapy knowledge must be organized in such a way as to incorporate both basic and applied science. Such knowledge will further the capabilities of the profession to address and solve problems of individuals with disability, and therefore meet very real societal needs. Kielhofner asserts that it is our practice which is our reason for being, and that research and theory must therefore serve practice.

> I think the basic sciences are learning the lesson of relevance. I would hate to see our scholars so wooed by the sirens of the hallowed academic halls that we forget the hard lessons of relevance gleaned by generations of therapists laboring in clinics with persons who have such pressing problems. (G. Kielhofner, personal communication, August, 1992)

> In the end it may be most appropriate to identify occupational therapy scholarship as *occupational therapy science*, which incorporates both a *basic occupational science* and an *applied therapeutic science* (both re-

flected in conceptual models of practice). They are dual and interrelated elements of the knowledge that will be necessary for the future of occupational therapy. (Kielhofner, 1992, p. 289)

REFERENCES

Baron, K.B. (1991). The use of play in child psychiatry: Reframing the therapeutic environment. *Occupational Therapy in Mental Health, 11*, 37–56.

Barris, R. (1982). Environmental interactions: An extension of the model of human occupation. *American Journal of Occupational Therapy, 36*, 637–644.

Barris, R., Kielhofner, G., Burch-Martin, R., Gelinas, I., Klement, M., & Schultz, B. (1986). Occupational function and dysfunction in three groups of adolescents. *Occupational Therapy Journal of Research, 6*, 301–317.

Barris, R., Kielhofner, G., Levine, R.E., & Neville, A. (1985). Occupation as interaction with the environment. In G. Kielhofner (Ed.), *A model of human occupation: Theory and application* (pp. 42–62). Baltimore: Williams & Wilkins.

Barris, R., Kielhofner, G., & Watts, J. (1983). *Psychosocial occupational therapy: Practice in a pluralistic arena*. Laurel, MD: RAM Associates.

Barris, R., Kielhofner, G., & Watts, J. (1988). *Occupational therapy in psychosocial practice*. Thorofare, NJ: Charles B. Slack.

Bentz, C. (1984). *A measure of personal causation for mildly and moderately retarded adults*. Unpublished master's project, Virginia Commonwealth University.

Blakeney, A.B. (1985). Adolescent development: An application to the model of human occupation. In F.S. Cromwell (Ed.), *Occupational therapy and adolescents with disability* (pp. 19–40). New York: Haworth Press.

Borell, L., Sandman, P., & Kielhofner, G. (1991). Clinical decision making in Alzheimer's disease. *Occupational Therapy in Mental Health, 11*, 111–124.

Burton, J.E. (1989a). The model of human occupation and occupational therapy practice with elderly patients. Part 1: Characteristics of aging. *British Journal of Occupational Therapy, 52*, 215–218.

Burton, J.E. (1989b). The model of human occupation and occupational therapy practice with elderly patients. Part 2: Application. *British Journal of Occupational Therapy, 52*, 219–221.

Curtin, C. (1991). Psychosocial intervention with an adolescent with diabetes using the model of human occupation. *Occupational Therapy in Mental Health, 11*, 23–36.

DeForest, D., Watts, J.H., & Madigan, M.J. (1991). Resonation in the model of human occupation: A pilot study. *Occupational Therapy in Mental Health, 11*, 57–71.

Doble, S. (1985). *Inter-rater reliability and concurrent validity of a process skills assessment*. Unpublished master's thesis, Boston University, Boston.

Donohue, M.V., & McCreedy, P. (1989). Letter to the editor. *American Journal of Occupational Therapy, 43*, 774–775.

Duellman, M.K., Barris, R., & Kielhofner, G. (1986). Organized activity and the adaptive status of nursing home residents. *American Journal of Occupational Therapy, 40*, 618–622.

Elliott, M.S., & Barris, R. (1987). Occupational role performance and life satisfaction in elderly persons. *Occupational Therapy Journal of Research, 7*, 215–224.

Feibleman, J.K. (1969). Theory of integrative levels. In J.C. Coleman (Ed.), *Psychology and effective behavior.* Glenview, IL: Scott, Foresman.

Fronczek, Y. (1985). *A study of the compliance and roles, locus of control, and interests of the acute hand injured patient.* Unpublished master's thesis, Virginia Commonwealth University.

Gregory, M. (1983). Occupational behavior and life satisfaction among retirees. *American Journal of Occupational Therapy, 37*, 548–553.

Grogan, G. (1991a). Anger management: A perspective for occupational therapy. (Part 1). *Occupational Therapy in Mental Health, 11*, 135–148.

Grogan, G. (1991b). Anger management: Clinical applications for occupational therapy. (Part 2). *Occupational Therapy in Mental Health, 11*, 149–171.

Gusich, R.L. (1984). Occupational therapy for chronic pain: A clinical application of the model of human occupation. *Occupational Therapy in Mental Health, 4*, 59–74.

Gusich, R.L., & Silverman, A.L. (1991). Basava day clinic: The model of human occupation as applied to psychiatric day hospitalization. *Occupational Therapy in Mental Health, 11*, 113–134.

Harrison, H., & Kielhofner, G. (1986). Examining reliability and validity of the preschool play scale with handicapped children. *American Journal of Occupational Therapy, 40*, 167–173.

Kaplan, K. (1984). Short term assessment: The need and a response. *Occupational Therapy in Mental Health, 4*, 29–45.

Katz, N., Josman, N., & Steinmetz, N. (1988). Relationship between cognitive disability theory and the model of human occupation in the assessment of psychiatric and nonpsychiatric adolescents. *Occupational Therapy in Mental Health, 8*, 31–43.

Khoo, S.W., & Renwick, R.M. (1989). A model of human occupation perspective on the mental health of immigrant women in Canada. *Occupational Therapy in Mental Health, 9*, 31–49.

Kielhofner, G. (1975). *The evolution of knowledge in occupational therapy: Understanding adaptation of the chronically disabled.* Unpublished master's thesis, University of Southern California, Los Angeles.

Kielhofner, G. (1977). Temporal adaptation: A conceptual framework for occupational therapy. *American Journal of Occupational Therapy, 31*, 235–242.

Kielhofner, G. (1978). General systems theory: Implications for theory and action in occupational therapy. *American Journal of Occupational Therapy, 32*, 637–645.

Kielhofner, G. (1980a). *Evaluating deinstitutionalization: An ethnographic study of social policy.* Unpublished doctoral dissertation, University of Southern California, Los Angeles.

Kielhofner, G. (1980b). A model of human occupation. Part two. Ontogenesis from the perspective of temporal adaptation. *American Journal of Occupational Therapy, 34*, 657–663.

Kielhofner, G. (1980c). A model of human occupation. Part three. Benign and vicious cycles. *American Journal of Occupational Therapy, 34*, 731–737.

Kielhofner, G. (1982a). Qualitative research. Part one. Paradigmatic grounds and issues of reliability and validity. *Occupational Therapy Journal of Research, 2*, 67–79.

Kielhofner, G. (1982b). Qualitative research. Part two. Methodological approaches and relevance to occupational therapy. *Occupational Therapy Journal of Research, 2*, 150–164.

Kielhofner, G. (Ed.). (1983). *Health through occupation: Theory and practice in occupational therapy.* Philadelphia: F.A. Davis.

Kielhofner, G. (1984). An overview of research on the model of human occupation. *Canadian Journal of Occupational Therapy, 51*, 59–67.

Kielhofner, G. (Ed.). (1985). *A model of human occupation: Theory and application*. Baltimore: Williams & Wilkins.

Kielhofner, G. (1992). *Conceptual foundations of occupational therapy*. Philadelphia: F.A. Davis.

Kielhofner, G., & Barris, R. (1986). Organization of knowledge in occupational therapy: A proposal and a survey of the literature. *Occupational Therapy Journal of Research, 5*, 67–84.

Kielhofner, G., & Brinson, M. (1989). Development and evaluation of an aftercare program for young chronic psychiatrically disabled adults. *Occupational Therapy in Mental Health, 9*, 1–25.

Kielhofner, G., & Burke, J.P. (1977). Occupational therapy after 60 years: An account of changing identity and knowledge. *American Journal of Occupational Therapy, 31*, 675–689.

Kielhofner, G., & Burke, J.P. (1980). A model of human occupation. Part one. Conceptual framework and content. *American Journal of Occupational Therapy, 34*, 572–581.

Kielhofner, G., & Burke, J.P. (1985). Components and determinants of human occupation. In G. Kielhofner (Ed.), *A model of human occupation: Theory and application* (pp. 12–41). Baltimore: Williams & Wilkins.

Kielhofner, G., Burke, J., & Igi, C.H. (1980). A model of human occupation. Part four. Assessment and intervention. *American Journal of Occupational Therapy, 34*, 777–788.

Kielhofner, G., Harlan, B., Bauer, D., & Maurer, P. (1986). The reliability of a historical interview with physically disabled respondents. *American Journal of Occupational Therapy, 40*, 551–556.

Kielhofner, G., & Henry, A.D. (1988). Development and investigation of the occupational performance history interview. *American Journal of Occupational Therapy, 42*, 489–498.

Kielhofner, G., Henry, A., Walens, D., & Rogers, E.S. (1991). A generalizability study of the occupational performance history interview. *Occupational Therapy Journal of Research, 11*, 292–306.

Knapp, J. (1983). *A study of leisure values and life satisfaction among retirees*. Unpublished master's project, Virginia Commonwealth University.

Kuhn, T.S. (1962). *The structure of scientific revolutions*. Chicago: University of Chicago Press.

Labovitz, D.R., & Miller, R.J. (1986). Commentary: Organization of knowledge in occupational therapy: A proposal and a survey of the literature. *Occupational Therapy Journal of Research, 6*, 85–92.

Lancaster, J., & Mitchell, M. (1991). Occupational therapy treatment goals, objectives, and activities for improving low self-esteem in adolescents with behavioral disorders. *Occupational Therapy in Mental Health, 11*, 3–22.

Lederer, J., Kielhofner, G., & Watts, J. (1985). Values, personal causation and skills of delinquents and non-delinquents. *Occupational Therapy in Mental Health, 5*, 59–77.

Lyons, M. (1983). *Employment and personal adjustment of mentally retarded persons: Towards an emic perspective of the relationship*. Unpublished master's thesis, Virginia Commonwealth University.

Mailloux, Z. (1980). *The relationship between self-esteem and visual motor integration praxis and student role performance in children with learning disabilities*. Unpublished master's thesis, University of Southern California, Los Angeles.

Neville-Jan, A., Bradley, M., Bunn, C., & Gehri, B. (1991). The model of human occupation and individuals with co-dependency problems. *Occupational Therapy in Mental Health, 11*, 73–97.

Oakley, F. (1987). Clinical application of the model of human occupation in dementia of the Alzheimer's type. *Occupational Therapy in Mental Health, 7*, 37–50.

Oakley, F., Kielhofner, G., & Barris, R. (1985). An occupational therapy approach to assessing psychiatric patients' adaptive functioning. *American Journal of Occupational Therapy, 39*, 147–154.

Oakley, F., Kielhofner, G., Barris, R., & Reichler, R. (1986). The role checklist: Development and empirical assessment of reliability. *Occupational Therapy Journal of Research, 6*, 157–170.

Pizzi, M. (1990). The model of human occupation with adults with HIV infection and AIDS. *American Journal of Occupational Therapy, 44*, 257–264.

Rogers, J.C., & Kielhofner, G. (1985). Treatment planning. In G. Kielhofner (Ed.), *A model of human occupation: Theory and application* (p. 140). Baltimore: Williams & Wilkins.

Salz, C. (1983). A theoretical approach to the treatment of work difficulties in borderline personalities. *Occupational Therapy in Mental Health, 3*, 33–46.

Scaffa, M.E. (1981). *Temporal adaptation and alcoholism.* Unpublished master's project, Virginia Commonwealth University.

Scaffa, M.E. (1991). Alcoholism: An occupational behavior perspective. *Occupational Therapy in Mental Health, 11*, 99–111.

Schaaf, R.C., & Mulrooney, L.L. (1989). Occupational therapy in early intervention: A family-centered approach. *American Journal of Occupational Therapy, 43*, 745–754.

Scott, M.B. (1982). *The validity of an Occupational Picture Interest Sort for mentally retarded adults.* Unpublished master's project, Virginia Commonwealth University.

Sepiol, J.M., & Froehlich, J. (1990). Use of the role checklist with the patient with multiple personality disorder. *American Journal of Occupational Therapy, 44*, 1008–1012.

Shakun, R. (1982). *The assessment of the reliability of the Occupational Picture Interest Sort for mentally retarded adults.* Unpublished master's project, Virginia Commonwealth University.

Sholle-Martin, S. (1987). Application of the model of human occupation: Assessment in child and adolescent psychiatry. *Occupational Therapy in Mental Health, 7*, 3–22.

Sholle-Martin, S., & Alessi, N.E. (1990). Formulating a role for occupational therapy in child psychiatry: A clinical application. *American Journal of Occupational Therapy, 44*, 871–882.

Smith, N., Kielhofner, G., & Watts, J. (1986). The relationships between volition, activity pattern, and life satisfaction in the elderly. *American Journal of Occupational Therapy, 40*, 278–283.

Smyntek, L., Barris, R., & Kielhofner, G. (1985). The model of human occupation applied to psychosocially functional and dysfunctional adolescents. *Occupational Therapy in Mental Health, 5*, 21–40.

Tigges, K.N., & Sherman, L.M. (1983). The treatment of the hospice patient: From occupational history to occupational role. *American Journal of Occupational Therapy, 37*, 235–238.

Watts, J.H., Kielhofner, G., Bauer, D., Gregory, M., & Valentine, D. (1986). The assessment of occupational functioning: A screening tool for use in long-term care. *American Journal of Occupational Therapy, 40*, 231–240.

Wieringa, N., & McColl, M. (1987). Implications of the model of human occupation for intervention with native Canadians. In F.S. Cromwell (Ed.), *Sociocultural implications in treatment planning in occupational therapy* (pp. 73–91). New York: Haworth Press.

Yelton, D., & Nielson, C. (1991). Understanding Appalachian values—Implications for occupational therapists. *Occupational Therapy in Mental Health, 11*, 173–195.

BIBLIOGRAPHY

1975

Kielhofner, G. (1975). *The evolution of knowledge in occupational therapy: Understanding adaptation of the chronically disabled.* Unpublished master's thesis, University of Southern California, Los Angeles.

1976

Cromwell, F.S., & Kielhofner, G. (1976). An educational strategy for occupational therapy community service. *American Journal of Occupational Therapy, 30,* 629–633.

1977

Kielhofner, G. (1977). Temporal adaptation: A conceptual framework for occupational therapy. *American Journal of Occupational Therapy, 31,* 235–242.

Kielhofner, G., & Burke, J.P. (1977). Occupational therapy after 60 years: An account of changing identity and knowledge. *American Journal of Occupational Therapy, 31,* 675–689.

1978

Kielhofner, G. (1978). General systems theory: Implications for theory and action in occupational therapy. *American Journal of Occupational Therapy, 32,* 637–645.

1979

Gillette, N., & Kielhofner, G. (1979). The impact of specialization on the professionalization and survival of occupational therapy. *American Journal of Occupational Therapy, 33,* 20–28.

Kielhofner, G. (1979). Temporal adaptation: A conceptual framework for occupational therapy. In O. Payton (Ed.), *Research: The validation of clinical practice* (pp. 210–222). Philadelphia: F.A. Davis. (Reprinted from *American Journal of Occupational Therapy,* 1977, *31,* 235–242.)

Kielhofner, G. (1979). The temporal dimension in the lives of retarded adults: A problem of interaction and intervention. *American Journal of Occupational Therapy, 33,* 161–168.

1980

Kielhofner, G. (1980). *Evaluating deinstitutionalization: An ethnographic study of social policy.* Unpublished doctoral dissertation, University of Southern California, Los Angeles.

Kielhofner, G. (1980). A model of human occupation. Part two. Ontogenesis from the perspective of temporal adaptation. *American Journal of Occupational Therapy, 34,* 657–663.

Kielhofner, G. (1980). A model of human occupation. Part three. Benign and vicious cycles. *American Journal of Occupational Therapy, 34,* 731–737.

Kielhofner, G., & Burke, J.P. (1980). A model of human occupation. Part one. Conceptual framework and content. *American Journal of Occupational Therapy, 34,* 572–581.

Kielhofner, G., Burke, J., & Igi, C.H. (1980). A model of human occupation. Part four. Assessment and intervention. *American Journal of Occupational Therapy, 34,* 777–788.

Kielhofner, G., & Takata, N. (1980). A study of mentally retarded persons: Applied research in occupational therapy. *American Journal of Occupational Therapy, 34,* 252–258.

1981

Kielhofner, G. (1981). An ethnographic study of deinstitutionalized adults: Their community settings and daily life experiences. *Occupational Therapy Journal of Research, 1,* 125–142.

Kielhofner, G., & Miyake, S. (1981). Therapeutic use of games with mentally retarded adults. *American Journal of Occupational Therapy, 35*, 375–382.

1982

Kielhofner, G. (1982). Theoretical foundations of occupational therapy. *Proceedings of the World Federation of Occupational Therapy*, 1265–1272.

Kielhofner, G. (1982). A heritage of activity: Development of theory. *American Journal of Occupational Therapy, 36*, 723–730.

Kielhofner, G. (1982). Qualitative research. Part one. Paradigmatic grounds and issues of reliability and validity. *Occupational Therapy Journal of Research, 2*, 67–79.

Kielhofner, G. (1982). Qualitative research. Part two. Methodological approaches and relevance to occupational therapy. *Occupational Therapy Journal of Research, 2*, 150–164.

Kielhofner, G., Barris, R., & Watts, J. (1982). Habits and habit dysfunction: A clinical perspective for psychosocial occupational therapy. *Occupational Therapy in Mental Health, 2*, 1–22.

Chao, R., Clark, F., & Kielhofner, G. (1982). Development of time concepts in mentally retarded adults and its relationship to mental age. *Proceedings of the Annual Piagetian Conference*, Los Angeles, California.

Vandenberg, B., & Kielhofner, G. (1982). Play in evolution, culture, and individual adaptation: Implications for therapy. *American Journal of Occupational Therapy, 36*, 20–28.

1983

Kielhofner, G. (1983). "Teaching" retarded adults: Paradoxical effects of a pedagogical enterprise. *Urban Life, 12*, 307–326.

Kielhofner, G. (1983). Occupation. In H. Hopkins & H. Smith (Eds.), *Willard and Spackman's occupational therapy* (6th ed.). Philadelphia: J.B. Lippincott.

Kielhofner, G. (Ed.). (1983). *Health through occupation: Theory and practice in occupational therapy*. Philadelphia: F.A. Davis.

Kielhofner, G., & Nelson, C. (1983). A study of patient motivation and cooperation/participation in occupational therapy. *Occupational Therapy Journal of Research, 3*, 35–46.

Kielhofner, G., Barris, R., Bauer, D., Shoestock, B., & Walker, L. (1983). A comparison of play behavior in nonhospitalized and hospitalized children. *American Journal of Occupational Therapy, 37*, 305–312.

Barris, R., Kielhofner, G., & Watts, J. (1983). *Psychosocial occupational therapy: Practice in a pluralistic arena*. Laurel, MD: RAM Associates.

1984

Kielhofner, G. (1984). An overview of research on the model of human occupation. *Canadian Journal of Occupational Therapy, 51*, 59–67.

Kielhofner, G. (1984). A paradigmatic view of rehabilitation. *Proceedings of the Second International Conference on Rehabilitation Engineering*, Ottawa, Canada.

Kielhofner, G., & Barris, R. (1984). Mental health occupational therapy: Trends in literature and practice. *Occupational Therapy in Mental Health, 4*, 35–50.

1985

Kielhofner, G. (Ed.). (1985). *A model of human occupation: Theory and application*. Baltimore: Williams & Wilkins.

Kielhofner, G. (1985). The demise of diffidence: An agenda for occupational therapy. *Canadian Journal of Occupational Therapy, 52*, 165–171.

Kielhofner, G. (1985). The model of human occupation: ett hjalpmedel for kliniskt uerksamma arbetsterapeuter. (C. Henriksson, Trans.). *Arbetsterapeuten (Swedish Journal of Occupational Therapy), 17*, 18–23.

Barris, R., & Kielhofner, G. (1985). Generating and using knowledge in occupational therapy: Implications for professional education. *Occupational Therapy Journal of Research, 5*, 113–124.

Barris, R., Kielhofner, G., & Bauer, D. (1985). Educational experience and changes in learning and value preferences. *Occupational Therapy Journal of Research, 5*, 243–256.

Barris, R., Kielhofner, G., & Bauer, D. (1985). Learning preferences, values, and student satisfaction. *Journal of Allied Health, 14*, 13–23.

Barris, R., Kielhofner, G., Levine, R.E., & Neville, A. (1985). Occupation as interaction with the environment. In G. Kielhofner (Ed.), *A model of human occupation: Theory and application* (pp. 42–62). Baltimore: Williams & Wilkins.

Lederer, J., Kielhofner, G., & Watts, J. (1985). Values, personal causation and skills of delinquents and non-delinquents. *Occupational Therapy in Mental Health, 5*, 59–77.

Neville, A., Kriesberg, A., & Kielhofner, G. (1985). Temporal dysfunction in schizophrenia. *Occupational Therapy in Mental Health, 5* (1), 1–20.

Oakley, F., Kielhofner, G., & Barris, R. (1985). An occupational therapy approach to assessing psychiatric patients' adaptive functioning. *American Journal of Occupational Therapy, 39*, 147–154.

Rogers, J.C., & Kielhofner, G. (1985). Treatment planning. In G. Kielhofner (Ed.), *A model of human occupation: Theory and application* (p. 140). Baltimore: Williams & Wilkins.

Smyntek, L., Barris, R., & Kielhofner, G. (1985). The model of human occupation applied to psychosocially functional and dysfunctional adolescents. *Occupational Therapy in Mental Health, 5*, 21–40.

1986

Kielhofner, G. (1986). A review of research on the model of human occupation. Part one. *Canadian Journal of Occupational Therapy, 53*, 69–74.

Kielhofner, G. (1986). A review of research on the model of human occupation. Part two. *Canadian Journal of Occupational Therapy, 53*, 129–134.

Kielhofner, G. (1986). A response to Sharrott's "An analysis of occupational therapy theoretical approaches for mental health." *Occupational Therapy in Mental Health, 5*, 17–23.

Kielhofner, G., & Barris, R. (1986). Organization of knowledge in occupational therapy: A proposal and a survey of the literature. *Occupational Therapy Journal of Research, 5*, 67–84.

Kielhofner, G., & Barris, R. (1986). Response to commentary: Organization of knowledge in occupational therapy: A proposal and a survey of the literature. *Occupational Therapy Journal of Research, 6*, 183–190.

Kielhofner, G., & Nelson, C. (1986). The nature and implications of shifting patterns of practice in physical disabilities occupational therapy. *Occupational Therapy in Health Care, 3*, 187–198.

Kielhofner, G., Harlan, B., Bauer, D., & Maurer, P. (1986). The reliability of an historical interview with physically disabled respondents. *American Journal of Occupational Therapy, 40*, 551–556.

Barris, R., & Kielhofner, G. (1986). Beliefs, perspectives, and activities of psychosocial occupational therapy educators. *American Journal of Occupational Therapy, 40*, 535–541.

Barris, R., Kielhofner, G., Burch-Martin, R., Gelinas, I., Klement, M., & Schultz, B. (1986). Occupational function and dysfunction in three groups of adolescents. *Occupational Therapy Journal of Research, 6*, 301–317.

Duellman, M.K., Barris, R., & Kielhofner, G. (1986). Organized activity and the adaptive status of nursing home residents. *American Journal of Occupational Therapy, 40*, 618–622.

Harrison, H., & Kielhofner, G. (1986). Examining reliability and validity of the preschool play scale with handicapped children. *American Journal of Occupational Therapy, 40*, 167–173.

Oakley, F., Kielhofner, G., Barris, R., & Reichler, R. (1986). The role checklist: Development and empirical assessment of reliability. *Occupational Therapy Journal of Research, 6*, 157–170.

Smith, N., Kielhofner, G., & Watts, J. (1986). The relationships between volition, activity pattern, and life satisfaction in the elderly. *American Journal of Occupational Therapy, 40*, 278–284.

Watts, J.H., Kielhofner, G., Bauer, D., Gregory, M., & Valentine, D. (1986). The assessment of occupational functioning: A screening tool for use in long-term care. *American Journal of Occupational Therapy, 40*, 231–240.

1988

Kielhofner, G. (1988). Occupational therapy base in occupation. In H. Hopkins & H. Smith (Eds.), *Willard and Spackman's occupational therapy* (7th ed.). Philadelphia: J.B. Lippincott.

Kielhofner, G., & Henry, A. (1988). Development and investigation of the occupational performance history interview. *American Journal of Occupational Therapy, 42*, 489–498.

Kielhofner, G., & Henry, A. (1988). Use of an occupational history interview in occupational therapy. In B. Hemphill (Ed.), *Mental health assessment in occupational therapy* (2nd ed.) (pp. 59–71). Thorofare, NJ: Charles B. Slack.

Barris, R., Kielhofner, G., & Watts, J. (1988). *Bodies of knowledge in psychosocial practice.* Thorofare, NJ: Charles B. Slack.

Barris, R., Kielhofner, G., & Watts, J. (1988). *Occupational therapy in psychosocial practice.* Thorofare, NJ: Charles B. Slack.

Barris, R., Oakley, F., & Kielhofner, G. (1988). The role checklist. In B. Hemphill (Ed.), *Mental health assessment in occupational therapy* (2nd ed.) (pp. 73–79). Thorofare, NJ: Charles B. Slack.

1989

Kielhofner, G., & Brinson, M. (1989). Development and evaluation of an aftercare program for young chronic psychiatrically disabled adults. *Occupational Therapy in Mental Health, 9*, 1–25.

Kielhofner, G., & Nicol, M. (1989). The model of human occupation: A developing conceptual tool for clinicians. *British Journal of Occupational Therapy, 52*, 210–214.

Fisher, A.G., Kielhofner, G., & Davis, C. (1989). Research values of occupational and physical therapists. *Journal of Allied Health, 18*, 143–156.

Kaplan, K., & Kielhofner, G. (1989). *The occupational case analysis interview and rating scale.* Thorofare, NJ: Charles B. Slack.

1990

Boyle, M.A., Dunn, W., & Kielhofner, G. (1990). Funding for research and training in professional occupational therapy education programs from 1985 to 1987. *Occupational Therapy Journal of Research, 10*, 334–342.

1991

Kielhofner, G., & Fisher, A. (1991). Mind-brain relationships. In A. Fisher, E. Murray, & A. Bundy (Eds.), *Sensory integration: Theory and practice* (pp. 30–38). Philadelphia: F.A. Davis.

Kielhofner, G., Henry, A., Walens, D., & Rogers, E. (1991). A generalizability study of the occupational performance history interview. *Occupational Therapy Journal of Research, 11*, 292–306.

Borell, L., Sandman, P., & Kielhofner, G. (1991). Clinical decision making in Alzheimer's disease. *Occupational Therapy in Mental Health, 11*, 111–124.

1992

Kielhofner, G. (1992). *Conceptual foundations of occupational therapy.* Philadelphia: F.A. Davis.

Kielhofner, G. (1992). The future of the profession of occupational therapy: Requirements for developing the field's knowledge base. *Journal of the Japanese Occupational Therapy Association, 11*, 112–129.

Munoz, J., Lawlor, M., & Kielhofner, G. (In press). Use of the model of human occupation in psychiatric practice. *Occupational Therapy Journal of Research.*

Chapter Eight

Claudia Allen

Mary V. Donohue

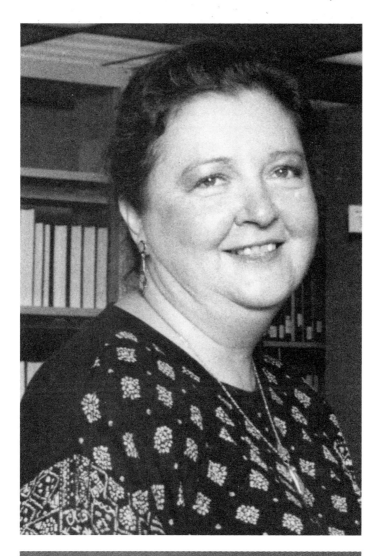

Claudia Allen

BIOGRAPHICAL SKETCH

Childhood

Claudia Allen was born in Oregon in 1941 and grew up on a farm in an environment where working with her hands, canning harvests, feeding animals, and doing crafts was part of everyday life. During the long summers she checked a dozen books at a time out of the library for hours of reading. She developed a talent for getting close to animals that helped her become a keen observer of behavior. To be quiet, to wait, to be patient are traits that she carries with her from relating to farm animals, and that help her in working with some disabled people when they are unable to express their needs. Allen perceives that cognitive levels can be observed across a continuum of animal species (C. Allen, personal communication, May 16, 1992).

Allen had a grandmother who was an artist. One afternoon a week in the summers was devoted to learning pastel painting, embroidery, and other handwork under her grandmother's tutelage. Influenced by her father, who would have liked to become a doctor, Allen thought for some time about becoming a dentist. It was through the interest she had in a blend of arts, crafts, and science that occupational therapy later appealed to her.

Education

Allen received a traditional American public school education with a college preparatory track in high school. Because she realized she needed work on her writing skills, she selected every writing class she could attend. At a recent class reunion, one of her teachers was truly amazed to learn that Allen had become an author! Allen and her high school sweetheart kept in contact during college, and in 1963, the year she graduated, they married.

During her freshman year at the University of Oregon, Allen realized that dentistry did not have the appeal she had anticipated. A fellow dormitory friend named Mary Foto told Allen about occupational therapy. Allen was intrigued by this field that clearly integrated art and science. During that summer she began looking around for an OT school.

She decided to attend San Jose State during an exciting era there. Mary Booth, Chair of the Department of Occupational Therapy, invited her entering students over for tea, giving their orientation to the field an environment for genteel ladies! Eleanor Mann was on the faculty; so was Doris Cunningham, who taught the psychiatry course as an analytic and intellectual exercise in an approach that Allen enjoyed. Gwen Wright, professor of kinesiology, received rave reviews from her students for teaching the subject matter as a course in logic (C. Allen, personal communication, May 16, 1992).

Professional Career

Allen began her career in occupational therapy at Widner Memorial School, where she learned about Ayres' theories while working with children who had polio. Together with a physical therapist, she used Frostig materials with five year olds in a summer program designed to give these children a head start for kindergarten. In an unairconditioned music room, they took the heavy long-legged braces off the children, put the children on mats, turned them around, used scooter boards, and had them crawl along strings on the floor. Without a formal design they had fortuitously provided an environment for a "comparison study" indicating that the children who had received therapy achieved better kindergarten starting points than those who had not received therapy.

Allen reports how difficult it was to work in a school where during the fall and spring sessions occupational therapists were only permitted to do pencil and paper work with the children in brief half-hour sessions. Meanwhile, the student population was shifting from children who had polio to children with cerebral palsy. The teachers and therapists had to adjust from teaching children who could keep up to expected educational norms, to teaching children with predictable falling-off points every three years, at the first, third, sixth, and ninth grades. About that time Allen visited Penthurst State Hospital, an acknowledged "snake pit," where some of the Widner children had gone to live:

> It was shocking and demoralizing to think that all of that effort had gone toward preparing the students for that, and that society was not really well equipped to deal with people with mental disorders. I think that had a very profound impression on me: no matter what anybody did, the special ed teachers, the OT's, PT's and speech pathologists could not help the students pass certain hurdles. So I think I got a real sense early on of what limitations there are that one can't overcome. (C. Allen, personal communication, May 16, 1992)

In the sixties, at a time when psychiatry still held out much hope for patients with mental illness, Allen took a position at Eastern Pennsylvania Psychiatric Institute (EPPI). There she worked in a uniquely stimulating intellectual environment. Each of the medical schools in Philadelphia had its own ward in this hospital, so that a variety of frames of reference were being practiced there.

> We had some very analytical people, we had Joe Wolkey who was very behavioral, we had Charlie Shagus who was an expert in biochemistry and had done some of the original work in the sixties on things like LSD, and then there was Birdwhistle who was talking about developing interplanted language, and Jay Hailey who was into family therapy. All

of those people eating in the same dining room together. (C. Allen, personal communication, May 16, 1992)

There were many disagreements that were noncombative in that accepting and nonrestrictive environment. Allen greatly enjoyed this exchange of theories and the interaction of unique personalities and lifestyles. There was also a wonderful library at EPPI, with a librarian who went to the ends of the earth to be helpful. At the time Allen assumed that all psychiatric patients and therapists enjoyed such a therapeutic and educational environment!

After several years at EPPI, Allen states: "I decided that I really didn't know what I was doing . . . and I decided that I needed to go to graduate school" (C. Allen, personal communication, May 16, 1992). She entered the master's program at New York University (NYU) where she studied with Gail Fidler, Anne Mosey, and Sue Fine. In the rich sixties, EPPI paid for her tuition, fees, and books, giving her a full salary with the agreement that she return to work for a year after graduation.

Professional Challenges

Upon returning to EPPI, Allen found that what she had learned at NYU and during her residency with the higher-level socioeconomic populations at New York State Psychiatric Institute did not apply to the average schizophrenic in a state hospital. While pondering this dilemma, she remembered that when she had first gone to EPPI it had struck her that many of the behaviors she observed were the same for schizophrenics as for children with cerebral palsy or mental retardation. The inability to follow more than one direction at a time was something both populations had in common (C. Allen, personal communication, May 16, 1992).

During that time her husband, Robert, shared with her the results of a study he heard presented in Grand Rounds at Temple University Hospital regarding Philip May's research comparing four different treatment approaches for psychiatric patients. The findings indicated the order of efficacy of treatment to be psychotherapy plus medication, medication alone, ECT (electroconvulsive therapy) alone, and, lastly, milieu therapy, of which occupational therapy was a part. Allen remembers being shocked and frightened at the implication that some of the things OTs claimed to do were not valid. This study made it appear that "medication was really 'doing it,' and that the rest of the therapies were 'icing on the cake,' and that we had better define our roles" (C. Allen, personal communication, May 16, 1992).

Allen was concerned not only for the patients but for the education of the students she was expected to mentor and supervise as part of the EPPI mission. This mobilized her to read extensively, covering every study she could obtain concerning psychopharmaceuticals and neurology, from Woodroff, Goodwin, and Guze's *Psychiatric Diagnosis* (1973) to the *Diagnostic and Statistical Manual of Mental Disorders III-Revised (DSM-III-R)* (Spitzer, 1987). While becoming immersed in this literature, she remained aware that psychotropic drugs are not cure-alls (C. Allen, personal communication, May 16, 1992).

In 1973 Allen moved to California, becoming Chief of Occupational Therapy at Los Angeles County/University of Southern California (USC) Medical Center. She accepted a teaching position in the Department of Occupational Therapy at USC in 1975. Mary Reilly, still a dominant force at USC in 1975, perceived Allen as a foreigner with a master's degree from NYU. Allen raised questions and was something of an irritant on the scene. She recalls, however, being positively influenced by exposure to systems theory and by the emphasis on social roles in the department at USC.

More recently, while Allen has been developing treatment goals, writing her books, developing Medicare regulations and guidelines (Allen, Foto, Sperling, & Wilson, 1989), and writing on documentation, the USC department has been developing its focus on occupational science. When asked about being in a department with historical emphasis on occupational behavior and systems theory, and now occupational science, Allen states that it is difficult on all faculty. "Pure science and clinical practice operate within different value systems, and we all struggle with the conflicts that emerge" (C. Allen, personal communication, September 28, 1992). As Allen continues to expand the understanding of the cognitive levels of intelligence with exploratory research on normal activity, her path may indeed converge with that of her colleagues in occupational science.

At this writing, Allen's dual clinical and academic position includes the title of Chief of Occupational Therapy in Psychiatry at the Los Angeles County/USC Medical Center and Instructor of Clinical Psychiatry and Behavioral Science at USC University Hospital. She is also a medical reviewer for Allied Health for Blue Cross of California. Her husband is now chief of a psychiatric unit at University Hospital and is also on the faculty at USC. They live in Pasadena, California, and have two daughters, one in high school and the other in college (C. Allen, personal communication, August 24, 1992).

Development of Theory

Although Allen is aware of occupational therapists' need to change their perspective, she is sensitive to the fact that "making these enormous shifts can be very tough" (C. Allen, personal communication, May 16, 1992). She traces the process of her own changing world view.

> When we got the first edition of Woodroff, Goodwin and Guze's *Psychiatric Diagnosis* (1973) out of St. Louis, which collected all of the

research studies that became the precursor for *DSM-III*—whoa, this is an entirely different ballgame! I think it's still difficult to turn ourselves around because we have got to get rid of the Cartesian split, and adopt a very different world view, adopt a very different understanding of the mind. And you just don't do that quickly. I have done that three times: I started out with a psychoanalytic view with Fidler and Mosey, went into a Piagetian view with assimilation and accommodation, which didn't work, and have now gone to a much more neuro-science, DNA kind of view. (C. Allen, personal communication, May 16, 1992)

Within this last theoretical perspective Allen is frustrated at the little hard data currently known with scientific accuracy and the distance we have yet to go in exploring neurodevelopment and psychopharmaceutical knowledge in order to understand the mind's abilities and disabilities.

In summarizing her early influences and mentors, Allen includes Ruth Weimer, Gail Fidler, Anne Mosey, Mary Kay Bailey, and Betty Tiffany (C. Allen, personal communication, August 24, 1992). It is clear, however, that Allen is an "original," both personally and as a thinker.

Allen is a charter member of the Fellows of the American Occupational Therapy Association (FAOTA) and was the Eleanor Clarke Slagle Lecturer in 1987. She was a keynote speaker representing the United States at the Tenth Congress of the World Federation of Occupational Therapists in 1988 in Australia.

THEORETICAL CONCEPTS

Neurobiological Bases of Cognitive Disability

Allen has long been concerned about the Cartesian split between "organic" and "functional" disorders that has separated neurological medicine from psychiatry during this century (Allen, 1985). She has stated that OT practice began by delivering services to psychiatric patients at a time when the empirical study of the brain was "thought to be impossible because the brain is so complex," but that neurobiological factors can no longer be excluded from occupational therapy models (Allen, 1982, p. 731). The first chapter of her first book (*Occupational Therapy for Psychiatric Diseases*), astonishing for the time, was entitled "Neuroscience Views of Routine Task Behavior." In it she argued that "a functional model of an emotional response to a task demand, based on a general description of total brain organization, is required for therapists to attain a holistic picture of an individual" (Allen, 1985, p. 182).

According to Allen, the evidence amassing in the literature of the past 30 years on psychopharmaceutical responses and the neurobiological bases of psychosocial disorders shows that the cause of psychiatric disorders cannot rest on psychodynamic explanations. In response to such evidence, Allen has shifted in her view of cognitive disabilities from a psychoanalytic and then a Piagetian orientation to a neurological orientation (Allen, 1987, 1988a; Allen, Earhart, & Blue, 1992). Her definition of cognitive disability as "a restriction in voluntary motor action originating in the physical or chemical structures of the brain and producing observable limitations in routine task behavior" speaks to her view of neurobiology as foundational to an understanding of the cognitive impairment underlying a cognitive disability (Allen, 1985, p. 31). This definition, and statements like "a cognitive disability is caused by a biologic defect" (Allen, 1985, p. 24), originally stirred up a great deal of controversy because they stood in sharp contrast to analytic perspectives that emphasized psychosocial causes. However, they are now widely accepted.

Cognitive Levels

In her Eleanor Clarke Slagle Lecture in 1987, Allen caused an uproar in some quarters when she stated that "specification has not been very popular in American occupational therapy; it is often ridiculed with labels such as the 'cookbook approach.' I think it is time to change that attitude. Accuracy, objectivity and measures of change in capacity that may be influenced by other factors all require specification" (Allen, 1987, pp. 372–373).

Allen explains that she had examined the five cognitive developmental levels of Piaget, the sensorimotor, preconceptual, intuitive, concrete operational, and formal operational phases, so as to describe the cognitive disabilities manifested by the behaviors or voluntary motor actions of patients treated in occupational therapy. Allen attempted to correlate each of Piaget's abstract cognitive levels with its external manifestations in behavior. Thus her schema represents an "occupational" or action-oriented interpretation of Piaget's cognitive levels.

Allen soon realized that she could not follow Piaget too closely: "If one assumes that the Piagetian hierarchy is only partially correct in describing the functional behavior of adults with mental disorders, then one must be prepared to look beyond the realm of the Piagetian hierarchy" (Allen, 1985, p. 328). Consequently, she revised her first formulations by winnowing the denotations and connotations of the labels most appropriate to represent the indications of intelligence that she had observed. Her current schema recognizes six distinct functional cognitive levels: automatic, postural, manual, goal-directed, exploratory, and planned action (Allen, 1985, 1988a; Allen, Earhart, & Blue, 1992). These concepts provide an ordinal scale of observable behaviors, thus enabling the development of a calibrated hierarchy of adequate specificity for measuring cognitive functions. Table 8-1 presents the culmination of this conceptual configuration. The first two cogni-

Table 8-1 Cognitive Levels

Attribute	Level I: Automatic Actions	Level 2: Postural Actions	Level 3: Manual Actions	Level 4: Goal-Directed Actions	Level 5: Exploratory Actions	Level 6: Planned Actions
Attention to sensory cues	Subliminal cues	Proprioceptive cues	Tactile cues	Visible cues	Related cues	Symbolic cues
Motor actions Spontaneous Imitated	Automatic None	Postural Approximations	Manual Manipulations	Goal-directed Replications	Exploratory Novelty	Planned Unnecessary
Conscious awareness						
Purpose	Arousal	Comfort	Interest	Compliance	Self-control	Reflection
Experience	Indistinct	Moving	Touching	Seeing	Inductive reasoning	Deductive reasoning
Process	Habitual or reflexive	Effect on body	Effect on environment	Several actions	Overt trial and error	Covert trial and error
Time	Seconds	Minutes	Half hours	Hours	Weeks	Past and future

Source: From *Occupational Therapy for Psychiatric Diseases: Measurement and Management of Cognitive Disabilities* (p. 34) by C. Allen, 1985, Boston: Little, Brown. Copyright 1985 by Little, Brown. Reprinted by permission.

tive levels, automatic actions and postural actions, most closely resemble Piaget's sensory-motor cognitive level; simple manual actions resemble Piaget's preconceptual level; and simple goal-directed actions resemble Piaget's level of intuitive thought. Exploratory actions and planned actions may be viewed as representing Piaget's concrete and formal operational levels, respectively.

Performance Modes of the Cognitive Levels

Allen has repeatedly indicated the need for specificity in standards of performance that can be used to evaluate cognitive disability levels (Allen, 1985, 1987; Allen, Earhart, & Blue, 1992), both for the sake of patients and in order to develop interdisciplinary credibility for observations in occupational therapy. The "performance modes" that she has identified for each of the cognitive levels in her schema supply this need (see Table 8-2).

Persons capable of automatic action only (level 1) are able to respond in a sensory manner to stimuli with movement of the head, eyes, tongue, arms, and legs, but are unable to maintain postural actions of sitting or walking. Individuals who have the ability of postural actions (level 2) can sit, stand, and walk, but may not know where they are going. People with the capacity for manual actions (level 3) can grasp and move their hands when objects are placed within reach, but may need instruction if several objects are present or if a number of steps are involved in utilization of the object. A distinction between levels 3 and 4 is that at level 3 the completion of a goal is only recognized after the task is "done"; there is no understanding of the "gestalt" of the action or anticipation of the finished product.

Goal-directed actions (level 4) manifest a cognitive ability to sequence steps independently through the parts of a simple, routine short-term task. This ability may rely on memory of steps practiced through months of repetition in order to learn a total activity pattern or to build a habit (Allen, Earhart, & Blue, 1992). Exploratory actions (level 5) reflect the mental ability to change the steps of an activity in a flexible manner. Learning by doing through a process of trial and error manifests the advantage of adaptability and the disadvantage of time-consuming or costly mistakes. Planned actions (level 6) reveal the intellectual capacity to anticipate results and to select courses of action that are projected as desirable. Covert thought processes may be revealed by pauses to stop and think before acting, by information gathering as preparation for action, or by requests to deliberate on alternatives before making a decision (Allen, Earhart, & Blue, 1992).

Allen comments that for the three lower performance levels, eating is usually the activity that is done best. In analyzing levels of learnings, Allen observes that true learning can take place at level 5, the exploratory level; practice is required for memory learning at level 4, the goal-directed level; and months of drill are necessary for structured memorization of actions at level 3, the manual level

Table 8-2 Modes of Performance within the Cognitive Levels

Cognitive Level	Performance Modes
Level 1: Automatic Actions	1.0 Withdrawing from noxious stimuli 1.2 Responding to positive stimuli 1.4 Locating stimuli 1.6 Rolling in bed 1.8 Raising body part
Level 2: Postural Actions	2.0 Overcoming gravity 2.2 Righting reflex/standing 2.4 Walking 2.6 Directed walking 2.8 Using grab bars/railings
Level 3: Manual Actions	3.0 Grasping objects 3.2 Distinguishing objects 3.4 Sustaining actions on objects 3.6 Noting effects on objects 3.8 Using all objects
Level 4: Goal-Directed Activity	4.0 Sequencing 4.2 Differentiating features 4.4 Completing goal 4.6 Personalizing 4.8 Rote learning
Level 5: Exploratory Actions	5.0 Making neuromuscular variations 5.2 Discriminating 5.4 Self-directed learning 5.6 Considering social standards 5.8 Consulting
Level 6: Planned Actions	(Not calibrated at this time)

Source: Adapted from *Occupational Therapy Treatment Goals for the Physically and Cognitively Disabled* (pp. 88, 89, 91, 94, 98) by C.K. Allen, C.A. Earhart, and T. Blue, 1992, Rockville, MD: American Occupational Therapy Association. Copyright 1992 by the American Occupational Therapy Association.

(Allen, Earhart, & Blue, 1992). Allen gives an extended example utilizing her schema for the task of food preparation.

Allen gives an extended example utilizing her schema for the task of food preparation. At performance mode 3.8, an individual may be trained to make a simple sandwich. At performance mode level 4.4, some persons with disabilities can prepare simple, well-learned dishes, follow a fixed diet, and shop for routine items, but they go to the store repeatedly to purchase immediate needs only. At performance mode level 5.2, people may be expected to know how to shop, wash, prepare, cook, and store food properly, with awareness of spoilage problems and ability to check quality of produce, but may impulsively change a shopping list and fail to follow dietary precautions in their meandering, exploratory style (Allen, Earhart, & Blue, 1992).

Allen believes that at cognitive levels 1 through 5 humans share sensorimotor processes with other species, but that the cognitive abilities of level 6 are uniquely human. Many of the activities of everyday life are done at lower levels of cognition because it is human nature to conserve energy when doing routine tasks. Also, when people are fatigued or lacking motivation, they are content to operate at lower levels, on automatic pilot. However, the intellectual competence of the individual without a cognitive disability includes the capacity to function at level 6 when the need or desire arises (Allen, Earhart, & Blue, 1992).

Cognitive levels 4 and 5 are perplexing to therapists wishing to determine whether lack of motivation or inability causes problematic behaviors of lack of participation or of effort. Allen admits that motivational explanations cannot always be eliminated. For that reason, when carrying out assessment of the cognitive levels, it is advisable to permit the patient to choose the activity (Allen, 1985, 1988a; Allen, Earhart, & Blue, 1992). It should also be pointed out that because about 20 percent of the nondisabled population operates for the most part at level 5, it is not always possible to determine whether an evaluation of a disabled person perceived as a level 5 is a temporary or usual mode of function (C. Allen, personal communication, May 16, 1992; Allen, 1985) (see Table 8-3).

Diagnoses Associated with Cognitive Levels

In her chapter in *Mental Health Focus* (1988a), Allen discusses the cognitive levels as they relate to various populations with whom occupational therapists work. She indicates the subsidiary divisions of each cognitive disabling impairment within the larger six levels (see Table 8-3).

Assessment of Cognitive Levels

Initially Allen began assessment of patients through clinical observation to develop face validity for the cognitive levels. She insists that occupational therapists should never abandon the strengths of their own clinical observation skills no matter how technical or stratified the format of formal assessments they utilize (C. Allen, personal communication, May 16, 1992).

Allen and other occupational therapy colleagues have developed numerous methods for evaluation of the cognitive levels. The first of these was the Allen

Table 8-3 Diagnoses Associated with Cognitive Disability Levels

Cognitive Level	Diagnoses
Level 1: Automatic Actions	Organic brain syndrome Severe dementia Recent traumatic brain injury Cardiovascular accidents Occasional psychiatric disorder
Level 2: Postural Actions	Dementia Cardiovascular accidents Traumatic brain injury Severely psychotic disorders
Level 3: Manual Actions	Dementia Traumatic brain injury Cardiovascular accidents Developmental disabilities Acute manic episodes Acute schizophrenic episodes
Level 4: Goal-Directed Actions	Mild dementia Traumatic brain injury Cardiovascular accidents Developmental disabilities HIV/AIDS Acute manic episodes Acute depressive episodes Chronic schizophrenic disorders
Level 5: Exploratory Actions	Affective disorders in remission Good-prognosis schizophrenic disorders Personality disorders Early-onset dementia Usual level of function for about 20% of persons with no distressing disability or symptomatology
Level 6: Planned Actions	Affective disorders in full remission Good prognosis schizophrenic disorders Acute brain syndromes, cleared Usual level of function for most "normal" persons

Source: Information from *Mental Health Focus* (pp. 3-28–3-32) by S. Robinson, ed., 1988, Rockville, MD: American Occupational Therapy Association.

Cognitive Levels (ACL), a craft-oriented leather-lacing task that incorporates three levels of difficulty in stitches. It has been used clinically since 1973 and is now produced by S&S Worldwide for evaluative purposes. It has three versions: the original, the expanded (ACL-E), and the problem-solving ACL. Allen has accepted the use of a large version of the leather-lacing sample, the Large ACL (LACL) developed by Kathy Kehrberg, for use in geriatric assessment (Kehrberg, Kuskowski, Mortimer, & Shoberg, in press). Allen emphasizes that users always need to check patients for visual impairment before beginning screening with the ACL. Josman and Katz (1991) developed a problem-solving version of the ACL (the ACL-PS) that permits much level 5 exploratory behavior before instructing the patient in the stitches and provides an opportunity for the patients to correct a deliberate error in the stitches. Allen saw the conceptual value of this addition, which removed the ceiling effect of the earlier ACL, and she incorporated this improvement in 1990, renaming the test the ACL-90. The ACL-90 incorporates several steps of problem solving to provide challenges for individuals with higher cognitive levels and additional discriminatory power through a refinement of intervals within the test (Allen, Earhart, & Blue, 1992). "The range of scores is 3.0 to 5.8, which seems to be more logically related to what leather lacing can measure" (Allen, Earhart, & Blue, 1992, p. 33).

Allen now considers the ACL to be a quick screening tool (Allen, Earhart, & Blue, 1992; C. Allen, personal communication, May 16, 1992). She believes that an assessment should begin with an interview to determine the individual's functional history, then screen with the ACL, and finally utilize the comprehensive Routine Task Inventory (RTI) (Allen, Earhart, & Blue, 1992), which aims at analyzing a basic and broad spectrum of independent living activities. Allen also encourages clinicians to develop their own assessment for activities that they constantly use in certain groups by calibrating them through the hierarchies of the performance modes of the cognitive levels (see Table 8-2).

> [The ACL] is so fast to administer, and so easy, that it goes into research designs very well. But it is still this fast little thing. The real power is in the RTI, not in the ACL. The real power is not in the leather lacing; it's in the activities of daily living pattern of performance, and people don't get that. They get hung up on this test. And maybe it's just an evolutionary process. Maybe it takes a year of administering the test before you get a Gestalt of what the performance modes are really all about. We now feel more comfortable with our clinical observation scores than with our ACL scores, and if there is a disparity, we take our clinical score over the ACL score. I keep telling people that they've got to get to that point. They can't stay wedded to that one little thing, [the leather lacing]. So the ACL is the best documented and the best investigated, but the least valid. I want people to get to where they trust their own judgment, and their own ability to assess from observing performance, because the natural performance is our ace in the hole. (C. Allen, personal communication, April 16, 1992)

It is clear, then, that despite the widespread use and improvement of the ACL, Allen now prefers the RTI, a more comprehensive evaluation tool that can serve as a precise indicator of goals to be addressed through discussion, problem solving, training, or drilling. Cognitive disabilities are often hidden, and can have a more pervasive impact than obvious physical disabilities. Therefore, Allen has argued that the evaluation instrument for their assessment needs to be more detailed and hierarchical in its calibrations in order to provide a well-documented picture of the disabled person (Allen, Earhart, & Blue, 1992). The RTI, with its multiple levels of distinctions of cognitive/behavioral indicators, provides this specificity.

Table 8-4 gives an outline of the four major kinds of disability that are analyzed through the RTI: self-awareness disability, situational awareness disability, occupational role disability, and social role disability (Allen, Earhart, & Blue, 1992, p. 36). Allen uses the International Classification of Impairments, Disabilities and Handicaps (ICIDH) format (World Health Organization [WHO], 1980) to define these disabilities. "Self-awareness disability is a mental disturbance in the ability to meet the natural demands of one's body"; "situational awareness disability is a mental disturbance of the capacity to register and understand relationships be-

---

Table 8-4 Activities Analyzed on RTI-2 as Behavior Disabilities

10.	Self-awareness disability	12.	Occupational role disability
.0	Grooming	.0	Planning/doing major role activities
.1	Dressing	.1	Planning/doing spare-time activities
.2	Bathing	.2	Pacing and timing actions
.3	Walking/exercising	.3	Exerting effort
.4	Feeding	.4	Judging results
.5	Toileting	.5	Speaking
.6	Taking medications	.6	Following safety precautions
.7	Using adaptive equipment	.7	Responding to emergencies
.8	Other	.8	Other
.9	Unspecified	.9	Unspecified
11.	Situational awareness disability	13.	Social role disability
.0	Housekeeping	.0	Communicating meaning
.1	Preparing/obtaining food	.1	Following instructions
.2	Spending money	.2	Contributing to family activities
.3	Shopping	.3	Caring for dependents
.4	Doing laundry	.4	Cooperating with others
.5	Traveling	.5	Supervising independent people
.6	Telephoning	.6	Keeping informed
.7	Adjusting to change	.7	Engaging in good citizenship
.8	Other	.8	Other
.9	Unspecified	.9	Unspecified

tween objects and persons within the context of daily living"; "occupational role disability is a mental disturbance of the ability to organize and participate in routine activities connected with the occupation of time, not only confined to the performance of work"; and "social role disability is a mental disturbance in the ability to meet social expectations when interacting with other people" (Allen, Earhart, & Blue, 1992, p. 349). Within each area, Allen lists eight basic activities of daily living essential for discrimination of safety and independence. She describes each of the four disability areas and their activities in detail. As she indicates in *Occupational Therapy Treatment Goals for the Physically and Cognitively Disabled* (Allen, Earhart, & Blue, 1992, p. 40), "This book is designed to give you feedback about the accuracy of your activity analysis so that you can confidently analyze any activity that is important to your patient." Extended examples that Earhart details in Chapter 6 of the book include the activities of sanding, staining, gluing, polishing/cleaning, cutting, sewing, measuring, and mixing ingredients, all of which are calibrated through the levels of the performance modes for each activity.

In describing the evaluation of human cognitive levels, and in delineating the process of developing a schema of performance modes for cognitive assessment, Allen states that

> things are pretty clear all though level four, but level five is a serious concern, and we really don't understand the difference between [difficulties in] problem-solving at level five when that's a disability or when it's normal [for that individual]. And we're having tremendous trouble with level six because the hierarchy from motor behavior and through symbolism as Piaget delineated it simply doesn't work. So we don't have a view of a hierarchy of normal learning that is really working. We have to develop our own.

> The surprising thing is that we have some very bright left-hemisphere dominant people who score 5.2 or 5.4 on the ACL, and function that way with their *hands*, my husband being one, who is very good conceptually, but becomes a level five on me routinely. There are some people who just don't problem-solve with their hands. . . . Perhaps the capacities of the left-dominant abstract thing became level 6, and may be hemispheric. I don't know what we are doing" [in human mentation]. [She goes on to speculate that] it may be units of the brain or verbal monitor role. All of that stuff is fouled up between 5.4 and whatever goes into level 6. We just stopped at 6.0 in this last book. It just got too confusing. (C. Allen, personal communication, April 16, 1992)

APPLICATIONS TO OCCUPATIONAL THERAPY PRACTICE

In 1985, Allen discussed the question, "Can occupational therapy services change the cognitive level?" She gave the answer of no, and admitted that this was a shocking reply (Allen, 1985, p. 31). Occupational therapists, she stated, needed "to switch from trying to change the patient to changing the activity" (Allen, 1985, p. 27). In 1992, Allen still speaks of cognitively impaired patients' general inability to move beyond their cognitive level, even with intensive training.

> It was very frustrating for me because clearly the thing to do is . . . to try to move a person to the next level. If we had a learning theory that worked, we could do it. But we can't seem to do it. We can't seem to make it work. Even with the new book, with 52 modes of performance, we just can't do it.

For example, if the patient is performing cognitively at a level 4.4 in the performance modes,

> . . . every time you give them a 4.6 cue, they ignore it. They don't know what to do with it, or they reject it, or they just don't see it. And we still come up against these brick walls. I think it goes back to having no good theory about learning. Maybe it's in the DNA, in that genetic stuff, and if the DNA is all fouled up, you just can't go on. (C. Allen, personal communication, August 24, 1992)

In her 1992 book, however, Allen acknowledged that some diagnostic groups of patients, such as those with affective disorders or good-prognosis schizophrenia, may experience a remission, thus changing cognitive levels. Other more chronic patients can solidify gains within a cognitive level through training and drilling, making movement upward within the performance modes. And although some patients, such as those with dementia, may manifest a decline in cognitive levels as part of the natural progression of their disease, others can be stabilized through a reasonably stimulating activity program to maintain their cognitive level of function, thus preventing deterioration (Allen, Earhart, & Blue, 1992).

Given these limitations, "change is made by getting the patient to do everything that he or she would like to do within his or her range of ability" (Allen, Earhart, & Blue, 1992, p. 23). The occupational therapist first identifies the patient's range of ability by assessing cognitive level, then selects and modifies tasks to bring them within that range. Allen emphasizes that the tasks selected should appeal to the patient and in fact be pleasant (Allen, 1985, p. 368). She has summarized these and other links between her theory of cognitive levels and the practice of occupational therapy in a list of nine propositions (Allen, 1985, p. 368; see Table 8-5).

Table 8-5 Summary of Propositions

Proposition

1. The observed routine task behavior of disabled patients will differ from the observed behavior of nondisabled populations
2. Limitations in task behavior can be hierarchically described by the cognitive levels
3. The choice of task content is influenced by the diagnosis and the disability
4. The task environment can have a positive or a negative effect on a patient's ability to regulate his or her own behavior
5. Patients with cognitive disabilities attend to those elements of the task environment that are within their range of ability
6. Therapists can select and modify a task so that it is within the patient's range of ability through the application of task analysis
7. An effective outcome of occupational therapy services occurs when successful task performance is accompanied by a pleasant task experience
8. Steps in task procedures that require abilities above a person's level of ability will be refused or ignored
9. The assessment of the cognitive level can contribute to the legal determination of competency

Source: Reprinted with permission from C.K. Allen, *Occupational therapy for psychiatric diseases: Measurement and management of cognitive disabilities.* Copyright 1985, Boston: Little Brown, p. 368.

Allen's approach to treatment of the cognitively disabled is in keeping with her broader views on OT treatment in general as she expressed them in her Eleanor Clarke Slagle Lecture "Activity: Occupational Therapy's Treatment Method" (1987). In this lecture, Allen stated that "therapeutic activity compensates for disability by utilizing remaining capabilities to accomplish desirable activities with satisfactory results" (1987, p. 574). She emphasizes the emotional satisfactions of successful activity and the occupational therapist's role of helping the disabled patient to obtain or regain these satisfactions. She points out, for example, that "activity actualizes a person's strengths" and that ". . . people with spinal cord injuries who are the most productive do not express their loss in physical terms; the greatest loss is expressed as a loss in activity" (1987, p. 573). Although activity is valued by everyone, it "is especially important to disabled people because their opportunity to engage in successful activity is limited" (1987, p. 574).

Allen has asserted that "safety in doing ordinary activities is the primary treatment goal" (Allen, Earhart, & Blue, 1992, p. 339) in working with patients who have any type of cognitive disability. She refers to the cognitive levels as a functional safety scale because lack of attention to cues is the principal problem of the cognitively disabled.

When a patient is discharged, "expected outcome is a recommendation of the least restrictive environment that the patient can function in safely at the time of discharge" (Allen, Earhart, & Blue, 1992, p. 20). The Allen Cognitive Levels have proven to be useful for making this determination. Allen indicates, for example, that a person who stabilizes at a 3.5 level most likely needs 24-hour supervision. A patient remitting at a 4.5 level does not need such supervision but has deficits that prevent "efficient and error-free performance of high level ADL's" (Allen, Earhart, & Blue, 1992, p. 49).

Allen has pointed out that the safety of the cognitively disabled patient is a legal issue in which occupational therapists are necessarily involved.

> What is the difference between looking at a person in the simulated environment versus the real environment? . . . How much can you predict in those carefully controlled situations as to what patients are going to do in an uncontrolled environment where a lot of out of the ordinary things happen? It's not going to be an either or kind of thing, but a weighted, multi-regression analysis kind of prediction. We really need to go into that kind of depth to really understand what we are doing when we get into these legal questions. . . . We have to prepare ourselves for that. Ultimately is it "child" custody or not? Where do we draw the line, and what factors determine where we draw the line? Really tough questions. (C. Allen, personal communication, May 16, 1992)

Allen herself has contributed to the clarification of these questions by drawing on *Black's Law Dictionary* (1979) and the *ICIDH* (WHO, 1980) to establish clear, common legal definitions of such concepts as competence, capacity, reasonable care, negligence, reasonable thought, prudent and diligent behavior, incapacitated status, and custody (Allen, Earhart, & Blue, 1992). "Our patients are mostly involuntary. We are faced with those kinds of legal questions daily" (C. Allen, personal communication, May 16, 1992). Allen has also provided distinctions between impairment and disability, recovery and remediation, and environmental compensations and social assistance by drawing on official health definitions put forth by WHO in *ICIDH* (WHO, 1980) and in the more recent *International Classification of Diseases* (Karaffa, 1992).

From the beginning, Allen's work has been guided by practical considerations. Her schema of cognitive levels and performance modes and her construction of the RTI were to a great extent responses to the dilemma of writing satisfactory progress notes for Blue Cross and Medicaid. As Allen noted, one "serious deficiency in the basic science literature" was that of classifications too broad in scope to detect the distinctions of varying cognitive disability levels or the small refinements therapists made to accommodate patients' disabilities. Because Allen had to make subtle changes in cognitively impaired patients visible, she teased apart the six cognitive levels, stretching them out so they could indicate a patient's change within the larger levels from one performance mode level to another. She then incorporated these distinctions into the RTI to make assessments of functioning as highly calibrated as possible.

The need to justify OT services to third-party payers has also contributed to Allen's emphasis on safety as the primary goal in treating the cognitively disabled.

> . . . the way to get out of being boxed in by Medicare to the self-care activities, to look at a broader view of the activities that people are going to do, is to emphasize safety. That's our key to getting paid if we are looking at the quality of life—a very practical approach. (C. Allen, personal communication, April 16, 1992)

Allen is also practical in another way. Her publications are filled with down-to-earth guidelines for clinical assessment, task analysis and accommodation, and preparation for the environment to which persons with cognitive disabilities are returning. Both her books utilize graded case examples to teach occupational therapy students and practitioners how to incorporate her concepts, propositions, and philosophy into their practice. Through leading questions, she enables the reader to ferret out pertinent facts within the cases to evaluate and provide direction for possible change or accommodation.

RESEARCH ON ASSESSMENT TOOLS

Allen Cognitive Level

In 1978, Moore tested the original Allen Cognitive Level (ACL) leather-lacing task for interrater reliability of five pairs of occupational therapists with 32 subjects. These therapists had had extensive experience in administering the ACL test for several years at the USC Medical Center. A high level of interrater reliability emerged: .99 (Moore, 1978). In this same study, Moore looked at the validity of placing patients in an occupational therapy group according to ratings by six occupational therapists based on general clinical observation. The placement/ratings by the therapists of the patients was within a close range, such as between group levels 3 and 4 versus 5 and 6. The resulting correlation between the ratings of the patients for general clinical group levels, and performance level on the ACL was r = .76 (Moore, 1978). The Brief Psychiatric Rating Scale, the Block Design of the Wechsler Adult Intelligence Scale (WAIS), and the Hollingshead Two-Factor Index of Social Position were used to check on concurrent validity (Allen, Earhart, & Blue, 1992, p. 32).

The version of the ACL to be used with populations where little change is expected is an extended assessment referred to as the ACL-E. The ACL-Extended was developed to expand the ratings of the ACL by lengthening the score sheet. This enabled therapists to evaluate populations with little potential for change in cognitive level by using more numerous graded intervals. The interrater reliability for this test was established by Newman (1987) as .95 (n = 21). Test-retest reliability was .75 based on Spearman rank correlation (Newman, 1987). Eight subtests on the WAIS were significantly correlated to the ACL-E.

The ACL has been used to assess patients with schizophrenia, depression, and dementia and to compare them to normal controls. Figure 8-1 shows comparison of scores among these four groups using the ACL. The partially overlapping histograms are found in the position relative to each other that most clinicians would

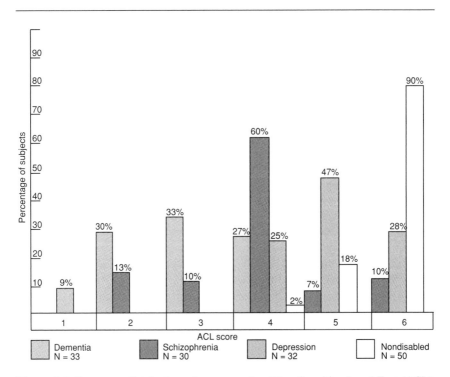

Figure 8-1 Frequency distribution of scores on the Allen Cognitive Level Test (ACL). *Source:* Reprinted with permission from Allen, C.K., *Occupational therapy for psychiatric diseases: Measurement and management of cognitive disabilities.* Copyright 1985, Boston: Little Brown, p. 369.

expect, giving the results clinical or face validity. The majority of patients with dementia are found in levels 1 to 4. The schizophrenic patients range from levels 2 to 6, with over half of this diagnostic group being found in level 4. Average scores of depressed patients fell in levels 4 to 6, with about 50 percent in level 5. Nondisabled individuals stretched from levels 4 to 6, with 80 percent ranking in level 6 (Allen, 1985, p. 369).

Allen has openly invited occupational therapists to test out the validity and reliability of the ACL through additional studies. In 1988, Katz, Josman, and Steinmetz reported from Israel that in a study of 20 psychiatric adolescent patients and matched healthy controls, a signficant difference was found in cognitive levels of the two groups (p < .01). None of the controls scored under level 5 on the ACL and half of them scored at level 6. By contrast, the patients had a wide range of cognitive skills, with 25 percent below level 5, 50 percent at level 5, and 25 percent at level 6 (Katz, Josman, & Steinmetz, 1988).

The validity of these results was strengthened by comparison with results of another cognitive measure, the Class Inclusion subtest of the Riska Object Classification (ROC) Test: p < .0001. "All subjects in the control group fully understood class inclusion relations, compared with only 60% of the patients" (Katz et al., 1988, p. 35).

Routine Task Inventory Test

In 1984, Allen, along with Earhart, Heyings, and Heimann, began to describe patient behavior through the Routine Task Inventory (RTI). Examining the RTI statistically in a study of 41 patients with Alzheimer's disease, Heimann found significant interrater reliability (r = .98) and test-retest reliability (r = .91), with an internal consistency alpha coefficient of .94 (Heimann, Allen, & Yerxa, 1989). Test-retest reliability for the RTI was replicated in a population with senile dementia (n = 20) as r = .99 by Wilson, Allen, McCormack, & Burton in 1989. Wilson et al. carried out validity studies, finding levels of correlation of r = .56 with the ACL and r = .61 with the Mini-Mental State (MMS; n = 20).

Cognitive Performance Test

In 1985, Theresa Burns began developing a Cognitive Performance Test (CPT) to provide a standardized ADL assessment for functional levels manifested in Alzheimer's disease based on Allen's cognitive levels of processing information. Burns selected six tasks, entitled Dress, Shop, Toast, Telephone, Wash, and Travel. Studies of reliability and validity of the CPT have been carried out at the Minneapolis VA Medical Center's Geriatric Research, Education and Clinical

Center (GRECC). External validity for 77 patients was measured in contrast to the Mini-Mental State Examination (MMSE: r = .67) and two caregiver's measures, Instrumental Activities of Daily Living, r = .64 and the Physical Self-Maintenance Scale, r = .49. Inter-rater reliability for 18 patients at 4 weeks was .91, and test-retest reliability for 36 patients at 4 weeks was .89 (Burns, 1992, pp. 1, 46–50). Burn's analysis of activities of daily living within the CPT is similar to Earhart's Analysis of Activities (Allen, Earhart, & Blue, 1992, pp. 126–305) based on Allen's modes of performance.

Modes of Performance

Since Allen has developed the "Modes of Performance within the Cognitive Levels" (1992), she has called for testing of these levels, which appear to have conceptual or face validity. "The task that needs to be done right away is establishing the interrater reliability of the modes of performance" (Allen, Earhart, & Blue, 1992, p. 101). Allen's goal in achieving reliability is to develop sufficient agreement in perception of the modes of performance to permit average therapists in practice to score the Inventory in the same way. Obviously, an accurate sequencing of the performance modes in cognitive development steps is essential, as Allen indicates. She has pointed out that Rasch analysis tools "hold promise for being able to investigate the validity of the sequence as well as the distances between the modes" (Allen, Earhart, & Blue, 1992, p. 102).

CRITIQUE OF ALLEN'S THEORY AND FRAME OF REFERENCE

In both of her books, Allen (Allen, 1985; Allen, Earhart, & Blue, 1992) has presented a holistic approach to occupational therapy. She has categorized the primary health problems treated by occupational therapists across traditional subspecialties as cognitive or noncognitive disabilities, regardless of the boundaries of typical areas of practice.

In the newest text, Tina Blue has set up a comparison of the Allen Cognitive Levels with the Rancho Cognitive Levels, which also builds a bridge across physical and mental assessments of cognitive losses (C. Allen, personal communication, August 24, 1992). Blue matches the Rancho levels of No Response, Generalized Response, and Localized Response with Allen's level 1, Automatic Actions; the Rancho Confused Agitated and Confused-Inappropriate levels with Allen's levels 2 and 3, Postural Actions and Manual Actions; the Rancho Confused-Appropriate and Automatic-Appropriate levels with Allen's level 4, Goal-Directed Activity; and the Rancho Purposeful-Appropriate level with Allen's level

5, Exploratory Actions. This comparison provides a clinical clarification of the two systems from divergent parts of the field of occupational therapy that are reconverging in the cognitive domain. Allen's cognitive levels seem more useful due to their greater clarity, simplicity, and ease of recall based on their correspondence to Piaget's well-known, though abstract, cognitive levels.

Early critiques of Allen's work focused on her apparently iconoclastic position of a neurological base for psychiatric disorders, her skepticism about patients' abilities to change their cognitive levels, and the definitions of some of her concepts. Most of these earlier problems that occupational therapists had with Allen's views have now been resolved. In some instances, Allen has shifted to a new position through development of her perceptions and assessment tools. Neurobiological world views have now become a central perspective. Allen has expanded the cognitive levels so that patients and therapists can clearly perceive the small, incremental steps that patients may achieve through cognitive drilling, training, learning, problem solving, or remission.

Most of Allen's earlier troublesome definitions have been expanded to the point of universality of conceptualization. For example, Allen's earlier definition of cognitive disability seemed to omit an important element. Allen stated that "a cognitive disability is a restriction in voluntary motor action originating in the physical or chemical structures of the brain and producing observable limitations in routine task behavior" (Allen, 1985, p. 31). Criticisms noted the omission of a phrase indicating the additional or initial restriction in covert mental processes, which may remain covert for long periods of time until implemented as actions. It was pointed out that "restrictions in voluntary motor action" were synonymous with "limitations in routine task behavior." A suggestion was made to include a phrase indicating that the restrictions were due to a cognitive impairment. Allen's adoption in 1992 of an *ICIDH* distinction between disability (concerned with global, functional limitations) and impairment (existing at the organ level) has helped to resolve some of the lack of clarity in the original statement (Allen, Earhart, & Blue, 1992, p. 345).

Similarly, while Allen indicates that sensory cues can be inner or outer, the definition of voluntary motor actions as "a behavioral response to a sensory cue that is guided by the mind" could have gained from the addition of the modifiers "internal or external" sensory cues.

More recently, in discussing learning, Allen (Allen, Earhart, & Blue, 1992) presents an explanation of the speculative sensorimotor models that the mind uses to improve premeditated performance options. The statement that "the speculation is done in reference to perceivable problems presented by material objects; the supposition is concrete rather than abstract" needs explanation (Allen, Earhart, & Blue, 1992, p. 340). For the sake of communication, the antecedent for the word "supposition" needs clarification, while the concept of "abstract" needs defining. Explaining why tangible and imagined are not in opposition or mutually exclusive, and indicating, by contrast, what kind of cognitive models *do* include imperceptible problems and intangible properties of objects would assist the reader.

In his 1992 text, *Conceptual Foundations of Occupational Therapy*, Kielhofner focuses his discussion of Allen's Cognitive Disabilities Model on concerns voiced about her earlier work: that occupational therapists must not inadvertently limit patients' opportunities to learn; insistence that research must be done to support or refute Allen's claim that learning does not occur within levels 1–4; and the need for research into issues of motivation and its effect on performance. Since Kielhofner and Allen published their 1992 texts almost simultaneously, Kielhofner may not be aware that Allen has gradually developed her model to include these issues. Kielhofner himself notes Allen's concern for motivation as far back as 1985 in her emphasis on the patient's selection of desirable activities. He does have a point, with which Allen would no doubt agree, that lack of change in patients may be partially attributable to the paucity of resources for patients in the current health care delivery system (Kielhofner, 1992). Kielhofner calls for further research comparing the relative importance of motivational factors with cognitive functional factors as contributors to the rehabilitation process.

Placed in perspective of the totality of Allen's work, these issues of concern are minor. Allen is to be admired not only for her expansion of Piaget's ideas into the functional realm of voluntary motor actions, but for her further refinement of providing performance modes to solve both conceptual and clinically pragmatic problems. Allen has opened a door of opportunities to empirical research in the psychosocial area of occupational therapy. She has enabled occupational therapists to understand what many have been doing intuitively in placing patients into cognitive levels. She has provided the field with six new concepts—automatic, postural, manual, goal-directed, exploratory, and planned actions—in an organized schema that has clinical and concurrent validity. She has established a model that lends itself to development of the realms of higher planning and problem solving. She has been open to suggestions and modifications by colleagues and researchers. She has even welcomed the consideration of a combination of the model of human occupation with cognitive disability theory (Allen, 1988b, pp. ix, x). And, primarily, she has brought disparate elements of the field of occupational therapy into greater integration.

Cognitive disability theory can help us understand human cognitive levels in general. Just as Piaget examined the mistakes his children made in order to get a glimpse of their covert and overt cognitive processes within sequential levels of thought, so too, Allen is enabling occupational therapists to examine varying cognitive process performance modes through levels of disability in voluntary motor actions of their patients so that they may better comprehend normal adult exploratory, problem-solving, and planned cognitions. As Allen remarked in summing up the presentation of her work in *Mental Health Focus* (1988a, p. 24): "The history of this frame of reference has only just begun."

REFERENCES

Allen, C.K. (1982). Independence through activity: The practice of occupational therapy. *American Journal of Occupational Therapy, 36*, 731–739.

Allen, C.K. (1985). *Occupational therapy for psychiatric diseases: Measurement and management of cognitive disabilities.* Boston: Little, Brown.

Allen, C.K. (1987). Activity: Occupational therapy's treatment method. 1987 Eleanor Clarke Slagle lecture. *American Journal of Occupational Therapy, 41*, 563–575.

Allen, C.K. (1988a). Cognitive disabilities. In S. Robinson (Ed.), *Mental health focus* (pp. 3–18—3–33). Rockville, MD: American Occupational Therapy Association.

Allen, C.K. (1988b). Preface. The development of standardized clinical evaluations in mental health. *Occupational Therapy in Mental Health, 8*, ix–x.

Allen, C.K., Earhart, C.A., & Blue, T. (1992). *Occupational therapy treatment goals for the physically and cognitively disabled.* Rockville, MD: American Occupational Therapy Association.

Allen, C.K., Foto, M., Sperling, T.M., & Wilson, D. (1989). Outpatient occupational therapy Medicare part B guidelines (DHHS Transmittal No. 565). In *Health insurance manual.* Baltimore, MD: Health Care Financing Administration.

Black's law dictionary (5th ed.). (1979). St. Paul, MN: Western Publishing.

Burns, T. (1992). "Part III: The Cognitive Perception Test: An approach to cognitive level assessment in Alzheimer's disease." In C.K. Allen, C.A. Earhart, & T. Blue (Eds.), *Occupational therapy treatment goals for the physically and cognitively disabled* (pp. 46–50). Rockville, MD: American Occupational Therapy Association.

Heimann, N.E., Allen, C.K., & Yerxa, E.J. (1989). The Routine Task Inventory: A tool for describing the functional behavior of the cognitively disabled. *Occupational Therapy Practice, 1*, 67–74.

Heying, L.M. (1983). *Cognitive disabilities and activities of daily living in persons with senile dementia.* Unpublished master's thesis, University of Southern California, Los Angeles.

Josman, N., & Katz, N. (1991). Problem-solving version of the Allen Cognitive Level (ACL) Test. *American Journal of Occupational Therapy, 45*, 331–338.

Karaffa, M.C. (1992). *International classification of diseases* (4th ed.). Los Angeles: Practice Management Information Corporation.

Katz, N., Josman, N., & Steinmetz, N. (1988). Relationship between cognitive disability theory and the model of human occupation in the assessment of psychiatric and nonpsychiatric adolescents. *Occupational Therapy in Mental Health, 8*, 31–43.

Kehrberg, K.L., Kuskowski, M.A., Mortimer, J.A., & Shoberg, T.D. (in press). Validating the use of an enlarged, easier-to-see Allen Cognitive Level Test in geriatrics. *Physical and Occupational Therapy in Geriatrics.*

Kielhofner, G. (1992). *Conceptual foundations of occupational therapy.* Philadelphia: F.A. Davis.

Moore, D.S. (1978). *An occupational therapy evaluation of sensorimotor cognition: Initial reliability, validity, and descriptive data for hospitalized schizophrenic adults.* Unpublished master's thesis, University of Southern California, Los Angeles.

Newman, M. (1987). *Cognitive disability and functional performance in individuals with chronic schizophrenic disorders.* Unpublished master's thesis, University of Southern California, Los Angeles.

Spitzer, R.L. (Ed.). (1987). *Diagnostic and statistical manual of mental disorders. III-Revised. (DSM-III-R).* Washington, DC: American Psychiatric Association.

Wilson, D.S., Allen, C.K., McCormack, G., & Burton, G. (1989). Cognitive disability and routine task behaviors in a community based population with senile dementia. *Occupational Therapy Practice, 1,* 58–66.

Woodroff, W.A., Goodwin, D.W., & Guze, S.B. (1973). *Psychiatric diagnosis.* New York: Oxford Press.

World Health Organization. (1980). *International classification of impairments, disabilities and handicaps (ICIDH).* Geneva: Author.

BIBLIOGRAPHY

1982

Allen, C.K. (1982). Independence through activity: The practice of occupational therapy. *American Journal of Occupational Therapy, 36,* 731–739.

Allen, C.K., & Mendel, W.M. (1982). Chronic illness and staff burnout: Revised expectations for change in the supportive-care model. *International Journal of Partial Hospitalization, 1,* 191–201.

1985

Allen, C.K. (1985). *Occupational therapy for psychiatric diseases: Measurement and management of cognitive disabilities.* Boston: Little, Brown.

1987

Allen, C.K. (1987). Activity: Occupational therapy's treatment method. 1987 Eleanor Clarke Slagle lecture. *American Journal of Occupational Therapy, 41,* 563–575.

Allen, C.K., & Allen, R.E. (1987). Cognitive disabilities: Measuring the social consequences of mental disorders. *Journal of Clinical Psychiatry, 48,* 185–191.

1988

Allen, C.K. (1988). Cognitive disabilities. In S. Robinson (Ed.), *Mental health focus* (pp. 3–18—3–33). Rockville, MD: American Occupational Therapy Association.

Allen, C.K. (1988). Preface. The development of standardized clinical evaluations in mental health. *Occupational Therapy in Mental Health, 8,* ix–x.

Allen, C.K. (1988). Occupational therapy: Functional assessment of the severity of mental disorders. *Hospital and Community Psychiatry, 39,* 140–142.

1989

Allen, C.K. (1989). Treatment plans in cognitive rehabilitation. *Occupational Therapy Practice, 1,* 1–8.

Allen, C.K. (1989). Psychiatry. In T. Malone (Ed.), *Physical and occupational therapy: Drug implications for practice.* Philadelphia: Lippincott.

Allen, C.K., Foto, M., Sperling, T.M., & Wilson, D. (1989). Outpatient occupational therapy Medicare part B guidelines (DHHS Transmittal No. 565). In *Health insurance manual*. Baltimore, MD: Health Care Financing Administration.

Heimann, N.E., Allen, C.K., & Yerxa, E.J. (1989). The Routine Task Inventory: A tool for describing the functional behavior of the cognitively disabled. *Occupational Therapy Practice, 1*, 67–74.

Wilson, D.S., Allen, C.K., McCormack, G., & Burton, G. (1989). Cognitive disability and routine task behaviors in a community based population with senile dementia. *Occupational Therapy Practice, 1*, 58–66.

1991

Allen, C.K. (1991). *Change within the Allen cognitive level 3, 4 and 5*. Paper presented at the annual conference of the American Occupational Therapy Association, Houston, TX.

1992

Allen, C.K. (1992). Cognitive disabilities. In N. Katz (Ed.), *Cognitive rehabilitation: Models for intervention and occupational therapy*. Boston: Andover Medical Publishers.

Allen, C.K., Earhart, C.A., & Blue, T. (1992). *Occupational therapy treatment goals for the physically and cognitively disabled*. Rockville, MD: American Occupational Therapy Association.

OCCUPATIONAL THERAPY ASSESSMENTS

1988

Earhart, C.A., & Allen, C.K. (1988). *Cognitive disabilities: Expanded activity analysis*. Colchester, CT: S&S/Worldwide.

1990

Allen, C.K. (1990). *Allen Cognitive Level Test Manual* (with kit included). Colchester, CT: S&S/Worldwide.

1991

Josman, N., & Katz, N. (1991). Allen Cognitive Level Test Problem-Solving (ACL-PS) test. *American Journal of Occupational Therapy, 45*, 331–338.

1992

Allen, C.K., Kehrberg, K., & Burns, T. (1992). *Evaluation instruments*. In C.K. Allen, C.A. Earhart, & T. Blue, *Occupational therapy treatment goals for the physically and cognitively disabled* (pp. 31–84). Rockville, MD: American Occupational Therapy Association.

In Press

Kehrberg, D., & Schoberg, T. (In press). *Large Allen Cognitive Level Test. (LACL)*. Minneapolis, MN: VA Medical Center, GRECC.

Chapter Nine

Theory Analysis

Kay F. Walker

Theory analysis provides a means to examine the unique features of a theory and, when applied to several theories in a field, can be used to identify major theoretical endeavors of that field. Because a theory is an attempt to explain, predict, or clarify phenomena, analysis of several theories in a profession serves to illuminate the field's major theoretical efforts.

In this chapter, the works of Claudia Allen, Jean Ayres, Gail Fidler, Gary Kielhofner, Lela Llorens, Anne Mosey, and Mary Reilly are analyzed in terms of (1) the theorists' backgrounds, (2) the processes of theory development, (3) the major premises posited by the theorists, (4) the clinical application of the theories, (5) the scope and complexity of the theories, and (6) the theorists' efforts to validate and disseminate the theory. Progress made by these theorists in the development of theory for occupational therapy is explored through the identification of areas of theoretical agreement and areas where theory development is needed. The status of theory development for OT practice in adult physical dysfunction is also discussed.

Theory analysis may include the evaluation of theory through the use of checklists (Chinn & Jacobs, 1983), models (Meleis, 1985), or frameworks (Duldt & Giffin, 1985). Theory evaluation can help therapists to select theory for practice, students to analyze theory for learning, and writers to synthesize theory for theory development. However, evaluation of the strengths and weaknesses of a theory is idiosyncratic to the perspective of the analyzer. To one person a theory may be judged as parsimonious and clinically useful, whereas to another that same theory may seem vague and of little value.

Therefore, in this chapter, which compares seven OT theories, the relative merits and flaws of the seven theories are not discussed. The purpose of this final chapter is not to assess the theories, but rather to review and compare them for their contribution to the contemporary status of theory in occupational therapy.

BACKGROUND OF THEORISTS

A theorist's background influences her or his career development and hence theory development. Statements of theoretical positions reflect very individualized perceptions that have been shaped by the person's life experiences and the prevailing social climate, national events, and professional issues of the time in which the person has lived. Examination of a theory against a backdrop of the theorist's life and times reveals important influences that contributed to the person the theorist became and therefore to the theory that was developed. The backgrounds of the seven theorists included in this book are reviewed from a historical perspective (see Table 9-1).

1910 to 1950

1910 to 1950—National Events

During the years 1910 to 1950, the United States was involved in World War I (1917–1918) and World War II (1939–1945). In these years, the 19th amendment to the Constitution was ratified, ensuring women's voting rights (1920). Citizens suffered through the stock market crash (1929) and the "Great Depression" (1930–1939). In 1947, the polio epidemic threatened the lives and health of many Americans (Hopkins, 1988; Reed & Sanderson, 1980).

1910 to 1950—Occupational Therapy

The OT profession was established in 1917, and its growth was influenced by the two world wars. During the period 1910–1950, educational training developed from non-degree training courses to master's degree programs, a journal was established, the populations treated in OT changed, and individuals who would go on to make major theoretical contributions to OT were born.

By the time the United States entered World War I, the National Society for the Promotion of Occupational Therapy had been organized, with its membership numbering 47 physicians, social workers, nurses, artists, and teachers. The United States' involvement in World War I provided an impetus for expansion of occupational therapy as OT reconstruction aides were trained to work with the wounded soldiers. In the next five years, training programs were designed, training manuals written, and a journal, *Archives of Occupational Therapy*, published (1922). With the increase in the number of training programs for occupational therapists came the establishment of educational standards (1923) and, by 1939, the registration examination.

World War II greatly stimulated the growth of the field and influenced the direction of OT treatment. In 1937, there were twice as many occupational therapists in psychiatric settings as in general hospital and orthopedic facilities, but the war-

Table 9-1 Historical Perspectives 1910–1950

	National and OT Events		*Theorists*
National events	World War I (1914–1918) 19th Amendment ratified (1920) Stock market crash (1929) Great Depression (1930–1939) World War II (1939–1945) Polio epidemic (1947)	**Fidler**	Born 1916, Spencer, Iowa Oldest of 4 children Debating team, sports in high school BA education and psychology (1938) Aide in state mental hospital U Penn OT certificate (1942), White Institute of Psychiatry and Psychology (1947–1951) First publication, *AJOT* (1948)
Occupational therapy events	National Association for Promotion of Occupational Therapy formed (1917) Reconstruction aides trained for WWI *Archives of OT* (1922). Later, *OT and Rehabilitation* (1925) and finally *American Journal of OT* (1947) War emergency courses for WWII Educational standards (1923) More OTs in psychiatry in 1937 but increase in physical disabilities OT with WWII Registration examination (1939)	**Reilly**	Born 1916, Boston, MA Strict girls' school Boston University OT Certificate 1940 U.S. Army Medical Dept. (1941–1955) First paper, *OT & Rehab* (1943)
		Ayres	Born 1923, California farm Childhood illnesses First publication, *AJOT* (1949)
		Llorens	Born 1933, Shreveport, LA Pre-Civil Rights era
		Mosey	Born 1938 3rd of 7 children
		Allen	Born 1941, Oregon farm
		Kielhofner	Born 1949, Oran, Missouri farm

time need for occupational therapy in the treatment of the injured soldier resulted in increased development of treatment techniques in physical disabilities. The number of OT programs increased from 5 to 18 during the period 1940–1945, and the population of therapists nearly doubled between 1941 and 1946. OT graduate education began with the establishment of the first OT master's degree program in 1947 at the University of Southern California (Hopkins, 1988; Reed & Sanderson, 1980).

1910 to 1950—The Theorists

Both Fidler and Reilly were born in 1916, one year before the United States entered WW I and before occupational therapy was organized as a profession. The independent and goal-oriented nature of the careers of these two women was becoming more socially acceptable by the time Fidler and Reilly were growing up. Women had secured the right to vote and, because of the wars, had been initiated into previously male vocations, such as military nursing and civilian assembly line work. In addition, early school experiences seem to have fostered the independence of both Fidler and Reilly. Fidler's high school sports and debating team activities provided outlets for independent expression, and Reilly's early schooling in a strict scholastic girl's school contributed to her lifelong interest in scholarly pursuits. As college graduates in the late 1930s, Fidler and Reilly found OT training through the established one-year certificate programs.

Early employment experiences influenced the directions of Fidler's and Reilly's careers. Fidler's first job was in psychiatry, setting her lifelong focus on mental health occupational therapy. Her first publication in 1948 concerned psychological evaluation of OT activities. After one year of working with children, Reilly worked for 14 years in the U.S. Army Medical Department in physical disabilities and she co-authored her first publication there in 1943 (Light & Reilly, 1943). Her enduring concern with the nature of the profession was evidenced in this first publication in which she addressed the relationship of occupational therapy to physical therapy.

Ayres was born in 1923 and thus was influenced by national and professional forces similar to those affecting Fidler and Reilly. However, Ayres' childhood on a farm in California during the Depression years, her battles with childhood illnesses, and her struggles with family issues seem to have been key elements in the development of her characteristic determination and independence. She obtained her OT education from the University of Southern California (USC) in 1945 at the time when the country's first OT master's degree was being developed there by Margaret Rood. This academic climate promoting the obtaining of advanced degrees may have influenced Ayres' use of scientific research methodology for theory development, and Rood's neurophysiologic theories may have promoted Ayres' use of neuroscience in her theory. Ayres' first OT job was in a psychiatric

Table 9-2 Continued Historical Perspective 1950–1980s

	1950–1960	1960–1970	1970–1980	1980–1992
National Events	Korean War begins (1951) VR Act of 1954 Federal money for health professions training	Civil Rights movement Kennedy, Johnson administrations Vietnam War Medicare	Watergate Women's movement Ecology issues P.L. 94-142 Education for All Handicapped Children's Act	Corporate health care Inflation Federal money cutbacks Information age
Occupational Therapy Events	Shift from acute to chronic care as medicine controls polio, TB, etc. WFOT formed (1952) Therapeutic use of self in OT psychiatry Improved rehab techniques	OT shortages—roles absorbed by other professions OT in the community Group techniques & object relations in OT psychiatry Entry MA at USC (1964) AOTA-business; AOTF-research Theory: Reilly—occupational behavior Ayres—sensory integration Llorens—developmental	Accountability in health care AOTA practice standards OT licensure Specialty sections Mosey's frames of reference for OT practice	Research emphasis OT doctoral degrees Training programs: TOTEMS; SCOPE; ROTE; PIVOT Governmental representation Role delineation Kielhofner et al—model of human occupation

continues

Table 9-2 Continued

	1950–1960	1960–1970	1970–1980	1980–1992
Fidler	*Intro to Psychiatric OT* (1954) Coordinator AOTA Mental Health Institute (1952–1955) Instructor, U. Penn; Dept Mental Health (1955–1957) Supervision workshops, Columbia U	ECS lecture (1965) *OT: A Communication Process in Psychiatry* (1963) Directorships: NY Neuropsych. Inst., Activities Therapy; NYU OT MA in psychiatry	Associate Director AOTA (1971–1975) Adjunct appts. several universities Consultant to hospitals Administrator, state mental health	AOTA Award of Merit Consultancies NYU, NY Mental Health CEO—hospital *Recapturing Competence: A System's Change for Geropsychiatric Care* (1992)
Reilly	UCLA Neuropsychiatric Institute (1959–1968) Intrinsic motivation theory of B. Smith	ECS Lecture (1962) USC OT Faculty, Graduate Director & Program Chair	*Play as Exploratory Learning* (1974) Retired (1977)	Charter member AOTF Academy of Research (1983) Article on client vs patient (1984)
Ayres	MA OT USC (1954) USC Faculty (1954–1968)	ECS Lecture (1963) AOTA Award of Merit (1965) PhD USC (1961) Postdoctoral work Brain Research Institute (1964–1965) USC special ed. faculty (1966–1977)	*Sensory Integration and Learning Disorders* (1972) Sensory Integration Tests USC OT faculty (1976–1988) Private foundation research money Ayres Clinic opened	Charter member AOTF Academy of Research (1983) Retires from Ayres Clinic (1984) *Developmental Dyspraxia & Adult Onset Apraxia* (1985) AOTF A. Jean Ayres Award Created (1987) Died, December 16, 1988 *Sensory Integration & Praxis Tests* (1989)

Llorens			
BS OT W Michigan U (1954) Lafayette Clinic Pediatric Psychiatry, influence of research team (1958–1968)	First publication, *AJOT* (1960) Instructor Wayne State (1960–1968) MA Wayne State (1962) *Developing Ego Functions* Llorens & Rubin (1967) OT consultant (1968–1971) ECS Lecture (1969)	U FL faculty (1971–1976) U FL Chair (1976–1982) PhD Walden U (1976) *Consultation in the Community* (1973) *Application of Developmental Theory* (1976)	San Jose State OT Chair (1982–present) *OT Sequential Client Care Record* AOTA Award of Merit (1986) AOTF Meritorious Service Award (1989)
Mosey			
BS OT U Minn (1960) MA OT NYU (1965) PhD NYU (1968) NY Neuropsychiatric Institute (1962–1966) Instr OT Columbia U (1966–1968) First publication, *AJOT* (1968) *OT Theory and Practice* (1968)	NYU OT chair (1972–1980) *3 Frames of Reference for Mental Health* (1970) *Activities Therapy* (1973)	*OT: Configuration of a Profession* (1981) ECS Lecture (1985) *Psychosocial Components of OT* (1986) *Applied Scientific Inquiry in the Health Professions—An Epistemological Orientation* (1992)	

continues

Table 9-2 Continued

	1950–1960	1960–1970	1970–1980	1980–1992
Allen		BS OT San Jose St U (1963) 1st jobs in pediatrics & adult psychiatry in PA MS OT NYU (1968)	Moved to California (1973) USC faculty Chief OT at Los Angeles County, USC Medical Center	Chief of OT Psych LA/USC Med Ctr USC faculty Medical reviewer for Allied Health-Blue Cross of California OT for Psychiatric Diseases: Measurement & Management of Cognitive Disabilities (1985) Cognitive Disabilities: Expanded Activity Analysis (1987) ECS Lecture (1987) Allen Cognitive Level Test Manual (1990) OT Treatment Goals for the Physically & Cognitively Disabled (1992)
Kielhofner		Monastic college for 2 years Vietnam conscientious objector Hospital recreation job	BA Psychology St. Louis U (1971) MS OT USC (1975) DPH USC (1979) First publication, AJOT (1976) Neuropsychiatric Institute, Los Angeles (1975–1979) USC OT faculty (1977–1979) VCU OT faculty (1979–1984)	Charter member AOTA Academy of Research (1984) Boston U OT faculty (1984–1986) U Ill OT chair (1986–present) Health through Occupation (1983) Psychosocial OT (1983) Model of Human Occupation (1985) A Jean Ayres Award (1988) Conceptual Foundations of OT (1992)

setting, where she published her first journal article in 1949 on the use of crafts with electroshock patients.

Born in 1933, Llorens grew up in the South before the Civil Rights movement, at a time when racial segregation was the norm. Llorens' personal situation and her father's goal-oriented childrearing practices seem to have been major contributing factors to her ambitions to surpass the usual limited expectations for black females in the South and to achieve independent career success.

Mosey was born in 1938 and grew up in a large Irish family where she was the third of seven children. Claudia Allen was born in 1941 and grew up on a farm in Oregon. Kielhofner, the youngest of the seven theorists, was born in 1949 into an extended farm family. By the time Kielhofner was born, Fidler and Reilly were experienced therapists, Reilly and Ayres had each published an article in OT journals, Llorens was beginning college, and Mosey was in high school. While Kielhofner was still a youngster, these other authors would go on to develop theories that he would later study before developing his own theory. These events occur in the next period to be discussed, 1950–1992 (see Table 9-2).

1950 to 1992

1950 to 1992—National Events

Major events in the United States during this period included involvement in the Korean war in the early 1950s and, in the 1960s, the Civil Rights movement, protests against U.S. involvement in the Vietnam War, the "Great Society" of the Johnson administration that provided federal funding for social and health programs, the establishment of Medicare, and the first walk on the moon. The 1970s saw the Watergate scandal, the modern-day women's movement, concern with ecology, and the passage of the Education for all Handicapped Children's Act of 1974. Inflation, cutbacks in federal spending, the "information age," and corporate health care characterized the 1980s.

1950s—OT Events and the Theorists

During the 1950s, improved OT techniques for physical disabilities were developed through federally funded rehabilitation programs. The focus shifted from acute care, such as bedside therapy for the injured soldier, to more chronic care as the war ended and medical science conquered such diseases as tuberculosis and polio. The World Federation of Occupational Therapists was formed. Occupational therapy in psychiatry focused on the therapeutic use of self, and Fidler's psychodynamic and psychoanalytic theories for the field in psychiatry were developed. Fidler and her husband (a psychiatrist) co-authored the book *Introduction to Psychiatric Occupational Therapy*, published in 1954. Her leadership in mental health occupational therapy was recognized in her appointment as coordinator of AOTA's Psychiatric Study Project 1955–1957 (Hopkins, 1988).

During the 1950s, the other theorists were involved in formative experiences that influenced the direction of their careers and theory development. From 1959 to the mid-1960s, Reilly was at the University of California at Los Angeles Neuropsychiatric Institute, where her mentor, B. Smith, influenced her thinking on intrinsic motivation. Ayres completed her master's degree in occupational therapy in 1954, worked with children with cerebral palsy, and was appointed to the USC faculty. Completing her OT education in 1953, Llorens worked in pediatric psychiatry at the Lafayette Clinic, where, over the course of the next ten years, she was involved in teaching, research, and clinical roles with colleagues and mentors who were influential in her career development. In the late 1950s, Mosey was in college, where she was influenced by Marvin Lepley, an early mentor; Allen was finishing high school; and Kielhofner was in grade school.

1960s—OT Events and the Theorists

In the 1960s, the number of occupational therapists did not keep up with the demands for OT services, and other disciplines absorbed roles created by the shortage of occupational therapists. Group techniques and object relationships were developed for mental health OT, occupational therapy in community-based settings was emphasized, and the American Occupational Therapy Foundation (AOTF) was established in 1965 to promote research.

OT theory developed further with the emergence of Reilly's occupational behavior theory, Ayres' sensory integration theory, and Llorens' developmental theory (Hopkins, 1988). Their contributions to theory development were recognized as each, including Fidler as well, was awarded Eleanor Clarke Slagle Lectureships in the 1960s. Reilly was honored as the Eleanor Clarke Slagle lecturer in 1962 and gave the lecture in which she stated her often-quoted OT premise: "Man, through the use of his hands, as they are energized by mind and will, can influence the state of his own health" (Reilly, 1962, p. 2). In 1963, Ayres lectured on perceptual motor development. Fidler's lecture in 1965 was on the teaching-learning process. In 1969, Llorens presented her developmental framework of occupational therapy in her Slagle lecture.

Fidler was professionally productive during the 1960s, publishing a book, *Occupational Therapy: A Communication Process in Psychiatry*, in 1963, directing professional education at New York State Neuropsychiatric Institute, and coordinating the master's program in mental health OT both at New York University (NYU) and Columbia University. Mosey was in school during the 1960s, completing her undergraduate OT degree in 1961, her OT master's degree in 1965, and her doctorate degree in 1968. She was influenced by Fidler, who was at the Neuropsychiatric Institute during the four years Mosey worked there and who was also director of the OT master's program at NYU when Mosey was a student there.

Allen completed her OT education in 1963 and was married that same year. She held her first OT jobs in pediatrics and adult psychiatry and in 1968 completed her master's degree. During these years, she studied and observed the functional problems of persons with chronic disorders which were later to become the focus of her theory development.

In 1960, Llorens published her first article; in 1962 she completed her master's work; and in 1967 she co-authored the book, *Developing Ego Functions* (Llorens & Rubin, 1967). During the 1960s, Ayres completed her doctoral work and engaged in postdoctoral studies at the Brain Research Institute, confirming her interest in the neurosciences. In the mid-1960s, Reilly served as chairperson and graduate faculty member at USC. Kielhofner's classical and rigorous scholarly background in a Catholic seminary high school fueled his ability and interest in writing. He completed high school and began college during the 1960s.

1970s—OT Events and the Theorists

In the 1970s, accountability was the watchword in health care, and the AOTA adopted several documents that addressed quality care in occupational therapy: (1) standards for practice in mental health, developmental disabilities, physical disabilities, and home health; (2) guidelines for administration and supervision; (3) a statement on referral; (4) revised essentials for accredited curricula; (5) a code of professional ethics; (6) an official definition of occupational therapy; and (7) uniform terminology guidelines. Occupational therapists were licensed in New York in 1976, and other states soon developed licensure laws. Specialization was recognized with the adoption of special interest sections in mental health, physical disabilities, developmental disabilities, sensory integration, and geriatrics. In OT theory, Mosey's emphasis on frames of reference for OT practice gained national recognition (Hopkins, 1988).

Two of Mosey's major works, *Three Frames of Reference for Mental Health* (1970) and *Activities Therapy* (1973), addressed the need for a frame of reference to guide practice, a need in keeping with the widespread concern that the field have standards, ethics, and defined practice guidelines. Mosey taught her theories to OT graduate and undergraduate students at NYU, where she also chaired the OT program for eight years during the 1970s.

In the 1970s, Fidler's publications addressed broad professional issues and reflected the concerns encountered in her work experiences as associate executive director of AOTA for five years, adjunct faculty to several universities, and consultant to hospitals and a state mental health agency.

The establishment of sensory integration as one of AOTA's special interest sections reflected the impact that Ayres' work was having on the field in the 1970s.

During this decade, Ayres served as an OT faculty member at USC and established the Ayres Clinic, training and teaching students in sensory integration therapy. Her research efforts were funded through grants from a private foundation. She authored two books during the 1970s, *Sensory Integration and Learning Disorders* (1972a) and *Sensory Integration and the Child* (1979).

Llorens continued the development of her framework for OT practice in her book *Application of a Developmental Theory for Health and Rehabilitation* (1976) and, reflecting the national trend for developing OT consultancy roles, edited the book *Consultation in the Community: Occupational Therapy in Child Health* (1973). She completed her doctoral degree during this decade and served as OT faculty member and then chair at the University of Florida.

In 1974, Reilly's book *Play as Exploratory Learning* was published; it was the culmination of the work-play theory of occupational behavior that she and her students had been developing for the three previous decades. Allen moved to California in 1973 and held a joint position as faculty at USC and OT director at USC Medical Center. Allen's focus on cognition and neurobiology contrasted with Reilly's occupational behavior theory that prevailed in the USC academic program. Allen was influenced by Reilly and, simultaneously, brought a different perspective to the faculty discussions. By the time Reilly retired from her faculty position at USC in 1977, she had influenced the thinking of many students over the years, most notably Gary Kielhofner. Kielhofner completed his bachelor's degree in psychology in 1971. In 1975, he received his master's degree in occupational therapy at USC, where the mentoring relationship he enjoyed with Mary Reilly was a major determining factor in the development of his theoretical formulations. Kielhofner went on to publish several papers, earn his doctorate degree, and serve as OT faculty member in two universities in the 1970s.

1980 to 1992—OT Events and the Theorists

The 1980s were characterized by an increased emphasis on research, study of OT personnel shortages (AOTA, 1985a), national training initiatives, increases in graduate education, entry-level role delineation concerns, political action, and human occupation theory. The AOTF's research initiatives included grants for OT research and sponsorship of (1) the research forum at the AOTA national conferences, (2) the publication *Occupational Therapy Journal of Research*, and (3) the honorary Academy of Research. The AOTA initiated continuing education courses in several areas: TOTEMS, Training: Occupational Therapy Management in Schools (1979); PIVOT, Planning and Implementing Vocational Readiness in Occupational Therapy (1985b); ROTE, the Role of Occupational Therapy with the Elderly (1986a); and SCOPE, Strategies, Concepts, and Opportunities for Program Development and Evaluation (1986b). In 1987, PATRA, Professional and Technical Role Analysis, was begun as a followup to the 1981 role delineation study. The AOTA Government and Legal Affairs Division successfully lobbied the passage of legislation affecting occupational therapy, such as Medicare amendments to provide increased funding for OT services.

The number of master's programs slowly but steadily increased in the 1980s (American Occupational Therapy Association [AOTA], 1985c), and the field resolved the debate of master's level entry into occupational therapy by encouraging (not mandating) the development of OT graduate education programs. Two students were graduated from the occupational therapy doctoral program at New York University in 1984, initiating the doctoral degree as the terminal degree in occupational therapy (AOTA, 1985c). The USC doctoral program in occupational science opened in 1989 with the intent to develop research and theory in the science of occupation in health and dysfunction (Brown, 1991). Texas Women's University opened the first OT doctoral program in a public university in 1993 (AOTA, 1993) and this, together with existing doctoral programs at NYU, Boston University, and USC, brought to four the number of OT doctoral programs in the nation.

In 1980, occupation was officially adopted as the major concern of occupational therapy (Hopkins, 1988). This event coincided with increasing interest in the human occupation model of Kielhofner and Burke, and Kielhofner's emergence as a leader in theory development for occupational therapy. Having completed his doctorate degree in 1979, Kielhofner assumed faculty positions at Virginia Commonwealth University and Boston University and became chair at the University of Illinois. In addition to journal publications, his first three books described the human occupation model. In 1983, Kielhofner edited *Health Through Occupation* and co-authored with Barris and Watts *Psychosocial Occupational Therapy* (Barris, Kielhofner, & Watts, 1983); in 1985 he edited *A Model of Human Occupation*. Kielhofner's contributions to the field were recognized by his appointment for charter membership in the AOTF Academy of Research in 1984 and the AOTF A. Jean Ayres Award for his contributions to theory in 1988. In his most recent book (1992), he reviewed conceptual foundations of OT.

In the mid- and late 1980s, Allen emerged as a new OT theorist. She published *Occupational Therapy for Psychiatric Diseases* in 1985 and co-authored *Cognitive Disabilities—Expanded Activity Analysis* in 1988. In 1987 she was awarded the Eleanor Clarke Slagle lectureship for her work in cognitive disabilities and chronic disorders; her address was entitled "Activity: Occupational Therapy's Treatment Method." Allen also co-authored a text on OT treatment of cognitive diseases (Allen, Earhart, & Blue, 1992) and published the *Allen Cognitive Level Test Manual* (1990).

From 1980 to 1992, the other theorists continued to be recognized nationally for their contributions to the field. They were productive in various ways, continuing to develop their theories, to pursue work activities, and, in some cases, to begin to gear down or refocus their pursuits as they approached retirement age. Fidler served as a consultant and administrator to mental health facilities and, in 1980, received the AOTA Award of Merit. She authored articles on the impact of occupational therapists' beliefs and values on the profession (1990) and on the changes in mental health practice (1991). In 1990, she accepted an offer to help an OT professional education program through difficult times and became interim program director there. In addition, she co-authored a book (Fidler & Bristow, 1992) on the development of a nursing home facility into a comprehensive geropsychiatric treatment and rehabilitation hospital.

Reilly was named to the Academy of Research in 1984. Although withdrawn from the field, she expressed her opinions about the use of the terms "client" versus "patient" in a 1984 article.

Mosey and Llorens continue their careers in academia. Mosey published *Occupational Therapy: Configuration of a Profession* in 1981 and *The Psychosocial Components of Occupational Therapy* in 1986. She was named the 1985 Eleanor Clarke Slagle Lecturer. Mosey's (1992a, 1992b) recent works focus on scientific inquiry and differentiating applied and basic scientific inquiry. She explored these issues further in her book on epistemology in health professions published by AOTA (Mosey, 1992a). Llorens became chairperson at San Jose State University in 1982, the same year that her book *Occupational Therapy Sequential Client Care Record Manual* was published. She was awarded the AOTA Award of Merit in 1986, the AOTF A. Jean Ayres Award in 1988, and the AOTF Meritorious Service Award in 1989. Llorens co-authored a book on research (Oyster, Hanten, & Llorens, 1987) and published articles in developmental theory for OT (1991), OT for elders (1988), and consultation (1992).

Occupational therapy suffered the loss of one of its greatest theorists upon Jean Ayres' death on December 16, 1988. Despite her long illness, Ayres had continued to be productive. She retired from the Ayres Clinic in 1984 to complete the Sensory Integration and Praxis Test, published in 1989. Eulogized in several ways after her death, she was also recognized before her death. In 1984 she was named to the AOTF Academy of Research, and in 1987 the AOTF created the A. Jean Ayres Award for outstanding research in her honor. Her last written work, published posthumously in 1991, was a co-authored chapter (Ayres & Marr, 1991) in the book *Sensory Integration Theory and Practice*. This comprehensive text continues Ayres' tradition of inquiry, critical literature analysis, and theorizing about how the brain processes sensation for human functioning.

DEVELOPMENT OF THEORY

The relationship of theory to practice and research can be examined by reviewing how the theory was developed. First, how does the theory begin? What is the

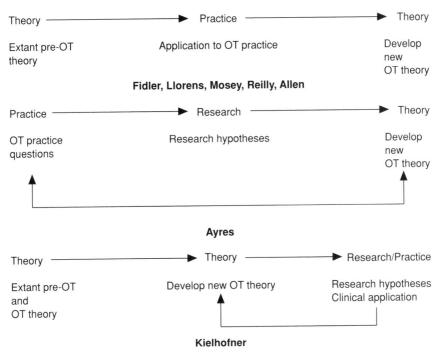

Figure 9-1 Three Theory Development Processes

impetus for the theorist to formulate the theory? What motivates the individual to assume the arduous task of committing formulations to writing? Is the writer driven by clinical questions, research findings, the need for theory in an area, or the desire for explanations of the profession? Second, what focus does the theory take? Is it specific to one clinical area, or does it address the entire field? Last, what is the role of research in the theory's development? Is the theory validated through research? These questions can be addressed by examining three processes of theory development adapted from Meleis (1985): the theory-practice-theory process, the practice-research-theory process, and the theory-theory-research/practice process (see Figure 9-1).

Theory-Practice-Theory Process

In the theory-practice-theory process, the theorist selects pre-OT theory (i.e., theory from other fields) and systematically applies it to OT practice to evolve primary OT theory, i.e., new theoretical formulations for occupational therapy.

The theory-practice-theory process is used when clinical questions pose problems for which the answers are not apparent in existing theoretical formulations. This process can be identified in Fidler's, Mosey's, Llorens', Reilly's, and Allen's work.

Fidler sought to develop a rationale for what her patients were doing in occupational therapy and whether it was helpful. Mosey, who was a student of Fidler, was inspired by Fidler's questioning of clinical practice theory definitions. Early in her career, Allen was influenced by Fidler's and Mosey's work, but saw OT being relegated to a nonscientific fringe service as psychiatry moved to treatment through medication and neurobiological explanations of mental illness. Llorens realized early in her clinical career that therapists could readily demonstrate the value of occupational therapy, but could not explain its value. She selected pre-OT theorists including Gesell, Piaget, Havighurst, Ericson, and Freud and systematically applied their theories to OT practice in formulating her developmental frame of reference. Reilly explained that the reductionist emphasis that she saw as a clinician ignored the importance of patient skills and competence.

These theorists were all troubled by the lack of sound explanations for OT, and they looked to other theoretical bases for relevant principles. Fidler embraced a psychoanalytic theory base; Mosey, a combination of pre-OT theories; Llorens, developmental theories; Reilly, a social psychology orientation; and Allen, cognitive development. These OT theorists all identified a need to clarify therapy rationale, and because OT theory was yet to be articulated, they looked beyond the field for relevant theory. They found new ways to apply existing theory from other fields in order to explain and conceptualize the rationale for OT practice.

Practice-Research-Theory Process

In the practice-research-theory process, the theorist identifies clinical practice questions and formulates theoretical hypotheses, conducts research aimed at answering questions and refuting or validating hypotheses, and uses research findings to develop and modify theory. This is the process used by Ayres in the development of her sensory integration theory.

In her efforts to formulate explanations and pose testable hypotheses about sensory integrative dysfunction, Ayres identified patient problems as the most challenging and motivating factor. She formulated her own ideas and consulted the neuroscience and neurobehavioral literature, designed and implemented research projects, and used the results of these studies to examine and modify her theory.

Theory-Theory-Research/Practice Process

The theory-theory-research/practice process uses existing pre-OT and primary OT theory to build new OT theory, which is then tested through research and clinical practice. This process is available to theorists when the field has developed sufficient primary theory—that is, theory developed by and for the field—so that the theorist can incorporate it in constructing new theory. Occupational therapy is just entering an era when this is possible because theory ground breaking has been done by such theorists as Fidler, Mosey, Llorens, Reilly, and Ayres.

Kielhofner's work is an example of the theory-theory-practice/research process. He and Burke used Reilly's occupational behavior paradigm (primary OT theory) and systems theory (pre-OT theory) to develop the model of human occupation (new OT theory). The recent work of Kielhofner and colleagues applies and tests this model through clinical practice and research.

Common Elements of Theory Development

Identification of three processes used to build theory in OT reveals several important common elements among the theorists reviewed. First, these OT theories emanate from a concern for OT practice. As a practice profession, occupational therapy has an urgent need to identify the unique theoretical underpinnings of services for patients and clients. Second, the pioneering efforts of Reilly, Fidler, Llorens, Mosey and, more recently, Allen bridged pre-OT and OT theory, making it possible for a second generation of OT theory to evolve. Third, research to test and validate OT practice and to build a body of knowledge for the profession is under way. The incorporation of research in theory building that is characteristic of Ayres' work is being increasingly emphasized in the work of Kielhofner and colleagues. Examining the processes by which theories are built illustrates common clinical practice concerns among the theorists, how theories build upon theories, and the relationship of research in contemporary OT theory development.

PREMISES

A review of the premises of the seven theorists is presented in Table 9-3. This review addresses the primary idea, conjecture, supposition, or position proffered by the theory and the key terms used in the theory. From this review of premises and key terms, similarities among the premises regarding activity, human competence, and OT clinical practice are identified.

Importance of Activities

The most obvious similarity among these seven theorists' premises is the focus on the importance of activities, tasks, and occupations for human functioning. Humans are not idle creatures—they are active, moving, stimulus-seeking beings who act on, interact with, and seek to alter their surroundings.

Table 9-3 Theorists' Premises and Terminology

Theorist	Premises	Terminology
Allen	Persons with disabilities will engage in activities to the extent that they have the cognitive capacity to do so. The degree of thought used to guide one's actions can be inferred by observing one's interactions with materials, objects, and people. OT adjusts activities so that they can be accomplished by persons with disabilities.	Cognitive levels Cognitive disabilities
Ayres	Learning occurs in the brain, and learning disabilities reflect neural dysfunction. Sensory integration supports neural functioning, and sensory integration dysfunction reflects neural dysfunction. Body senses and subcortical functions are important for visual, auditory, and cortical functions. Sensory integration therapy employs movement for its sensory-generating effects.	Sensory integration Tactile defensiveness Developmental dyspraxia Vestibular and bilateral integration dysfunction
Fidler	Purposeful activity and "doing" are the core of OT. Activity is a communication process for nonverbal communication and expression. Object relationships are used for exploration and mastery of the environment.	Object relation OT is a communication process Doing and becoming
Kielhofner	Humans are occupational beings who interact as open systems with the environment through the subsystems: volitional (personal causation, values, & interests); habituation (roles & habits); performance (motor, process, & communication/interpersonal skills). Humans interact with the environment in input-throughput-feedback processes. OT identifies and remedies problems in performance, habituation, and volitional subsystems to enhance occupational role functioning.	Model of Human Occupation (MoHo) Work-play continuum Occupational roles
Llorens	Humans develop chronologically and simultaneously in all areas of development. OT is a facilitation process for achievement and mastery of life tasks at various life stages. OT activities and interpersonal relationships are used to facilitate development.	OT is a developmental process Sequential Client Care Record (SCCR)

Mosey	OT treatment process recapitulates ontogenesis of development. Three frames of reference are useful in mental health OT: analytic, acquisitional, and developmental. Activities therapies use action-oriented interaction to promote mental health. Therapists should have a frame of reference for practice.	Recapitulation of ontogenesis Biopsychosocial model Activities therapy Epistemiology Scientific inquiry
Reilly	Humans are occupational beings who have an intrinsic need to act upon and master their environment. Occupational roles provide social meaning and belonging. Play is a precursor to occupational role and is important through life. OT uses occupations to restore abilities for role performance.	Occupational behavior Work-play continuum Occupational roles

Fidler posited that purposeful activity is the core of occupational therapy (Fidler & Fidler, 1978). She saw the use of activity as a communication process whereby thoughts and feelings are expressed nonverbally. Object relationships—that is, relationships with the nonhuman environment—are important for human development and functioning (Fidler & Fidler, 1963).

Mosey (1970) described the therapist's use of activity in various frames of reference for practice, rather than the nature of activity, tasks, and occupations for normal human function. Like Fidler, Mosey described activity therapies as those therapies that provide action-oriented interaction to help the patient with mental illness.

Activities, according to Llorens (1976), facilitate human growth and development by enabling one to explore the environment, establish relationships, acquire knowledge, and adapt successfully to one's world.

Ayres (1972a) described children's gross motor play activities in terms of sensory integrative properties and the organizing effects of movement in human neural functioning. Movement requires the integration of all the senses, is mediated at all levels of the neuroaxis, and generates important tactile, proprioceptive, kinesthetic, and vestibular sensations.

Taking a broad viewpoint, Reilly (1962) viewed humans as occupational beings who have an intrinsic need to act on and master their environment and to do so in ways that are in keeping with social role expectations. Meaning as a social being is derived through successful role performance whereby the individual is able to develop those skills necessary to meet role demands. One is satisfied with life and feels reinforced by one's society when one can perform in expected ways.

Building on Reilly's work, Kielhofner (1985) proposed that humans are occupational beings who interact as open systems with the environment. As open systems, humans are active, goal-directed, purposeful creatures who take in information and energy from the environment (intake), use this information or energy for self-maintenance or to initiate further interaction with the environment (throughput), act or produce interaction with the environment (output), and monitor and alter responses on the basis of feedback from the environment.

Concerned that activities are undervalued in OT and that their therapeutic value is hard to explain to those outside of OT, Allen (1987) sought to provide a philosophical framework to emphasize the value of activities as therapeutic. Convinced that humans engage in activity for a purpose and that humans use thoughts to guide activities, she proposed the levels of thought required to guide one's behavior in engaging in an activity. She used activities to explain cognitive deficits: "Disability is understood within the context of doing an activity" (Allen, 1987, p. 565).

In summary, Fidler said that "doing is becoming," Mosey advocated action-oriented interactions, Llorens described activity in the OT process of facilitating developmental progression, Ayres focused on the importance of movement for neutral integration, Reilly and Kielhofner described the occupational nature of humans, and Allen focused on the levels of thought necessary to perform activities.

Human Competence

These seven theorists agreed that, through action on and interaction with the environment, humans grow and develop those skills and abilities that enable them to be competent members of a society and to gain a sense of self and social worth.

Fidler (Fidler & Fidler, 1963) spoke of the interaction of competence, mastery, adaptation, and self-esteem. Through interaction with objects in the environment, humans respond to an innate drive to explore and master their environment. Through action-oriented experiences, humans test skills; clarify relationships; develop and integrate sensory, motor, cognitive, and psychological functions; become socialized to cultural norms and roles; and gain competence as social beings. The skills one develops through "doing" help one become competent in self-care, provide intrinsic gratification, and afford one the means to care for others. Skill development is influenced both by the environment and the individual's biological makeup.

Similarly, Mosey (1973) stated that, through engagement in activity, humans learn to perform life tasks necessary to meet their own needs and the demands of living in their community. Interaction with the nonhuman environment enables the individual to acquire the skills necessary for the performance of life tasks. Mosey defined life tasks as requiring not only the performance of manual skills but also interpersonal relationships, work roles, and recreation. In Llorens' (1970) outline of ten premises for the OT process, she states that humans naturally develop and master skills, abilities, and relationships simultaneously and chronologically across all areas of development (premises 1–4). This development is fostered by the interaction of the individual's genetic makeup and the environment (premises 5, 6).

Ayres' (1972a) sensory integration theory addressed the development of competence in humans in terms of learning and neural processes. She proposed that, because learning occurs in the brain and is dependent on neural processes, learning disabilities reflect dysfunction in neural functioning. The brain takes in information through the senses; thus integration and processing of sensory information are necessary for learning. The body senses (tactile, proprioceptive, kinesthetic, and vestibular) develop first and provide a basis for the development of visual and auditory systems. Subcortical functions develop first ontogenetically and phylogenetically and provide a basis for the development of cortical, conscious processes. Thus, Ayres considered the body senses and subcortical neural developmental processes to be important for the development of human competency.

Reilly (1974) viewed competency in terms of social role performance, particularly occupational role performance. Occupational roles develop in childhood through play, chores, and schooling as the child acquires the adaptive skills and interactive skills needed as a competent adult worker. Play and social recreation are important throughout life because they promote manipulatory and social skills necessary for role performance and provide socially accepted outlets for aggression.

In the human occupation model, Kielhofner (1985) proposed that the human open system includes three hierarchical subsystems: the volitional, habituation, and performance subsystems. The volitional subsystem addresses the human drive for competence and mastery and includes motivation and belief in one's ability to act (personal causation) and the development of interests and values. In the habituation subsystem, one develops habits and roles for efficient coping with daily life experience. Underlying the habituation subsystem is the performance subsystem, which includes motor, process, and communication skill development through symbolic, neurologic, and musculoskeletal components. These subsystems interact with the environment in an input-throughput-output feedback process, as noted above, to bring about occupational role functioning.

Allen (1987) stated: "Human functioning is the process of engaging in purposeful motor actions within a context of material objects and people" (p. 565). Interaction of individual and environment is seen in recommendations for adjusting the task parameters to enable the individual to perform. By defining what the patient needs to do to accomplish everyday tasks and what the therapist needs to do to adapt the task, Allen described cognitive levels needed for normal task performance.

In summary, these seven theorists proposed that human-environment interaction is the mechanism for the development of skills to master the environment and perform as competent members of a society. Fidler said that through doing one becomes competent. Mosey offered her organization of various frames of reference for conceptualizing skill development through activity. Llorens described interaction with the environment as crucial for human development. Ayres posed the relationship of learning to effective interaction with the environment through sensory systems and motor functioning. To Reilly, interaction with the environment in a play-work continuum was necessary for role skill development. Kielhofner viewed humans as open systems interacting with the environment for adaptive functioning. Allen defined the cognitive levels necessary to perform ordinary activities.

OT Clinical Practice

A third similarity of these OT theorists is the view that, just as activity is used to acquire skills, it can be used therapeutically to restore, regain, or renew skills.

To Fidler (Fidler & Fidler, 1963) occupational therapy in psychiatry was a communication process involving the psychodynamics of activities and therapeutic relationships. By engaging in activities, patients come to express their emotions and thoughts, learn to interact effectively with the nonhuman environment, and develop skills.

Mosey (1970) provided practical guidelines for the use of activity in therapy. She described the use of work-related, recreational, and creative tasks for improving psychosocial functioning. She promoted activities therapy as a way to use everyday interactions and activities to help persons function in the broader community.

Llorens (1970, 1976) described OT as a facilitation process that assists the individual to achieve and master the tasks of living presented at various life stages. The therapist functions as an enculturation agent to bridge the gap between the patient's functioning level and the level that is socially age-expected. Occupational therapy can facilitate the closure of developmental gaps and prevent further dysfunction through the judicious analysis, selection, and use of activities and interpersonal relationships (premises 9, 10).

Ayres' (1972a) sensory integrative therapy used carefully selected motor and sensory activities applied in a developmental sequence to elicit increasingly adaptive sensory and motor responding.

According to Reilly (1974), disease states run counter to the development of life role skills and result in role dysfunction and dissatisfaction. Occupational therapy promotes life satisfaction and self-actualization through the restoration of abilities needed for occupational role functioning.

Occupational therapy, according to Kielhofner (1985), addresses breakdowns in the human/environment open system interaction by identifying occupational role dysfunction and providing remediation at the subsystem level (performance, habituation, or volitional) required to restore or enhance occupational role functioning.

Allen (1987) selected disability as the focus of study and developed taxonomies of cognitive levels to delineate what is missing or lost from normal functioning in persons with disabilities. She described ways to adjust activities to a level that enables persons with disabilities to use their remaining capacities to achieve some degree of functioning.

Summary

Although these theorists present a variety of ideas and concepts that are enriched and embellished through their exploration of many issues in the profession, they repeatedly return to a few central themes: the view of humans as occupational beings, mastery of the environment through skill development, the ability of humans to affect their own state of health, and the therapeutic value of tasks, activi-

Table 9-4 Clinical Application of Theory

Theorist	Evaluation	Treatment	Patient Population and Setting

Allen	Allen Cognitive Level Test
	Routine Task Inventory
	Cognitive Disabilities Expanded
	    Activity Analysis
		Activities adjusted to cognitive level of
		    person w/disability
		Daily living skills
			Developed for adult mental health
			and expanded to adult physical
			dysfunction

Ayres	Southern California Sensory
	    Integration Tests
	Postrotary Nystagmus Tests
	Sensory Integration and Praxis Test
	Ayres' clinical observations
		Sensory integrative therapy with tactile,
		    proprioceptive, vestibular, and kines-
		    thetic emphasis
		Use of scooter boards, net hammock,
		    and suspended sings
			Children with learning disabilities in
			schools and community clinics

Fidler	Projective Diagnostic Battery Object History Play History Lifestyle Performance Profile Patient questionnaires Guidelines for program development	Activity analysis Prescriptive use of activities Task groups Nonverbal communication	Adult psychiatry in institutional and community settings
Kielhofner	Observation, history, interview, and projective assessments	Therapy principles for treatment planning	Applicable to all age and disability groups and settings, but roots are in psychosocial dysfunction

Llorens	Developmental Analysis, Evaluation
	    and Intervention Schedule
	    (DAEIS)
	Sequential Client Care Record
	    (SCCR)
		Age-appropriate activities
		Interpersonal relationships
			All developmental age groups,
			disabilities, and settings

Mosey	Survey Instruments: Group interaction, self-care, child care, work, and recreation Activity Configuration Questionnaires based on Fidler's	Use of groups Body image treatment Activities therapy	Adult and adolescent psychiatry in institutional and community settings
Reilly	Observation, history, and interview techniques	Use of arts, crafts, toys, games, and leisure activities	Applicable to all age and disability groups and settings, but focuses on adults in the community

ties, and occupations. It would appear that substantial work has been done to provide us with a working body of knowledge that can be confirmed through clinical practice and research, leading to refined theory building in occupational therapy.

CLINICAL APPLICATION

Evaluation Tools

Most of the theorists developed evaluation tools for OT practice, many of which were originally created for use in mental health occupational therapy. All of the theorists advocated the use of the therapist's observations and informal assessments (see Table 9-4).

Fidler constructed clinical observation tools for use in psychosocial evaluation: the Projective Diagnostic Battery, the Object History, the Play History, and the Lifestyle Performance Profile (1982). Mosey developed survey instruments for group interaction, self-care, child care work, and recreation. She also devised an activity configuration for analysis of time spent in various activities throughout the day and questionnaires based on Fidler's work (1973).

Llorens' framework (1976) for practice that spanned infancy through adulthood and aging advocated testing, evaluation, and observation to determine the developmental level of the patient. Reilly (1974) advocated the case method approach for patient treatment. Direct observations, testing, interview, and history taking were used for evaluation and clinical problem solving and to accommodate individual patient variations. Evaluation results were examined to identify patterns of success and failure, learning style, and level of function and to provide data for formulating an action plan.

Kielhofner (1985) edited a textbook that specifically applied the model of human occupation to five disability areas and included an assessment library of observation, history, interview, and projective assessment tools. The instruments (most were nonstandardized) were selected for applicability to the human occupation model, and many were in use before the publication of the model. Development of tools for the model is now under way.

In contrast to these theorists, Ayres devoted a substantial portion of her work to the development of standardized testing instruments for use in OT evaluation of children with learning disabilities. These tests include the Southern California Sensory Integration Tests (1972b), the Southern California Postrotary Nystagmus Test (1975), and, more recently, the Sensory Integration and Praxis Tests (1989). Sensory integration tests brought occupational therapy into the realm of psychometric testing, requiring therapists' adherence to standard administration and scoring procedures.

Allen's methods for evaluating human cognitive levels include the Allen Cognitive Level Test (ACL) (Allen, 1990) and the Routine Task Inventory (RTI)

(Allen, Earhart, & Blue, 1992). The ACL is used in conjunction with an interview to screen for the level of cognition the individual used in learning leather lacing. The RTI provides for detailed observation of the level of cognition used in performing daily living skills. Allen emphasized that the therapist's clinical observations play an important role in effective use of these evaluation instruments.

Treatment

OT treatment approaches developed by these theorists were predominantly based in mental health occupational therapy. Fidler's clinical contributions include her prescriptive use of activities, suggestions for the use of task groups, and use of activities in nonverbal communication and object relations work in mental health (Fidler & Fidler, 1954, 1963). Mosey regarded clinical practice as the scientific application of theory. The use of five types of groups (1973), treatment of distorted body image (1969), and guidelines for activities therapy in mental health (1973) comprise the specific treatment approaches she introduced.

Activities and relationships that are in keeping with the patient's age and life roles can be used to facilitate development, according to Llorens (1976). Her early work was in child psychiatry, although her developmental model is applicable across age and dysfunction categories.

Reilly's students applied her theory in various therapy settings, especially mental health, as described later in the section on dissemination.

Although so far primarily applied in psychosocial areas (Barris, Kielhofner, & Watts, 1983), Kielhofner's work (1985) provided a framework for conceptualizing OT evaluation and treatment across patient categories. Similarly, Allen's clinical work was in the area of mental health, but her recent book (Allen, Earhart, & Blue, 1992) includes application of the cognitive levels in physical dysfunction. Activities are analyzed for the cognitive processes requisite for accomplishing the task. The therapist selects, modifies, or adjusts the activity so that the patient can use existing cognitive abilities to accomplish the task.

An exception to these theories that began in mental health occupational therapy is Ayres' sensory integrative therapy. It uses equipment and devices aimed at generating bodily sensations of tactile, proprioceptive, kinesthetic, and vestibular systems. Ayres (1972a) developed the use of the scooter board, net hammock, and suspended swings of various types, which require adequate clinical space designed to accommodate this kind of equipment safely.

SCOPE AND COMPLEXITY

Scope addresses the range of the theory. Does it apply to all of occupational therapy or only to a part? Does it seek to explain the profession as a whole or to focus on one aspect of the profession? Is the theory a closed theory, or does it allow for expansion and further development? The review of complexity explores the number of concepts in each theory, the intensity of study needed to understand the theory, its implications, and the internal consistency of the theory.

Scope

As a group, these theories address the entire range of population ages, settings, and disabilities seen in OT practice, although the scope of each theory differs. Fidler's contribution to the body of knowledge in the field is perhaps most appropriately viewed in terms of various constructs for OT practice. She provided theoretical formulations for psychoanalytically based occupational therapy in psychiatry and expanded these to include new knowledge through the years. In addition, her work influenced the development of two other theorists reviewed in this book, Mosey and Llorens.

In scope, Mosey has helped articulate the wholeness of occupational therapy and its parts by presenting frameworks for viewing the profession and what we are using and doing. She provided (1) frameworks for structuring and thinking about the OT profession and its knowledge (1968, 1970, 1992a); (2) a taxonomy for identifying the elements of the profession (1981); and (3) therapy approaches for OT in mental health (1973, 1986).

Allen provided depth in a focused area of study, the level of cognition needed to perform tasks. She identified six levels of thinking that one uses and analyzed numerous ordinary tasks in terms of these levels. Allen described the cognitive requisites for performing a task, and conversely, the level of cognitive deficits that exists when an individual is unable to perform a task at a given level. Thus, her work is applicable across disability areas and diagnoses because it focuses on cognitive ability, regardless of the cause of the patient's problem.

The scope of Llorens' work included all of occupational therapy, but has been most applicable to pediatrics where more is known about developmental processes than in adulthood and aging. Llorens (1976) provided a way to conceptualize OT practice, to explain what occupational therapy is, and to be able to teach this to students. Because her work is a point of view for the field and embodies beliefs about the field, it could be considered a paradigm. However, Llorens presented her work more as a view of occupational therapy for practice than as a paradigm for the profession.

Sensory integration theory addressed a portion of the field of occupational therapy, occupational therapy for children with learning disabilities (Ayres, 1972a). Ayres' sensory integration theory was developed for the child who has no demonstrable neurological deficits but is having difficulty learning. It was not developed to address neurologic deficits, such as those encountered in mental retardation or cerebral palsy. Yet, principles for understanding sensory and motor functioning and for treatment have been found to be useful for several patient populations.

Reilly's work (1962) is considered a paradigm because she attempted to articulate the idea underlying the field of occupational therapy. She imposed order on multidisciplinary information to proclaim the particular features of the profession. Reilly's paradigm provides her grand-scale perception of the exciting uniqueness of occupational therapy.

Kielhofner's development of Reilly's paradigm stems from his position that there is a critical need to have a mutually agreed-on paradigm in OT. Going beyond Reilly, Kielhofner (1985) has provided a comprehensive model for dealing with the complexity of the occupational aspects of humans in a clinical situation. This model includes a framework for evaluation, treatment, and research.

Complexity

Fidler's work has been most valuable in articulating the constructs of object relationships, doing and becoming, competence, and mastery. These have not been reassembled into a complex and cogent theoretical framework that interrelates the various constructs, yet they express elements of OT practice. Fidler has consistently advocated the articulation of OT theory. She has stated that the fundamental concept underlying occupational therapy is viable, but that unless it is developed, it will be usurped by other professions.

Mosey progressively expanded and modified her theoretical contributions in a continued quest for a model for the profession. A prolific writer, Mosey's work has been complex. Her ideas have been presented in a logical and orderly way, though terminology in her synthesis works is sometimes awkward, perhaps due to the difficulty of clearly presenting distillations of the ideas of other theorists. Terminology in recent works has been clearly defined and used consistently. She has developed original ideas as her perceptions have been refined through her relentless examination of ideas underlying OT theory.

Allen described six cognitive levels from first-hand observations of how humans are able or unable to do tasks. Her rationale, definitions, task analyses, evaluations, and treatment applications provide a comprehensive yet practical way for therapists to think about the patient or client's thinking.

Llorens provided ten premises for OT practice that are succinctly stated, comprehensive, and internally consistent. She has continued to refine the application of these concepts in later works.

Ayres' complex theory of sensory integration requires knowledge of neuroscience and thoughtful study of the theory for thorough understanding. Her reliance on neuroscience literature requires the reader to have a background in neurophysiology and neuropsychology. Concepts are consistently and logically presented, building on one another. Terminology is well developed and used consistently throughout.

Although Reilly's ideas were simply and consistently presented, an understanding of her theory requires thoughtful study and careful reading of her writings and that of her students. Because the theory is a macroview of the profession, some readers may find it difficult to bring it from the realm of the theoretical to the practical.

Kielhofner's work on the model of human occupation demonstrated his belief in the need to develop a comprehensive theory for occupational therapy that could be developed through research. Thorough study is necessary to grasp the model in its complexity. His development of new meanings for existing terms and his introduction of new terms into the field have led to some confusion and criticism (Labovitz & Miller, 1986).

In summary, these seven theorists demonstrate a valiant commitment to writing the ideas that form the basis for the profession and the principles that guide OT intervention. Fidler presented constructs for OT practice; Mosey, conceptual frameworks for the profession, for OT practice in mental health, and for theory building; Allen, analyses of the cognitive ability needed to perform tasks; Llorens, a conceptualization of the OT practice process; Ayres, a research-based theory for OT practice in pediatrics; Reilly, a paradigm; and Kielhofner, a paradigm and a comprehensive practice model. The theories are intricate and complex in their own ways and are deserving of careful study for appreciation of the depths of knowledge offered.

DISSEMINATION, VALIDATION, AND FURTHER DEVELOPMENT

Throughout their careers, the seven theorists have consistently disseminated their ideas, hypotheses, and findings through writings, teachings, and presentations. They have also attempted to validate their theories and develop their ideas further through research and clinical application (See Table 9-5).

Dissemination

Estimating from the bibliographies in the preceding chapters of this text, this group of theorists have written 25 books and 240 articles and other scholarly writings. All of them have served as OT educators, and most of them have shared their ideas through workshops and presentations. Fidler has written 4 books and 22 articles and has disseminated her ideas through workshops, lectures, clinical teaching, supervision, and service to the AOTA. Mosey has written 6 books and 15 papers and has disseminated her concepts through OT graduate education and workshops. Many of Llorens' 76 publications and much of her teaching in work-

Table 9-5 Theory Dissemination, Research, and Application/Development of Theory by Others

Theorist	Books and Articles	Presentations	Research	Application/Development of Theory by Others
Allen	Cognitive disabilities Assessment of cognitive levels	Clinical teaching of: Assessment	Cognitive levels	Assessment of cognitive levels
Ayres	Sensory integration theory SI dysfunction Testing and treatment	Workshops, OT education, Clinical teaching of: Sensory integration Treatment	Sensory integration Learning disabilities Autism, aphasia	Sensory Integration International Adult psychiatry Aphasia Mental retardation Cerebral palsy Hyperactivity
Fidler	OT psychiatry OT theory Activities Professional issues	Workshops, Clinical teaching of: Group process OT psychiatry Program design Management Activities		
Kielhofner	Human occupation theory and application	OT education, Workshops	Human occupation Psychosocial problems Adolescents Delinquency Elderly Mentally retarded adults Assessment and instrument development	Learning disabilities Alcoholism Adults w/mental retardation Spinal cord injury Elderly Assessment and instrument development

continues

Table 9-5 Continued

Theorist	Books and Articles	Presentations	Research	Application/Development of Theory by Others
Llorens	Development theory for OT OT in child psychiatry Consultation in community Black culture OT record system CPM dysfunction	OT education of: Developmental theory	Emotional disturbance—children OT record system AOTF	
Mosey	OT theory OT psychiatry Activity	OT education, Workshops of: Frames of reference Activity		
Reilly	Work-play continuum OT education OT profession	OT education of: Play Work OT education OT profession		Roles Play Work Interests Motivation Curriculum design Temporal adaptation Occupational behavior theory Assessment

shops and graduate and undergraduate OT programs reflect aspects of her developmental theory. Ayres published 3 books, 52 articles, 22 test instruments, and 4 professional films. She informed students and therapists about sensory integration theory through workshops and clinical training in her Ayres Clinic. Reilly's theories have been disseminated through her writings (16 articles and 1 book) and through her students' works. As a scholar, Reilly's goal was to enable students to learn to think critically, utilize logical thought processes, and develop qualitative, quantitative, and historical perspectives. Kielhofner, who has produced 55 papers and 5 books, is the most prolific writer for his age of the theorists reviewed and the only example of dissemination through extensive collaborative authorship. He also teaches in workshops and classrooms. Allen, the newest of the theorists reviewed, has published 8 articles and 3 books and developed 2 test instruments.

Validation

Validation efforts vary among these theorists: some have validated their ideas empirically through years of clinical practice, some have conducted research, and some have stimulated others to do research.

Fidler derived her ideas from, and tested them through, clinical practice. Although she has not conducted research, she advocated that occupational therapists study activities according to a standardizing process to search for the meaning of activity and its application in the field.

Similarly, Allen developed her taxonomy of cognition for task performance from her clinical practice. In the practice arena, she and colleagues have developed test instruments and conducted research.

Mosey advocated research to test theories and theoretical foundations, but has not conducted research herself. She proposed research as indirectly related to practice and to practice frames of reference. The role of research in theory building should be to contribute to the theoretical base and body of knowledge. Through their modification of the theoretical base, research findings then trickle down to frames of reference for practice. Thus, clinical practice is based on theoretical foundations that are modified by research.

Llorens' nearly two decades of clinical practice contributed to the formulation of her ideas for a developmental theory of occupational therapy. She conducted research in child psychiatry and the use of her OT record system and has been instrumental in promoting research through her leadership role in the AOTF as well. Her Sequential Client Care Record (SCCR) and case study methods are clinical research data gathering tools, and she has coordinated their use with therapists in various states in the nation.

To construct sensory integration theory, Ayres conducted numerous research projects. The most prolific researcher of these seven theorists, Ayres' research efforts span more than two decades. Her work includes test instrument development and treatment efficacy studies with learning disabled children and, more recently, with autistic and aphasic children.

The focus of OT research, according to Reilly, should be to study the nature of occupation from a developmental perspective. Thus research should focus on achievement, creativity, aptitude, and interest patterns in relationship to occupations and activities. Because of Reilly's influence, a tradition of OT scholarly productivity has endured at USC for many years, and Reilly's students have been responsive to that tradition.

With the model of human occupation now well described, Kielhofner and his colleagues and students are undertaking research based on the model. This research is aimed at the development of assessments and testing of treatment based on the model.

Development of the Theory by Others

Further application, research, and development have occurred in sensory integration theory, occupational behavior theory, human occupation theory, and cognitive disability theory. Ayres' sensory integration theory has spawned more research efforts by clinicians and students than has any other theory to date. Therapists have applied the treatment principles to several patient populations, including children with mental retardation and other developmental disabilities and hyperactive, aphasic, autistic, and adult psychiatric patients. Supporters of her work established what is now Sensory Integration International (SII), a nonprofit corporation that supports sensory integration research and disseminates the theory. The faculty of SII comprises therapists from throughout the nation who conduct workshops to teach sensory integration theory and test administration and interpretation to occupational therapists in the United States and abroad.

Reilly's students have been instrumental in researching and applying her theory through (1) the development of survey, interview, observation, and history tools; (2) the description of roles and occupational stages, the influence of interests and motivation, and the play-work continuum; and (3) sequences and variables for clinical practice for use with adolescents with delinquent behaviors, geriatric patients, and persons with physical disabilities, mild mental retardation, and psychiatric disorders Her ideas about OT curricula have been incorporated into curriculum designs based on occupation (Levine, 1984). Her work profoundly influenced the development of Kielhofner's ideas.

The model of human occupation has stimulated research in the last decade, most of it since 1980. Kielhofner's students and colleagues have researched the model of human occupation with several patient groups, including children with learning disabilities, alcoholics, adults with retardation, persons with spinal cord injury, and the elderly. Other research efforts have addressed assessment and instrument development.

Although their work has influenced the thinking of occupational therapists, Fidler's, Mosey's, and Llorens' theories have not been developed through an identifiable body of research or through an identified group of researchers, and Allen's theory is just beginning to receive research attention. However, these theorists' works are cited in the literature when reference is made to basic ideas of occupational therapy and have been included in theory compilations (Clark & Allen, 1985; Kielhofner, 1992; Reed, 1984). Like Reilly, these theorists synthesized OT theory from theories in other fields and made it possible to develop theory from within the field, as Kielhofner has done.

All of these theorists generously shared their ideas through written and spoken communications. They have contributed their hypotheses and conceptualizations to the rest of the profession for use, examination, and improvement.

THEORY FOR PRACTICE IN PHYSICAL DYSFUNCTION

A review of seven major OT theories presented in this book reveals gaps in OT theory development concerning the two main patient treatment areas that comprise OT practice. Patients treated in OT are generally classified as (1) adolescent, adult, and aging persons with physical disabilities or psychosocial dysfunction and (2) infants and children with developmental or pediatric problems. The theories of Fidler, Mosey, Reilly, Allen, and Kielhofner focus on adolescents and adults with psychosocial dysfunction. Llorens' and Ayres' theories are considered pediatric theories. Llorens' developmental theory and, more recently, Kielhofner et al.'s model of human occupation encompass all OT clinical areas, including psychosocial dysfunction and physical disabilities and all age groups. Allen's theory of cognitive disability addresses adults with psychosocial dysfunction and, recently, adults with physical dysfunction.

However, theory originating in OT practice with adolescent, adult, and aging persons with physical disabilities is limited. This is interesting, considering that persons with physical disabilities comprise more than 83 percent of the patients served by occupational therapists (American Occupational Therapy Association, 1990).

This is not to say that OT practice in physical dysfunction is non-theory-based, for it is. Pre-OT theories of Rood, Bobath, Brunnstrom, and Knott and Voss underlie OT evaluation and treatment in this area. These theories were developed by physical therapists as pragmatic clinical applications of neuroscience and neurophysiology. Farber (1982) synthesized these treatment rationales in her model of neurorehabilitation for persons with central nervous system dysfunction.

Arnadottir (1990) applied theories of neurobehavior in her tool for assessing how cognitive perceptual deficits interfere with the performance of daily activities.

In addition, OT textbooks have been organized in the following ways: (1) to reflect three conceptual categories for OT evaluation and treatment in physical disabilities—neurodevelopmental, biomechanical, and rehabilitative approaches (Trombly, 1989); (2) to reflect the OT process in physical disabilities (Pedretti & Zoltan, 1990); and (3) to define the rationale and procedures for treatment in rehabilitation (Abreu, 1981). These textbooks incorporate theoretical and practical knowledge from anatomy, neuroscience, kinesiology, physical science, muscle physiology, and medicine and combine this with OT principles of activity analysis, self-care, and functional adaptation to provide a rich array of techniques for OT intervention in physical disabilities. Thus therapists have available a variety of treatment approaches and theoretical rationales to address the numerous human conditions encountered in physical disabilities practice.

Future development of theory for practice in physical dysfunction may take several directions: application of existing theory from pre-OT theory (Arnadottir, 1990; Farber, 1982); refinement of existing ways of organizing knowledge in physical dysfunction (Abreu, 1981; Pedretti & Zoltan, 1990; Trombly, 1989); initiation of new theoretical frameworks (Sabari, 1991); application of cognitive theory (Allen et al., 1992); and incorporation of physical dysfunction in the model of human occupation (Kielhofner, 1985). Whether these existing frameworks are sufficient to provide the theoretical bases for OT practice in physical dysfunction or whether researchers must develop additional theory in physical dysfunction, just as Fidler and Mosey developed theory for psychosocial dysfunction, is a question for the future.

Perhaps one or more of the current directions in the field holds promise for theory development in physical dysfunction, including clinical reasoning (Mattingly, 1991; Parham, 1986; Rogers, 1983), human performance (Christiansen & Baum, 1991), and occupational science (Clark et al., 1991).

COMMENT

It is interesting to speculate about what determines whether a theoretical formulation becomes widely adopted in the field. Does a theory come to have widespread and established acceptance solely on its merit and the merit of its postulates, research, and clinical application, or are there other factors involved? Perhaps the popularity and acceptance of a theory may be related to the persona of the theorist as a leader in the field as well as to the theoretical content. The sociopolitical climate of the field and trends in OT's national office may contribute to spotlighting one work to the exclusion of another. Publications in the *American Journal of Occupational Therapy* may gain the attention of OTs more than publications in other journals or in books. Workshops and presentations that supplement written works may be important for therapists to learn about the theory and the theorist first-hand. The textbooks and reading assignments that educators select influence OT students' exposure to theoretical material. As the field grows, theories will proliferate, as they have already done since the first edition of this book in 1988. Future theories will need to be true to the traditions of OT and yet reflect contemporary practice if they are to remain useful for explaining, interpreting, and guiding OT practice, education and research. From the array of ideas and viewpoints that will be forthcoming in the future, discerning therapists will consider the theoretical soundness of an idea to be equally as important as the popularity of that idea.

CONCLUSION

Lewin (1947) described three stages of theory development: (1) speculative, in which theory is proposed to explain phenomena; (2) descriptive, in which research is used to quantify phenomena and test theory; and (3) constructive, in which new theory is devised through revision of existing theory and through the use of facts versus speculation. Occupational therapy theory development is now at stages one and two.

Fidler, Mosey, Llorens, Ayres, Reilly, Kielhofner, and Allen have all proposed rationales for the profession's existence and/or explanations of OT practice. Through her efforts to quantify sensory integrative phenomena and to test her ideas, Ayres' research has brought OT theory into stage two. Other theorists have contributed to this stage. Fidler and Mosey have been research advocates. Llorens, through her SCCR, provided a method for clinical case study data collection. Reilly's students conducted research for instrument development and to explain constructs of occupational behavior theory. Kielhofner and colleagues have engaged in research on the model of human occupation. Allen and cohorts have conducted studies of her evaluation methods. Theories described in this book have begun to be validated through research.

Although the field of occupational therapy has begun a serious attempt to specify phenomena of concern, much remains to be done to test the theories described in this book and to validate frames of reference and theoretical formulations that exist in the field but are beyond the scope of this book. In this book alone are contained innumerable research ideas, and within its literature possible research directions are limitless. Occupational therapy is on the threshold of developing research traditions, identifying research processes, and claiming research areas that will help us begin to test our ideas scientifically. This era will give us the research know-how and clearer descriptions of "what OT is" that will serve as a basis for bringing OT theory development to stage three: theory construction.

Hudson's thoughts, as expressed in the *American Journal of Occupational Therapy* in 1954, on the nature of research, provide a challenge to each of us as occupational therapists: "It is exciting to realize that we are all on a scientific frontier that has hardly been penetrated—that the opportunities for individual contribution to knowledge are endless" (Hudson, 1954, p. 150).

REFERENCES

Abreu, B.C. (1981). *Physical disabilities manual.* Raven Press: New York.

Allen, C.K. (1985). *Occupational therapy for psychiatric diseases: Measurement and management of cognitive disabilities.* Boston: Little, Brown.

Allen, C.K. (1987). Activity: Occupational therapy's treatment method. *American Journal of Occupational Therapy, 41,* 563–575.

Allen, C.K. (1990). *Allen Cognitive Level Test manual.* Colchester, CT: S&S/Worldwide.

Allen, C.K., Earhart, C.A., & Blue, T. (1992). *Occupational therapy treatment goals for the physically and cognitively disabled.* Rockville, MD: American Occupational Therapy Association.

American Occupational Therapy Association. (1979). *TOTEMS: Training Occupational Therapy Management in the Schools.* Rockville, MD: Author.

American Occupational Therapy Association. (1985a). *Occupational therapy manpower: A plan for progress.* Rockville, MD: Author.

American Occupational Therapy Association. (1985b). *PIVOT: Planning and Implementing Vocational Readiness in Occupational Therapy.* Rockville, MD: Author.

American Occupational Therapy Association. (1985c). *Education data survey.* Rockville, MD: Author.

American Occupational Therapy Association. (1986a). *ROTE, Role of Occupational Therapy with the Elderly.* Rockville, MD: Author.

American Occupational Therapy Association. (1986b). *SCOPE, Strategies Concepts, and Opportunities for Program Development and Evaluation.* Rockville, MD: Author.

American Occupational Therapy Association (1990). *1990 Member data survey.* Rockville, MD: Author.

American Occupational Therapy Association. (1993). TWU establishes PhD program in occupational therapy. *OT Week, 7* (1), 12.

Arnadottir, G. (1990). *The brain and behavior: Assessing cortical dysfunction through activities of daily living (ADL).* St. Louis: C.V. Mosby.

Ayres, A.J. (1949). An analysis of crafts in the treatment of electroshock patients. *American Journal of Occupational Therapy, 3,* 195–198.

Ayres, A.J. (1963). The development of perceptual motor abilities as a theoretical basis for treatment of dysfunction. *American Journal of Occupational Therapy, 6,* 221–225.

Ayers. A.J. (1972a). *Sensory integration and learning disorders.* Los Angeles: Western Psychological Services.

Ayres, A.J. (1972b). *Southern California Sensory Integration Tests.* Los Angeles: Western Psychological Services.

Ayres, A.J. (1975). *Southern California Postrotary Nystagmus Test.* Los Angeles: Western Psychological Services.

Ayres, A.J. (1979). *Sensory integration and the child.* Los Angeles: Western Psychological Services.

Ayres, A.J. (1985). *Developmental dyspraxia and adult onset apraxia.* Torrance, CA: Sensory Integration International.

Ayres, A.J. (1989). *Sensory Integration and Praxis Tests.* Los Angeles: Western Psychological Services.

Ayres, A.J., & Marr, D.M. (1991). Sensory Integration and Praxis Tests. In A.G. Fisher, E.A. Murray, & A.C. Bundy (Eds.), *Sensory integration: Theory and practice* (pp. 203–229). Philadelphia: F.A. Davis.

Barris, R., Kielhofner, G., & Watts, J.H. (1983). *Psychosocial occupational therapy.* Laurel, MD: Ramsco.

Brown, E.J. (1991). Occupational science: What will it mean to OT? *Advance for Occupational Therapists*, January 7, 1991.

Chinn, P.L., & Jacobs, M.K. (1983). *Theory and nursing—A systematic approach.* St. Louis: C.V. Mosby.

Christiansen, C., & Baum, C. (1991). *Occupational therapy: Overcoming performance deficits.* Thorofare, NJ: Charles B. Slack.

Clark, F.A., Parham, D., Carlson, M.E., Frank, G., Jackson, J., Pierce, D., Wolfe, R.J., & Zemke, R. (1991). Occupational science: Academic innovation in the service of occupational therapy's future. *American Journal of Occupational Therapy, 45*, 300–310.

Clark, P.N., & Allen, A.S. (1985). *Occupational therapy for children.* St. Louis: C.V. Mosby.

Duldt, B.W., & Giffin, K. (1985). *Theoretical perspectives for nursing.* Boston: Little, Brown.

Earhart, C.A., & Allen, C.K. (1988). *Cognitive disabilities: Expanded activity analysis.* Colchester, CT: S&S/Worldwide.

Farber, S.D. (1982). *Neurorehabilitation: A multisensory approach.* Philadelphia: W.B. Saunders.

Fidler, G.S. (1948). Psychological evaluation of occupational therapy activities. *American Journal of Occupational Therapy, 1*, 284–287.

Fidler, G.S. (1982). The lifestyle performance profile: An organizing frame. In B. Hemphill (Ed.), *The evaluation process in psychiatric occupational therapy* (pp. 43–47). Thorofare, NJ: Charles B. Slack.

Fidler, G.S. (1990). Reflections on choice. *Occupational Therapy in Mental Health, 10*, 77–84.

Fidler, G. S. (1991). The challenge of change to OT practice. *Occupational Therapy in Mental Health, 11*, 1–11.

Fidler, G.S., & Bristow, B. (1992). *Recapturing competence: A system's change for geropsychiatric care.* New York: Springer.

Fidler, G.S., & Fidler, J.W. (1954). *Introduction to psychiatric occupational therapy.* New York: Macmillan.

Fidler, G.S., & Fidler, J.W. (1963). *Occupational therapy: A communication process in psychiatry.* New York: Macmillan.

Fidler, G.S., & Fidler. J.W. (1978). Doing and becoming: Purposeful action and self-actualization. *American Journal of Occupational Therapy, 32*, 305–310.

Hopkins, H.L. (1988). An historical perspective on occupational therapy. In H.L. Hopkins & H.D. Smith (Eds.), *Willard and Spackman's occupational therapy* (7th ed.) (pp. 16–42). Philadelphia: J.B. Lippincott.

Hudson, B. (1954). What is research? *American Journal of Occupational Therapy, 8*, 140–141, 150.

Kielhofner, G. (Ed.). (1983). *Health through occupation: Theory and practice of occupational therapy.* Philadelphia: F.A. Davis.

Kielhofner, G. (Ed.). (1985). *A model of human occupation.* Baltimore: Williams & Wilkins.

Kielhofner, G. (1992). *Conceptual foundations of occupational therapy.* Philadelphia: F.A. Davis.

Labovitz, D.R., & Miller, R.J. (1986). Commentary: Organization of knowledge in occupational therapy: A proposal and a survey of the literature. *Occupational Therapy Journal of Research, 6*, 85.

Levine, A.E. (1984, May). *A design for an entry-level curriculum based on occupation.* Paper presented at the meeting of the American Occupational Therapy Association Commission on Education, Kansas City, Missouri.

Lewin, K. (1947). *Principles of topological psychology.* New York: McGraw-Hill.

Light, S., & Reilly, M. (1943). The correlation of physical therapy and occupational therapy. *Occupational Therapy and Rehabilitation, 22*, 171–175.

Llorens, L.A. (1970). Facilitating growth and development: The promise of occupational therapy. *American Journal of Occupational Therapy, 24*, 93–101.

Llorens, L.A. (Ed.). (1973). *Consultation in the Community: Occupational therapy in child health.* Dubuque, Iowa: Kendall-Hunt.

Llorens, L.A. (1976). *Application of a developmental theory for health and rehabilitation.* Rockville, MD: American Occupational Therapy Association.

Llorens, L.A. (1982). *Occupational therapy sequential client care record manual.* Laurel, MD: Ramsco.

Llorens, L.A. (Ed.) (1988). *Health care for ethnic elders: The cultural context.* Proceedings of Stanford Geriatric Education Center Conference, 1988. Available from: Stanford Geriatric Education Center, 703 Welch Road, Palo Alto, CA 94305.

Llorens, L.A. (1991). Performance tasks and roles throughout the life span. In C. Christiansen & C. Baum (Eds.), *Occupational therapy: Overcoming human performance deficits* (pp. 45–68). Thorofare, NJ: Charles B. Slack.

Llorens, L.A. (1992). Program consultation for children and adults. In E. Jaffe & C.F. Epstein (Eds.), *Occupational therapy consultation: Theory, principles and practice* (pp. 356–363). St. Louis, MO: C.V. Mosby.

Llorens, L.A., & Rubin, E.Z. (1967). Developing ego functions in disturbed children: occupational therapy in milieu. Detroit: Wayne State University Press.

Mattingly, C. (1991). What is clinical reasoning? *American Journal of Occupational Therapy, 45*, 979–987.

Meleis, H.I. (1985). *Theoretical nursing: Development and progress.* Philadelphia: J.B. Lippincott.

Mosey, A.C. (1968). Recapitulation of ontogenesis: A theory for practice of occupational therapy. *American Journal of Occupational Therapy, 22*, 426–432.

Mosey, A.C. (1969). Treatment of pathological distortion of body image. *American Journal of Occupational Therapy, 3*, 413–416.

Mosey, A.C. (1970). *Three frames of reference for mental health.* Thorofare, NJ: Charles B. Slack.

Mosey, A.C. (1973). *Activities therapy.* New York: Raven Press.

Mosey, A.C. (1981). *Occupational therapy: Configuration of a profession.* New York: Raven Press.

Mosey, A.C. (1985). A monistic or pluralistic approach to professional identity. *American Journal of Occupational Therapy, 39*, 504–509.

Mosey, A.C. (1986). Psychosocial components of occupational therapy. New York: Raven Press.

Mosey, A.C. (1992a). *Applied scientific inquiry in the health professions: An epistemological orientation.* Rockville, MD: American Occupational Therapy Association.

Mosey, A.C. (1992b). The issue is: Partition of occupational science and occupational therapy. *American Journal of Occupational Therapy, 46,* 851–853.

Oyster, C.K., Hanten, W.P., & Llorens, L.A. (1987). *Introduction to research: A guide for the health science professional.* Philadelphia, PA: J.B. Lippincott.

Parham, L.D. (1986). Applying theory to practice. In American Occupational Therapy Association (Ed.), *Target 2000, Occupational Therapy Education* (pp. 119–122). Rockville, MD: American Occupational Therapy Association.

Pedretti, L.W., & Zoltan, B. (Eds.). (1990). *Occupational therapy practice skills for physical dysfunction.* St. Louis: C.V. Mosby.

Reed, K.L. (1984). *Models of practice in occupational therapy.* Baltimore: Williams & Wilkins.

Reed, K.L., & Sanderson, S.R. (1980). *Concepts of occupational therapy.* Baltimore: Williams & Wilkins.

Reilly, M. (1962). Occupational therapy can be one of the great ideas of 20th century medicine. *American Journal of Occupational Therapy, 1,* 1–9.

Reilly, M. (1974). (Ed.). *Play as exploratory learning.* Beverly Hills, CA: Sage Publishers.

Reilly, M. (1984). The issue is—The importance of the client versus patient issue for occupational therapy. *American Journal of Occupational Therapy, 38,* 407–408.

Rogers, J.C. (1983). Eleanor Clarke Slagle Lectureship, 1983: Clinical reasoning: The ethics, science, and art. *American Journal of Occupational Therapy, 37,* 601–616.

Sabari, J.S. (1991). Motor learning concepts applied to activity-based intervention with adults with hemiplegia. *American Journal of Occupational Therapy, 45,* 523–530.

Trombly, C.A. (1989). *Occupational therapy for physical dysfunction.* Baltimore: Williams & Wilkins.

Index